HOW TO Install and Tune NITROUS OXIDE Systems

Bob McClurg

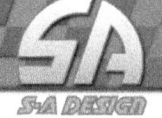

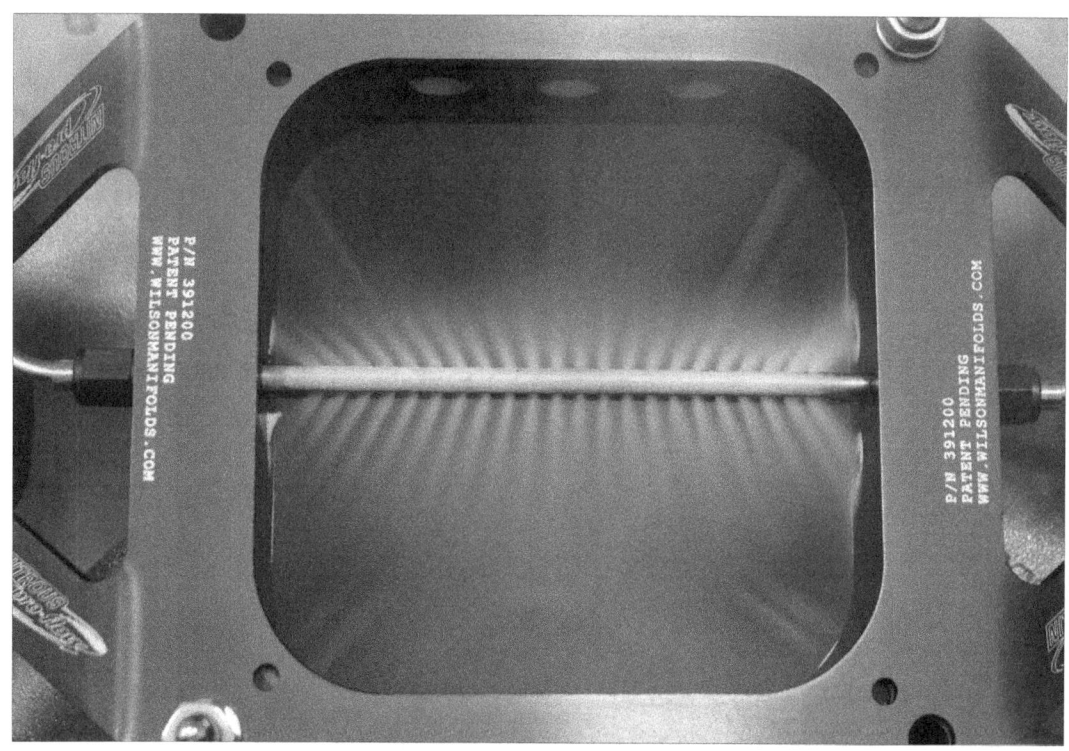

CarTech®

CarTech®

CarTech®, Inc.
39966 Grand Avenue
North Branch, MN 55056
Phone: 651-277-1200 or 800-551-4754
Fax: 651-277-1203
www.cartechbooks.com

© 2012 by Bob McClurg

All rights reserved. No part of this publication may be reproduced or utilized in any form or by any means, electronic or mechanical, including photocopying, recording, or by any information storage and retrieval system, without prior permission from the Publisher. All text, photographs, and artwork are the property of the Author unless otherwise noted or credited.

The information in this work is true and complete to the best of our knowledge. However, all information is presented without any guarantee on the part of the Author or Publisher, who also disclaim any liability incurred in connection with the use of the information and any implied warranties of merchantability or fitness for a particular purpose. Readers are responsible for taking suitable and appropriate safety measures when performing any of the operations or activities described in this work.

All trademarks, trade names, model names and numbers, and other product designations referred to herein are the property of their respective owners and are used solely for identification purposes. This work is a publication of CarTech, Inc., and has not been licensed, approved, sponsored, or endorsed by any other person or entity. The Publisher is not associated with any product, service, or vendor mentioned in this book, and does not endorse the products or services of any vendor mentioned in this book.

Edit by Scott Parkhurst
Layout by Monica Seiberlich

ISBN 978-1-61325-187-4
Item No. SA194P

Library of Congress Cataloging-in-Publication Data

McClurg, Bob.
  How to install and tune nitrous oxide systems / by Bob McClurg.
     p. cm.
  ISBN 978-1-934709-34-4
  1. Nitrous oxide injection systems (Fuel systems) 2. Automobiles--Motors--Fuel injection systems. 3. Automobiles, Racing--Motors--Fuel injection systems. I. Title.

TL214.F78M33 2012
629.25'3--dc23

2011030

Written, edited, and designed in the U.S.A.
Printed in the U.S.A.

Front Cover:
A Hogan sheet-metal tunnel-ram-style intake manifold, outfitted with port nitrous injection by Nitrous Supply, is test fired.

Title Page:
A Wilson Nitrous Pro-Flow plate is tested on the bench. Its angled spray jets distribute nitrous evenly throughout the intake manifold.

Back Cover Photos

Top Left:
Over the past 40 years, the crossbar-design N_2O plate has been accepted as the standard of the industry. It resembles a 1/2- to 1-inch-thick 4-barrel carburetor spacer plate. The brass, aluminum, or stainless-steel crossbar, featuring a series of finely drilled holes or sprayers, is fed by fuel and N_2O jet ports located at opposite ends.

Top Right:
Installing a single-stage, single-carbureted nitrous oxide system can be done at home using common shop tools, but it's advisable that you start with a healthy engine and a properly working carburetor first.

Middle Left:
The NOS 200- to 400-hp Big Shot Single Stage N_2O system is geared toward the really serious street/strip enthusiast. Advertised as the World's Most Powerful Single-Stage Plate Nitrous System, power output is adjustable in increments from 200 to 400 hp.

Middle Right:
Edelbrock Nitrous offers a 100-150-200-250-hp 2x4 Performer RPM single-stage dual-plate application for either the square-bore or Holley-type 4500-series carburetors.

Bottom Left:
This Nitrous Supply Universal Supercharger Show Plate Kit for the GMC 6.71 to 8.71 supercharger and its aftermarket variants is bolted on depending on distributor location/clearance and optimum solenoid placement. Made out of 1/2-inch thick polished aluminum, it uses stainless-steel lines and red and blue nozzles.

Bottom Right:
Test firing this Nitrous Supply–prepared Hogan 2x4 big-block Chevrolet fogger intake is an awesome sight. This particular setup incorporates a set of NS Mutha Fogga 360-degree nozzles and one of its .250-inch orifice-equipped Slayer high-yield solenoids.

OVERSEAS DISTRIBUTION BY:

PGUK
63 Hatton Garden
London EC1N 8LE, England
Phone: 020 7061 1980 • Fax: 020 7242 3725
www.pguk.co.uk

Renniks Publications Ltd.
3/37-39 Green Street
Banksmeadow, NSW 2109, Australia
Phone: 2 9695 7055 • Fax: 2 9695 7355
www.renniks.com

CONTENTS

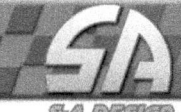

Acknowledgments 4
About the Author 5
Introduction 6

Chapter 1: Single-Stage Single-Plate Systems 10
    Carburetor Plate Kits 11
    Nitrous Oxide and Fuel Jets 11
    Nitrous Oxide Solenoids 12
    Project: NOS Solenoid Rebuild 14
    Nitrous Lines and Carburetor Supply Lines 20
    Nitrous Oxide Filter 20
    Nitrous Oxide Bottles 20
    Electrical Components 21
    Fuel Pumps and Fuel Pressure Regulators 21
    Project: Nitrous Supply Powerstar 8001 for
       350 Chevy Small-Block Installation 23
    Project: Edelbrock Performer 70001 Big-Block Chevrolet
       Single-Plate Nitrous Kit Installation 34

Chapter 2: Single-Stage Dual-Plate Carbureted Systems ... 39

Chapter 3: Two-Stage Single-Plate Systems 42

Chapter 4: Single-Stage Nitrous Supercharger Systems ... 45
    Project: Nitrous Supply/Weiand 6.71
       Supercharger Kit Installation 46

**Chapter 5: Hidden Single-Stage Systems:
    Top Shot and Friends** 49
    Top Shot 49
    Street Heat 49
    Sneaky Pete 50
    The Stealth Nozzle 50

Chapter 6: Nitrous Fogger 52

Chapter 7: Multi-Stage Systems 55
    Project: Nitrous Supply Two-Stage
       Nitrous 2x4 Intake Buildup 58

**Chapter 8: Bad-Ass 540-ci Merlin III
    Nitrous Big-Block Buildup** 66
    Fortifying the Engine 67
    Intake Manifold 70
    Project: Wilson Manifolds & Nitrous Pro-Flow
       Merlin III Two-Stage Plate and Fogger Intake Buildup ... 70
    The Supporting Cast 73
    Project: Final Assembly 75
    One Year Later 83

Chapter 9: EFI, Wet and Dry 85
    Wet-Plate Systems 85
    Wet-Manifold Systems 88
    Dry-Manifold Systems 89
    Electronic Fuel Injectors 94
    Project: Nitrous Express 2010 Camaro SS
       Single-Stage Plate Installation 97
    Project: Bullitt Reloaded 101
    Project: Nitrous Express Dodge Challenger
       SRT8 Fly-By-Wire Stage 1 EFI Kit Installation ... 112

Chapter 10: Nitrous Accessories 120
    Accessory Nitrous Jetting 120
    Advance-Design Nitrous Plates 121
    Super Solenoid 121
    Ignition Systems 122
    Nitrous Controllers 124
    Spark Plugs 126
    Nitrous Oxide Bottles and Tanks 127
    Bottle Valves and Openers 127
    Remote Bottle Control 128
    NOS Pinch Valve Kit 129
    Blow-Down Tube 129
    Lines—Nitrous Oxide and Fuel 129
    Fuel Pumps and Systems 130
    Purge Systems 130
    High-Flow Sprayer Nozzles 131
    Nitrous Oxide Filling Stations 133
    Nitrous Gauges 133
    Project: ZEX Bottle Pressure Gauge Installation ... 133
    Bottle Blankets 135
    Project: Nitrous Express GENX2 Bottle
       Warmer Installation 135
    Another Way of Doing It 137

**Chapter 11: Commonly Asked Questions
    About Nitrous Oxide** 140
    By Mike Thermos, CEO of Nitrous Supply

Source Guide 143

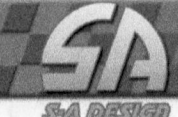

DEDICATION

To my father, Robert H.S. McClurg, who labored long and hard to provide me with a good education. This book is also dedicated to my son, Jonathan Meyer, who inherited my talent for putting thoughts into words and my grandson, Brandon Bregel, who inherited my love of fast cars and photography.

ACKNOWLEDGMENTS

I wish to thank the following individuals and/or companies, without whose help this book may not have been possible: ARP Fasteners/Holland Communications; Jim Beatty and Ricky Hults, ATI, Inc.; Chase Augustin, C.A.R.S.S. LLC; Aaron Mick, Competition Cams; Ron Beaubien and Nick D'Agostino, Diamond Pistons; John Verburg, Ferrea, Inc.; Rob Gavel, Jr., Redline808.com; Ron and Becky Hammel, 10,000 RPM Speed Equipment; Steven Heye, Heatshield Products; Denny and April Duquette, Island Performance & Offroad; Danny Jesel, Jesel, Inc.; Shane Pochaeon and Derek Scott, Lunati Power, Inc.; Don Meziere, Meziere Industries; Steve Morrison and Ken Sink, Milodon, Inc.; Barbara Miller, Moroso Performance; Mike Abney, Randall Mathias, Fred Smith, Mike Golightly and Mike Wood, Nitrous Express; Barry and Robin Grant and Adam Campbell, Barry Grant, Inc., and NitrousWorks; James and Tana Galante, RaceTrans.com; Sue and Victor Moore, Moore Good Ink; Todd Ryden and Joe Pandro, MSD; Mark Honsowetz and Jason Snyder, Edelbrock Nitrous Systems; Jay McFarland, Holley Performance Products, Inc.; Tom Boroner, Lucas Oil Products; Don Sarian, Sarian Graphics; Mike Slover, Slover's Porting Service; John Williams, Trend Performance; Mike Thermos, Wady Hammam, Mike Flynn, Bill Thurmon, and Scott Cochran, Nitrous Supply.com; Brad Lagman, Robert Bieschke, Mike Consolo, and James Gumabao, QMP Racing Engines; Keith Wilson, Rob Junior Klein, Wilson Manifolds & Nitrous Pro-Flow; Bill Mitchell and Bill Mitchell, Jr., World Products; Trent Goodwin, ZEX Nitrous Products.

About the Author

Sixty-something photojournalist Bob McClurg grew up in the 1950s in Southern California, where the sport of hot rodding, and particularly drag racing, was gaining a strong footing. Bob's earliest automotive influences included hanging around the local Ford and Chevrolet dealers, which were located on Chapman Avenue in his hometown of Orange. Across the street from Selman Chevrolet's OK Used Cars was Towne Barber Shop, where Bob earned pocket money sweeping up and shining shoes. Its magazine rack was always well stocked with copies of *Hot Rod*, *Car Craft*, and *Motor Trend* magazines, which the 10-year-old youngster constantly pored over between shoe shines. One of Bob's customers was the future NHRA Competition Director, the late Jack Hart, who operated Hart Texaco and Hart Automotive one block over. He used to hang around Jack's shop, and ask a lot of questions. Most of the time he was chased away by the help, but every now and then, Jack gave him a little encouragement!

McClurg wrote his first legitimate newspaper article on traffic safety while in the 5th grade at St. John's Lutheran School, and brought it to the editor of the *Orange Daily News*. About the same time, Bob's uncle Victor sent him his old Argus C3 35-mm camera. At first, he wasn't sure about what to do with it. It was obvious to him that photography required basic math skills, and he didn't regard math as a strong subject.

Meanwhile, Bob occupied himself by racing slot cars, and entering model car contests. He also worked part time for a man named Roger Clausen who owned Gish's Toy Store.

He remembers Clausen talking nonstop about a guy named Garlits. One Saturday afternoon in 1963 Clausen finally took him to Lions Associated Drag Strip. "Big Daddy" Don Garlits was appearing in a four-way Top Fuel match race against Don "The Snake" Prudhomme, "TV" Tommy Ivo, and (as he remembers) Kenny Safford. The sights; the sounds; the smells—all sensations you never experience by just reading a car magazine—were absolutely incredible to young McClurg.

It took another year or so, but once McClurg became the yearbook photographer at Villa Park High School, things, if you'll excuse the pun, began to click. One Saturday night in 1964, Bob snuck out on the Lions Associated Drag Strip starting line with the yearbook's Yashica LM 2¼-inch camera in hand, and from then on, he spent Saturdays and Sundays going to Lions, Irwindale, and sometimes Carlsbad Raceway. Then, in August 1968, Orange County International Raceway opened its doors.

With all the publicity generated by the opening of the nation's first Super Strip, breaking drag racing into the local newspapers became much easier. Then a sponsored trip to the 1968 United States Nationals at Indianapolis, shooting ad photos for the Fram Corporation, changed everything. In April 1969, *Super Stock & Drag Illustrated* came calling, so 20-year-old Bob packed up his Nikons and Hasselblads and headed for the East Coast.

Eastern drag racing was a different ball game. You could go to the races practically every night of the week. Capitol Raceway, Budd's Creek, Aquasco, Cecil County, Suffolk Raceway, York U.S. 30—you name it, and there was always something going on somewhere. Between those races and the national events, it made for an exciting summer!

In the fall of 1969, McClurg headed back to the West Coast to pursue his education, but arrived just in time to take in the AHRA and NHRA Winter events, which provided him with some outstanding photos. Apparently, *Hot Rod* magazine editor Don Evans thought so too, because Bob enjoyed a string of "HRM Racing Galleries" published in 1970–1971. Eventually that led to a full-time position as photo editor at Petersen Specialty Publications (1976), which launched him into the photo editor's job at *Hot Rod* magazine in 1977.

As the 1970s closed, Bob made his living freelancing. Then in the early 1980s, Bob was coaxed to come back to Petersen Publishing Company, and eventually assumed the editorship at Petersen's *Kit Car* magazine. This was followed by a 14-year stint as the editor for McMullen & Yee's *Mustang Illustrated* and *Ford High Performance* magazines.

Of the nine books Bob McClurg has authored, five have been for CarTech, Inc./SA Design Books: *Diggers, Funnies, Gassers & Altereds*; *Drag Racing's Golden Era*; *How to Build Supercharged and Turbocharged Small-Block Fords*; *Fire, Nitro, Rubber and Smoke: Bob McClurg's Drag Racing Memories*; *Yenko: The Man, The Machine, The Legend*; plus this one.

INTRODUCTION

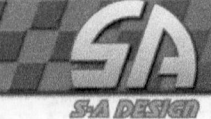

Wherever modern dentistry is practiced, the cryogenic gas known as nitrous oxide, composed of two parts nitrogen and one part oxygen (N_2O), has functioned as a viable pain killer and sedative for more than 170 years. However, when English chemist Joseph Priestley published his discovery in 1775, the scientist referred to the inert gas as "phlogistacated nitrous air," which he had created by heating iron filings dampened with nitric acid. N_2O's original use was anything but that of a medical nature.

Historically, nitrous oxide was first used around 1790 as a recreational drug by Englishman Humphrey Davy, who tested the substance on himself and friend Samuel Taylor Coleridge. These gentlemen of leisure discovered, at informal social situations called "laughing gas parties," that N_2O not only dulled the sensation of pain, it also had a mirthful, albeit hallucinogenic, effect on those who inhaled it.

In the 1840s, nitrous oxide was introduced in America by medical researcher Gardner Quincy Colton. The substance was first commercially manufactured in this country by Trenton, New Jersey's George Poe, inventor of the respirator and cousin to famed poet Edgar Allan Poe. Poe was the first to liquefy N_2O by carefully heating ammonium nitrate, which decomposed into N_2O and water vapor. Poe also discovered that the addition of various phosphates created a purer gas (like modern medical-grade nitrous oxide, for example) at lower brewing temperatures.

Dentist Horace Wells first used medical-grade nitrous oxide as a legitimate sedative because dentists, particularly in rural America, did not have access to an anesthesiologist. The gas enabled them to operate, yet maintain some form of communication with conscious patients. Today, medical N_2O is a controlled substance and is monitored by the Drug Enforcement Agency (DEA) and the Food and Drug Administration (FDA).

Nitrous Oxide's Widespread Use

Nitrous oxide has been used to treat severe depression and anxiety in mental patients. It can also be found in a bag of potato chips! An N_2O composition has been used as a propellant in aerosol spray cans like those used for cooking sprays, whipped cream, spray waxes, and bags of potato chips for years.

But this book is about boosting engine performance with industrial-grade nitrous oxide, or Nytrous Plus, which is the official trademarked name adopted in the mid 1980s by Nellore-Puritan-Bennett. The company, which has manufactured and marketed N_2O since 1913, acted upon a suggestion made by Nitrous Oxide Systems co-founder Dale Vaznaian. Nytrous Plus differs significantly from medical N_2O in that its composition features .01 percent sulfur-dioxide, which has been added to produce an unpleasant odor that prevents substance abuse.

A Genuine Power Adder

When used as a power adder, nitrous oxide can significantly enhance the performance potential of any internal combustion engine. However, N_2O does not actually burn, and is not a graded fuel.

INTRODUCTION

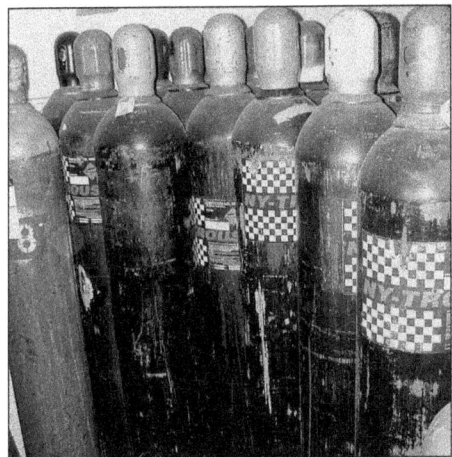

Industrial grade nitrous oxide or Nytrous Plus, which differs in purity from medical nitrous oxide, or High Purity N_2O, is the official trademarked name adopted in the mid 1980s by Nellore-Puritan-Bennett. This company has been engaged in manufacturing nitrous oxide since 1913, acting upon a suggestion by NOS founder Dale Vaznaian. Instead of being 100-percent pure, Nytrous Plus' chemical composition is 99.0-percent nitrous oxide and 0.01-percent sulpher dioxide, which was added to produce a foul odor, presumably to prevent potential substance abuse and death from asphyxiation.

In fact, N_2O is inflammable. When injected as a compressed liquid at 127 degrees F, it allows an engine to burn more air/fuel by dramatically dropping intake charge temperature, resulting in a denser and more enhanced internal combustion. What is basically being done here is the creation of a more user-friendly and oxygen-enriched atmospheric condition inside the cylinders of an engine. Here are the characteristics of Nytrous Plus:

- Molecular Weight: 44.02 g/mole
- Boiling/Condensation Point: 126.4 degrees F
- Melting/Freezing Point 131.8 degrees F
- Critical Temperature: 97.9 degrees F
- Vapor Pressure: 745 psig
- Vapor Density: 1.53 (Air = 1)
- Liquid Density at BP: 76.8 ft-lbs^3
- Specific Volume: 8.6957
- Gas Density: .115 ft-lbs^3

Hitler's Luftwaffe took great advantage of N_2O during World War II. Specifically intended to provide superior high-altitude performance with a quick getaway, N_2O-equipped fighter planes like the Messerschmitt-produced ME-109 routinely used N_2O. The Japanese Imperial Air Force kamikaze squadrons also used N_2O as a last-minute accelerant during suicide attacks on American warships.

Over the years, N_2O has also been tested as a rocket propellant, or an oxidizer in rocket engines. In 1914, American rocket pioneer Robert Goddard suggested the use of N_2O and gasoline for a liquid-fueled rocket. Actual use of N_2O with both solid fuel and liquid fuel/impulse rockets has been also used with great success. For example, the combination of N_2O and hydroxyl-terminated polybutadiene fuel was successfully used as a propellant in Spaceship One, which landed on the moon. Even amateur rocketeers use N_2O today on homemade rocket experiments.

Nitrous Oxide Performance Pioneers

Historically, the first high-performance automotive aftermarket retailer to introduce nitrous oxide to the automotive sector was Ron Hammel. His company, 10,000 RPM Speed Equipment, began selling nitrous in 1962.

Hammel recalls, "After moving from Spokane, Washington, to Southern California around 1958, I had worked for a number of drag racing teams including Jack Chrisman's Howard's Cams Special, so I kind of knew what dragster racing was all about. Around 1962–1963, I had been experimenting with nitrous oxide, and installed a small system on a Pacific Northwestern-based Top Fuel car called the *Top Hat Special*. The car was a good running car [before the nitrous], but it was just an average running car. Anyhow, we set Low E.T. and Top MPH during qualifying at the Bakersfield Fuel & Gas Championships, so I figured that the startling increase in performance had to be attributed to the juice."

Energized by what had happened, Hammel went back to where he worked, Tony Capanna's shop called Hot Rod City, and began doing development work on a series of 4-barrel-carbureted gasoline-burning engines. Then he began selling kits.

Hammel recounts, "In 1969, when the astronauts went to the moon, I told everyone, [and thought] maybe now they'll believe how good this stuff [nitrous oxide] really is! We did a lot of engine development (dyno) work, and learned about things like air/fuel ratio [AFR]. We learned how to set up an engine while lowering the exhaust temperature so that you didn't burn the darned thing up. Our development work even included Diesel engines. Basically, we worked at it until we got it right!"

Initially, 10,000 RPM's N_2O kits were based on mechanical throttle linkage systems. "From about 1969 to the early 1980s we sold a lot of kits," says Hammel. "Our first kits were all manually operated using the existing

INTRODUCTION

original equipment throttle linkage that came with the carburetor. We set up these mechanical systems to work at wide open throttle [WOT]. At WOT the system turned itself on. If you had anything less than WOT, the system turned itself back off."

However, the more 10,000 RPM became involved in the sale of nitrous kits, the more it found that various compromises, such as throttle kickdowns, were being made with the factory throttle linkage, so it became necessary to switch to electrically activated solenoids, which have now become an industry standard.

Arguably, the popularization of nitrous oxide as an automotive power adder would not have experienced such rapid growth and popularity had it not been for a couple of other factors: first, the resurgence of street racing in the 1970s, due in part to the closing of a number of popular drag strips across the country; and second, the overwhelming popularity of bracket racing and its various forms—Outlaw Street Car, Street Legal Drag, World's Fastest Street Car Competition, etc. This type of competition became a viable alternative to costly NHRA-, AHRA-, and IHRA-class racing. Of course a direct spin-off the widely accepted popularity of nitrous oxide, or so-called Throttle in a Bottle, was the establishment of a number of new nitrous-oxide-systems manufacturing companies. One of them was Compucar Nitrous Oxide Systems, founded in the early 1970s by Ron Ractoff, and later purchased by Ernest Wrenn. Another key player was Nitrous Oxide Systems, or NOS as it is widely known, co-founded in 1978 by Southern California drag racers Mike Thermos and Dale Vaznaian.

Enthusiast Publication Support

The overwhelming acceptance of N_2O also owes a great deal of its success as a viable yet affordable power adder to enthusiast publications like *Hot Rod, Car Craft, Popular Hot Rodding, Super Chevy, Muscle Mustang & Fast Fords, Super Stock & Drag Illustrated, Cars*, etc. Once discovered, magazine editors all across the country were singing N_2O's praises.

For example, *Hot Rod* magazine was one of the first enthusiast magazines to publish an in-depth article on N_2O in July of 1981. Automotive techno-writer David Vizard penned the article "Built to Stay Tough, Nitrous Small-Block Chevy Has Bottom End Punch and High-Speed Power."

Basing his engine build on a totally streetable, 350-ci four-bolt-main Chevrolet small-block, the main objective was to build an engine that averaged 25 mpg highway, and propel a 3,800-pound car down the quarter mile in the mid-11-second range. Vizard's 10.5:1 compression small-block 350 test engine featured a set of .030-inch-overbore Sealed Power pistons, a set of Motor Machine-prepared 350 Chevrolet connecting rods, a .010 re-sized Chevrolet 350 crank, Federal Mogul engine bearings, a Competition Cams 268-H grind hydraulic cam, and a Chevy 350 truck timing chain. It also received a set of G&G Porting 186-casting Chevrolet cylinder heads featuring a high-flow/high-velocity intake port with 2.02-inch intake valves and 1.60-inch exhaust valves. A set of Sealed Power lifters, 1.6:1-ratio Comp Cams rocker arms, and 1.5-inch NASCAR-type Comp springs were also

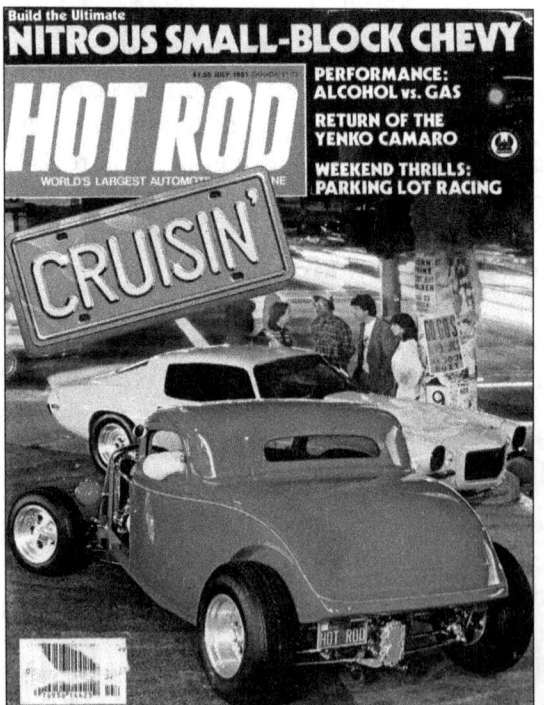

In Petersen Publishing Company's July 1981 issue of Hot Rod *magazine (today a Source Interlink publication), technical writer David Vizard conducted a three-way nitrous street engine shootout using an Internal Combustion Engines (I.C.E.) carbureted plate nitrous kit, an NOS carbureted plate kit, and a 10,000 RPM Speed Equipment–carbureted nitrous-plate-kit-equipped 350 small-block Chevrolet V-8 engine. Vizard also experimented with various-size carburetors, air cleaner stacks, and types of headers. NOS was the overall winner, producing 491 hp at 5,120 rpm and 562 ft-lbs of torque at 4,100 rpm on 92-octane pump gas. The high interest level created by this, the very first nitrous-oxide-kit shootout article published, popularized N_2O, and its proponents quickly nicknamed the inert gas "Throttle in a Bottle!"*

INTRODUCTION

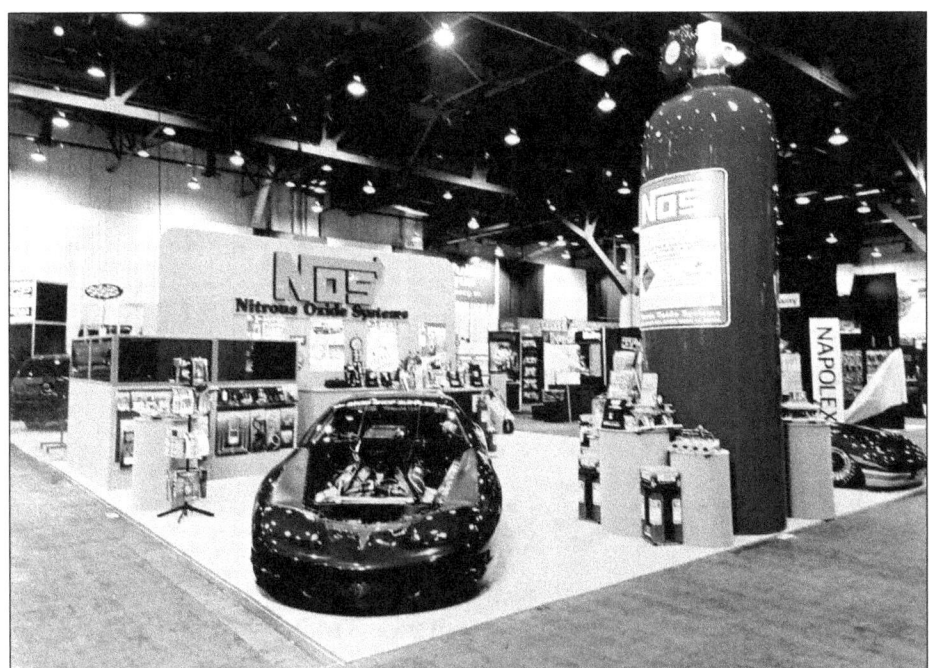

Nitrous Oxide Systems, Inc. (NOS), co-founded in the late 1970s by Mike Thermos and Dale Vaznaian popularized nitrous oxide for the street through an aggressive R&D program, which covers all makes and models of carbureted cars. That research eventually led to the first electronic fuel injection (EFI) kits for the modern-era small-block Ford EFI and Chevrolet TPI engines.

part of the combination. Induction was handled by an Edelbrock Victor Jr. 4-barrel manifold and a 730-cfm Internal Combustion Engines–prepared Holley 650 carburetor. It had a Melling oil pump and Cyclone headers; in other words, all over-the-counter internal components.

It is very interesting that Vizard tested not one, but a total of three different N_2O systems: a Nitrous Oxide Systems 1-inch 4-barrel carburetor plate kit, an Internal Combustion Engines (I.C.E.) Spray-Bar 1-inch spacer plate 4-barrel carburetor kit, and a 10,000 RPM 1-inch-spacer Stage II 4-barrel carburetor plate kit, tested using a Superflow 800 computerized chassis dyno.

After a series of dyno pulls testing different rocker arm ratios, air filters, and exhaust headers, Vizard and company were able to realize 376 hp and 404 ft-lbs on the engine alone (naturally aspirated).

With 92-octane fuel in the tank and 34 to 36 degrees of total timing advance, the Nitrous Oxide Systems kit proved to be the winner, producing 491 hp at 5,150 rpm and 562 ft-lbs at 4,100 rpm.

Still not through, Vizard and company substituted 102-octane So-Cal Orange race gas, re-set the timing at 39 to 40 degrees, and un-corked the headers in their test Camaro Z-28. Then they recorded 414 hp at 5,500 rpm and 412 ft-lbs on the engine, and 529 hp at 5,500 rpm with 570 ft-lbs at 4,000 rpm on the squeeze!

"That [*Hot Rod*] article was the first magazine article we ever did," says former NOS CEO Mike Thermos, "and it really put us on the map! I remember we built our first kit—a Holley 4-barrel, small-block Chevrolet application, using stuff out of hardware stores and hobby shops. However, once we got everything sourced out, things started going really well for us. Then the magazines got involved with our company, and that took us to the next level. We began advertising and that's when Nitrous Oxide Systems' business really took off!"

The key to Nitrous Oxide Systems' success is likely that the company has never rested on its laurels. The company has consistently refined its kits in an attempt to offer the best equipment on the market at an affordable price. NOS was one of the first aftermarket companies to develop N_2O street kits for EFI applications, beginning with the 5.0/5.8L Ford EFI small-blocks, and TPI-, LT1-, and LS-Series 350 small-block Chevrolet powerplants.

"Nitrous certainly has a home on the street," says Thermos. "That is where it was founded, and it offers a viable performance advantage over costly and sometimes illegal engine modifications. Of course, these days, modern electronics are certainly making things more and more involved, and the industry has to keep up with those trends or fall behind!"

Acquired in 1999 by Holley Performance Products, Inc., Nitrous Oxide Systems continues to be a recognized leader in the nitrous oxide industry, along with companies like Applied Nitrous Technologies, Compucar Nitrous Oxide Systems, Edelbrock Nitrous Systems, Induction Solutions, NANO Nitrogen Assisted Nitrous Oxide, Nitrous Express, Inc., Nitrous Outlet, Nitrous Supply (Thermos' newest venture), Wilson Pro Flow Nitrous, ZEX Nitrous Products, and numerous others. The result is a thriving and competitive nitrous oxide industry.

CHAPTER 1

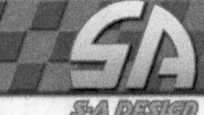

SINGLE-STAGE
SINGLE-PLATE SYSTEMS

When describing the obvious performance benefits from using nitrous oxide, substantial horsepower increases (from 50 to 350) are possible on your average small- or big-block Chevrolet, Ford, or Mopar V-8 engine, when equipped with a single-stage street/strip N_2O kit using a standard-flange Holley, Ford Motorcraft, or Autolite single 4-barrel carburetor; a dominator-flange-design Holley; or a spread-bore-design Carter Thermo-Quad, Rochester, or Edelbrock single 4-barrel carburetor. However, no matter what type or brand of carburetor used, it is vitally important to the overall performance of the system that you start with a good one; adding nitrous only compounds existing problems. Sticking floats, lazy power valves, partially clogged jets, and/or fuel metering rods that are in poor condition can result in sloppy throttle response, backfires, or more costly and permanent engine damage.

Carburetor size also matters. A carburetor that is too large runs rich at idle and lean at wide open throttle (WOT). If in doubt, contact any of the leading N_2O kit manufacturers' technical hot lines. They can assist you in selecting the right N_2O kit and recommend the right carburetor for the application.

Purchasing a factory blueprinted carburetor from either Holley Performance Products or Edelbrock Corporation not only provides peace of mind, it's also a viable alternative to costly rebuilds. Ordering a ready-to-install carburetor from a specialty

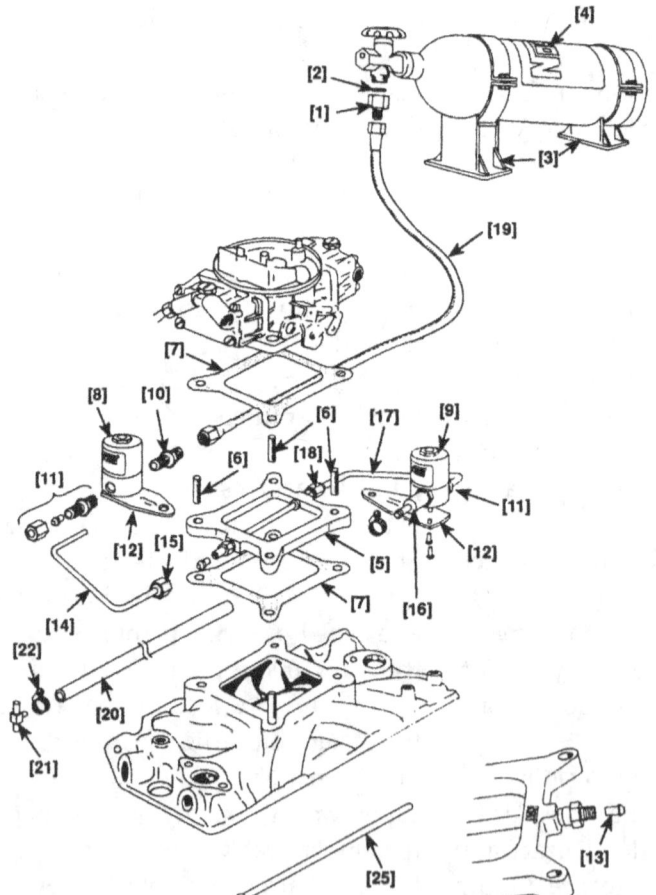

This diagram from Nitrous Oxide Systems, Inc., a division of Holley Performance Products, Inc., does a great job of showing the components used in the construction of a single-stage single-plate N_2O system and its installation on your average American-manufactured small-block or big-block V-8 engine. (Photo Courtesy Nitrous Oxide Systems, Inc.)

---

10   HOW TO INSTALL AND TUNE NITROUS OXIDE SYSTEMS

SINGLE-STAGE SINGLE-PLATE SYSTEMS

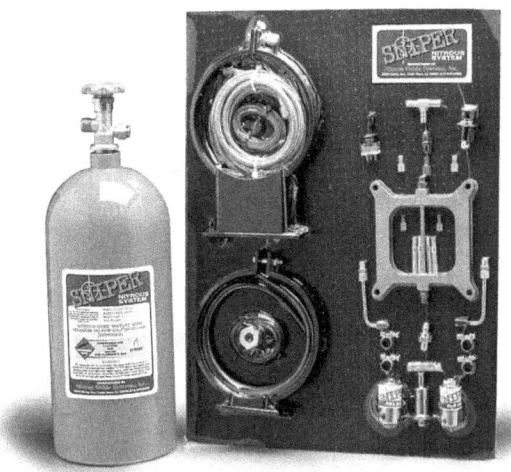

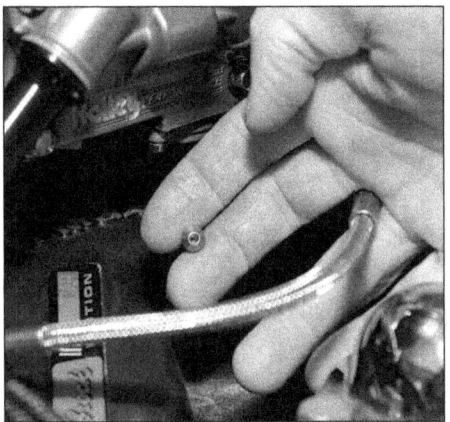

Nitrous Oxide Systems (NOS) Sniper is an entry-level, race ready single-stage street/strip nitrous oxide kit capable of delivering an adjustable 100 to 150 hp and is very affordably priced. When tested on a 355-ci small-block Chevrolet engine, Sniper produced an extra 163 hp and torque was increased by an astounding 165 ft-lbs. Sniper is available in either standard Holley/square bore, PN 07001NOS, or Quadrajet type applications PN 7004NOS, and comes complete with 10-pound tank and all accessories.

N_2O and fuel jets are both CNC manufactured from either brass or stainless-steel and are drilled, or inner-contoured, per each N_2O manufacturers' specifications in order to arrive at what is perceived to be the ideal rate of flow. Jet size ranges from .014 to .136 inch on average. Per application, a series of pre-selected jets are typically included in a single-carbureted street N_2O kit. For example, with Edelbrock Corporation's 50- to 100-hp Universal Big-Block Chevrolet Square Flange (nitrous) Kit (PN 70001), the grouping of three N_2O and fuel jets are perfectly matched to their counterparts.

shop, such as The Carburetor Shop, Braswell Carburetion, or Quick Fuel Technology (just to name three) is another choice.

Carburetor Plate Kits

The premise of a single-stage 4-barrel N_2O carburetor-plate kit, whether it's designed for the street or for competition use, didn't take a brain surgeon to figure out. The nitrous oxide plate itself looks like a standard 1/2- to 1-inch-thick 4-barrel carburetor spacer plate. In fact, I wouldn't be surprised if that's what its inventor originally adapted it from. Then along came the addition of fuel and N_2O jet ports accompanied by brass, aluminum, or stainless-steel spray bars. They feature a series of finely drilled holes running either north/south, or east/west, depending on carburetor type and throttle linkage design. When you activate the N_2O system, this combination of gasoline and N_2O gets mixed with the atomized fuel from the carburetor, and is distributed throughout the intake runners to the combustion chambers. Once

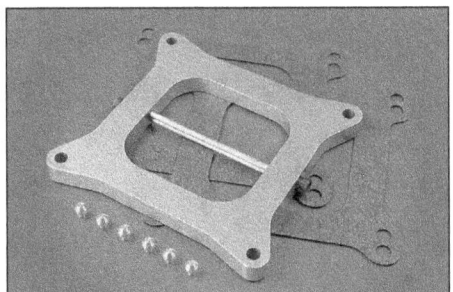

Over the past 40 years, the crossbar-design N_2O plate has been accepted as the standard of the industry.

lit, the byproduct is an instant and dramatic burst of power!

Not all single-stage carburetor plates are alike. In an ongoing attempt to improve on the basic 40-year-old design and perhaps gain a larger market share, some manufacturers (like Nitrous Express and ZEX Nitrous Products) have introduced advanced design nitrous plates, such as the ZEX Perimeter Plate, as standard equipment.

You may be asking, "Why a fuel port when there's already a carburetor?" The most obvious reason is the power adder concept itself, keeping in mind that N_2O enters the intake runners of an internal combustion engine at 127 degrees F.

The molecular density of N_2O is such that you need an additional shot of fuel—using a properly matched gasoline jet—to offset the nitrous charge and fire the cylinder. Otherwise, you have to run a huge carburetor jet, which affects overall fuel mileage and driveability under normal driving conditions.

Nitrous Oxide and Fuel Jets

Nitrous oxide and fuel jets are both power-matched to complement a particular N_2O kit or application. For example, with Edelbrock Corporation's 50- to 100-hp Universal Big-Block Chevrolet Square Flange

Kit (PN 70001), the N_2O and fuel jets (three per grouping) are perfectly matched to their counterparts, such as: Nitrous/Fuel 38/38 = 50, 46/46 = 75, 57/57 = 100 hp.

However, that may not always be the case. For example, with Nitrous Supply's Power Star Holley carburetor nitrous kit for the carbureted 350-ci small-block Chevrolet (PN 8001), jetting favors the nitrous side of the equation: Nitrous/Fuel 42/47 = 75, 47/53 = 100, 55/61 = 125, 63/71 = 150. Always pay close attention to the manufacturer's recommended jet specification sheet.

As a rule, nitrous jets are all CNC machined out of brass or stainless steel. Why both? Originally, it was to visually determine the difference between fuel (brass) and N_2O (stainless). However, in recent years some N_2O kit manufacturers have exclusively switched to precision-machined stainless steel jets to avoid corrosion issues. Sized or upgraded nitrous and fuel jets are available in master jet packs through participating N_2O kit manufacturers and/or retailers.

Nitrous Oxide Solenoids

Simply put, a solenoid is an electrically activated on/off valve that controls fuel flow (which could be either gasoline or alcohol) and nitrous oxide flow at the flick of a switch. When it comes to actual construction, some solenoids are manufactured out of stainless steel or aluminum. The higher quality the materials, the less trouble you're going to have in the long run, so it is always wise to check with the manufacturer first when buying a single-stage N_2O kit.

If there is such a thing as a heart and soul of a solenoid, it is the electric coil used to open and close the fuel orifice (see the illustration on page 14). Generally speaking, the coil is designed to operate at 20 percent of the maximum fuel operating pressure at WOT. The duty cycle of a

Tuning Tips

Here are a few tuning tips that I've found to be useful over the years:

- Start with a realistic nitrous calibration recommended by the manufacturer.
- When you are comfortable with the recommended power level, increase power by providing more fuel and more N_2O to the engine through jet changes. At the first sign of detonation, backfire, or misfire, always reduce the size of the nitrous jets first.
- As you add N_2O (and thereby create more heat in the cylinder), pull back ignition timing. One general rule is to retard the timing at top dead center (TDC) until you experience a notable loss of power. Then kick it up a couple of degrees.
- An ignition retard box like one from MSD is highly recommended and functions as a safety valve.
- However, if you don't have one of these boxes, set your ignition timing to a normal, non-nitrous setting so that your engine performs well when the N_2O system is turned off.
- After you have started with a properly adjusted carburetor, jetting should start on the rich side because it's safer, and power levels are not as seriously affected nor are internal engine components as seriously taxed if coming from a rich condition rather than coming from a lean one.
- When adding nitrous oxide to a highly modified engine (i.e., big cam, high-compression pistons, ported and polished heads, headers, etc.), it is also safer to start on the rich side when tuning-in the system. Two jet sizes up from stock is considered being on the safe side.
- Of course there's nothing like a good old-fashioned tune-and-test session down at the local drag strip to establish a creditable baseline. Again, start with a conservative jet size—perhaps one recommended by the nitrous kit manufacturer—and continue to tune your way up until you have achieved your fastest time.
- If in doubt, don't be afraid to consult with some of the more successful nitrous racers who are running similar combinations, and keep a notebook of your progress.
- Caution: Do not make multiple changes to the engine, such as timing, valve lash, etc., while you are in the process of establishing a workable carburetor-tuning baseline. Make one change at a time to determine its effect and worth.

SINGLE-STAGE SINGLE-PLATE SYSTEMS

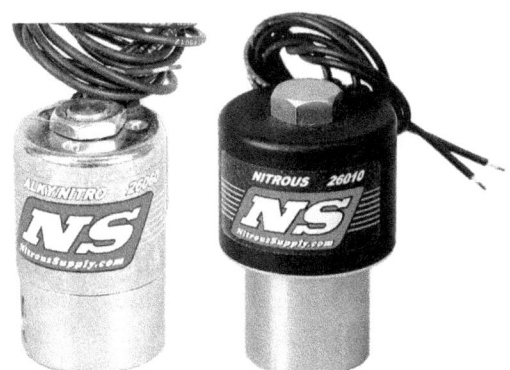

A solenoid is simply an electrically-activated on/off valve, which controls both fuel flow (gasoline or alcohol) and the flow of N_2O at the flick of a switch. Some solenoids are manufactured of stainless-steel, and some from aluminum. Suffice it to say, the higher quality the materials, the less trouble you're going to have in the long run, so it is always wise to check with the manufacturer before buying a single-stage N_2O kit.

high-pressure solenoid (which would always be the nitrous side) is generally no more than 30 seconds at 33 percent. Low-pressure solenoids (typically used on the fuel side) have a duty cycle duration of 5 seconds at 50-percent duty cycle.

Amperage draw varies. Most single-stage kits feature 8.5- to 10-amp nitrous and 4-amp fuel solenoids, which combine for a system draw of 12 amps. But a higher amperage draw is going to allow the coil to open at a higher pressure. However, the longer a coil is open, the more amperage it draws, and the hotter it gets!

Orifice size is also very important because it dictates flow capacity. Think of a solenoid as a huge jet. You want the solenoid to flow at maximum PSI. In fact, its flow rating should always be larger than the combined metering jets throughout the rest of the fuel system.

Plunger quality and seal quality, which control the hit (or intensity) is also very important and has a lot to do with the longevity of the solenoid(s). Again, be sure to consult with your manufacturer of choice before selecting a kit. Remember, a bargain kit may not be such a bargain when you balance it against long-term component reliability.

Never use the wrong solenoid for an application. That is the quickest way to cause serious damage to an engine! Generally speaking, fuel and nitrous solenoid mounting brackets on a single-stage-plate N_2O kit typically have the fuel solenoid located at the left rear carburetor stud, in the general vicinity of the fuel supply line and the N_2O solenoid being located at the left front carburetor stud. Mounting brackets vary depending on the level of sophistication and cost of the kit in question. Of course, you can always upgrade. Just to cite one example, Edelbrock Nitrous' optional CNC-machined Two-Solenoid Bracket(s) for square-flange Edelbrock Performer, Holley 4500, and Dominator carburetors are some of the nicest solenoid brackets I've seen.

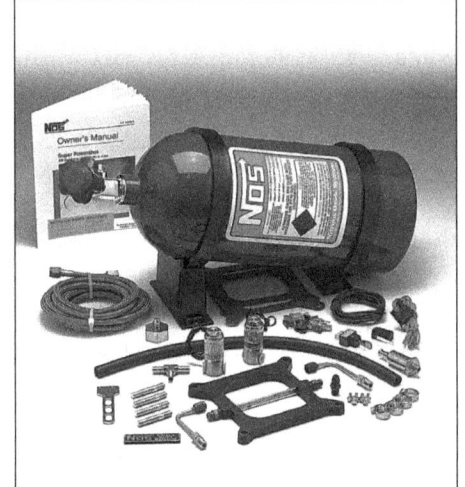

Nitrous Oxide Systems' non-adjustable Powershot N_2O kit (PN 05001NOS) for the Holley flange, and Q-Jet–type spread-bore flange (PN 05004NOS) offer up to 125 hp at the touch of a button. Note that there is also a Powershot Universal kit application (PN 05000NOS). For those who want more power and controllability, there's the 100-125-150-hp Super Powershot nitrous kits available in standard Holley 4V flange (PN 05101NOS), Q-Jet-type spread-bore flange (PN 05104NOS), and even a Holley 2300 2-barrel-flange application (PN 051056NOS).

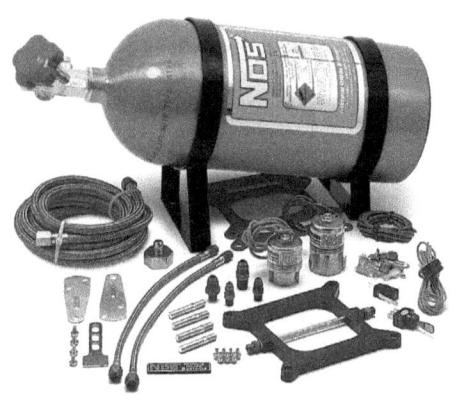

The NOS 200- to 400-hp Big Shot Single Stage N_2O system is geared toward the really serious street/strip enthusiast. Advertised as the World's Most Powerful Single-Stage Plate Nitrous System, power output is adjustable in increments from 200 to 400 hp. Available kits include the standard Holley 4V-flange (PN 02101NOS) and Holley Dominator-flange (PN 02102NOS). Nitrous Oxide Systems also offers five Cheater Upgrade Kits to convert Sniper (Powershot, and Super Powershot single-plate single-stage N_2O systems) to 200 to 400 hp!

CHAPTER 1

Project: NOS Solenoid Rebuild

Some nitrous oxide solenoids are rebuildable and some are not. Generally, the higher the quality of the solenoid, the greater the likelihood that it's rebuildable. The top-of-the-line solenoids manufactured by Nitrous Oxide Systems (NOS), Nitrous Express (NX), Nitrous Supply (NS), Wilson Manifolds & Nitrous Pro-Flow, ZEX, etc., are all rebuildable and rebuild kits are available.

If you are an active nitrous oxide racer, chances are pretty good that servicing your solenoids as part of overall trackside maintenance is normal. But for those who only occasionally use their N_2O systems, it is highly recommended that you check these solenoids at least once each year to avoid leaks or complete failure. Problem areas to look for include the following:

- The internal seal, which is an O-ring that surrounds the plunger and rides up and down on the stem of your solenoid, can deteriorate from wear and debris. These seals are usually designed to withstand up to 1,100 psi. However, they can get cut or pinched due to over pressurization. If it is a rubber seal, it can swell up. If it's a Teflon seal it can be beaten down into the seat at the base from excessive pressure and constant use.
- Nitrous plungers are also susceptible to the physical laws of nature, such as fluctuations in manifold pressure, fuel vapors, etc., and can swell up and in some cases disintegrate. This reduces the nitrous flow to your engine, causing excessively rich nitrous/fuel conditions and loss of power.
- Keeping in mind that lift on most N_2O solenoids is .050 to .060 inch max, excessive buildup of N_2O deposits from fuel vapors, lack of use, and poor filtration can seriously affect nitrous flow through the orifice. It's almost like having an impassible stalactite hanging down from the roof of a cave.
- Generally speaking, coils are trouble free unless they are left on too long. That's especially the case with the higher-pressure nitrous side. Most N_2O solenoid coils pull around 8.5 to 10 amps. Some heavier-duty/higher-capacity N_2O race coils may pull as much as 15 amps but, generally speaking, 8.5 to 10 amps is average for a single-stage Street/Strip nitrous kit.
- If a nitrous coil is left on (open) for 30 to 60 seconds, the heat buildup needs to be radiated away. A recommended cooldown period is generally 30 minutes between duty cycles, or the coil could ultimately fail.
- Another byproduct of an overheated nitrous coil is the creation of an open circuit. Quite typically, the average N_2O coil draws 1.2 to 1.4 ohms during duty cycle. If the coil is stuck in the open position, it either produces an excessive reading of more than 20 ohms or reads as a dead short.
- Fortunately, fuel solenoids are almost indestructible. Due to the chemical composition and temperature of gasoline, their resistance is much higher; up to 20 ohms. However, fuel plungers and seals are also susceptible to excessive pressure, contaminants, lack of use, and material buildup in the orifice from fuel percolation, dirt, or gummy fuel additives, etc., so it's sheer folly to not simultaneously rebuild the nitrous and fuel solenoids.

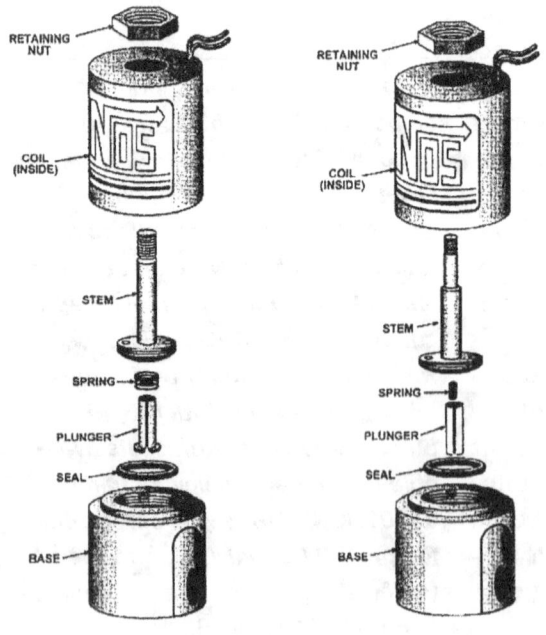

These exploded views of both an NOS PN 16000-16040 N_2O solenoid (left), and PNs -16020, -16050, and -16080 fuel solenoids (right) clearly illustrate the component makeup of each one. These are commonly used on almost all popular Holley/NOS street/strip N_2O kits, although the actual design is fairly universal. (Illustration Courtesy Holley/NOS).

SINGLE-STAGE SINGLE-PLATE SYSTEMS

Nitrous solenoid rebuild kits cost about $35 to $40 at participating nitrous retailers. Ideally, these kits feature a new spanner nut for each solenoid, new nitrous and fuel solenoid plungers, plunger springs, new O-ring seals, and highly detailed instructions. Actual rebuild time is largely dependent on the mechanical skills of the builder. About two hours per solenoid is average, and no special tools are required. Or you can pay a competent shop such as Nitrous Supply to perform the rebuild for you. Depending on type and size of nitrous and fuel solenoid, a service fee of about $40 to $60 is average. The following steps show 30-year N_2O veteran Mike Flynn of Nitrous Supply as he rebuilds a set of NOS N_2O Pro Shot (PN 16040), and Fuel Cheater solenoids (PN 16050), using an NOS Nitrous Solenoid Rebuild Kit (PN A-5141-S).

On/Off Solenoid Activation Micro-Switch

Obviously, nitrous solenoids and solenoid micro switches go hand-in-hand. Not all carburetor throttle linkage is alike, so most single-stage N_2O kits come with a universal micro-switch mounting bracket, which the installer can modify to best suit the application. For one such example, check out the owner-fabricated micro switch bracket used in "Project: Nitrous Supply Powerstar 8001 for 350 Small-Block Chevy Installation" on page 23. Again, most major N_2O kit manufacturers offer a complete line of optional specific-application micro-switch brackets to fit most popular styles and makes of carburetors.

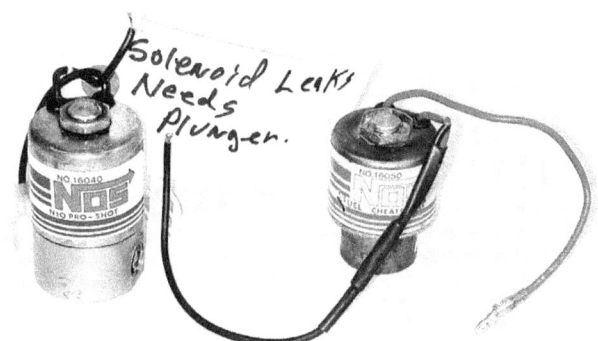

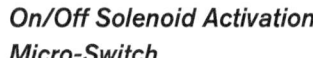 **With street applications, it's a good idea to check your N_2O solenoids at least once per year. When racing, it should be part of your routine maintenance schedule. Problem areas that you want to be looking out for** include the internal seal that rides up and down on the plunger, which can swell up, or get pinched or cut through normal use. The rubber seal inside the plunger can also be affected as it can swell up, under pressure. Checking the orifice for sediment buildup is another important step as well as checking the coil resistance. Typically, 1.2 to 1.4 ohms is ideal for a N_2O solenoid and 20 ohms is ideal for fuel solenoids. NOS Pro Shot N_2O (PN 16040) solenoid (left) and NOS Fuel Cheater (PN 16050) solenoids (right) are slated for rebuild. A visual inspection of both solenoids revealed a leaking problem due to bad seals, debris, and a cut seat. If professionally rebuilt by a shop like Nitrous Supply, cost for rebuilding a set of solenoids like these runs between $35 and $65.

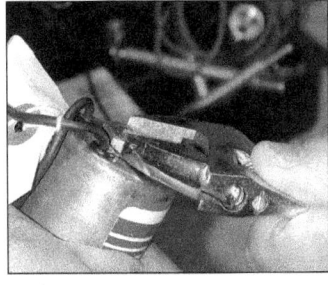

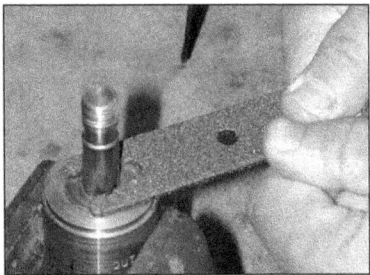

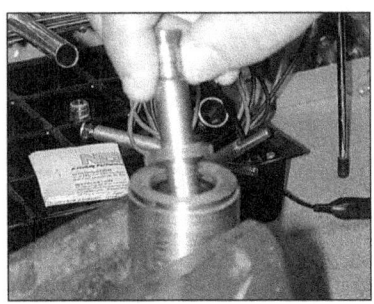

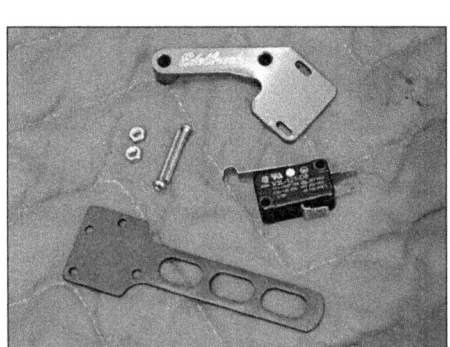

Begin by removing the retaining nut from the top of NOS (PN 16050) Fuel Cheater solenoid housing using a small crescent wrench. The sole purpose of this nut is to secure the coil cover to the solenoid.

After securing the solenoid base in a vice, being careful not to get too aggressive clamping it down, use a spanner-type wrench available from Nitrous Supply to remove the stem from the base.

N_2O solenoids and nitrous solenoid micro switches go hand-in-hand. The sole purpose of a micro switch is to activate the solenoids based on the position of the throttle. This is done by positioning the switch to come in at or near WOT using an adjustable micro switch bracket. Most single-stage N_2O kits come with a universal micro-switch mounting bracket that you can personally modify to best suit the application.

HOW TO INSTALL AND TUNE NITROUS OXIDE SYSTEMS

CHAPTER 1

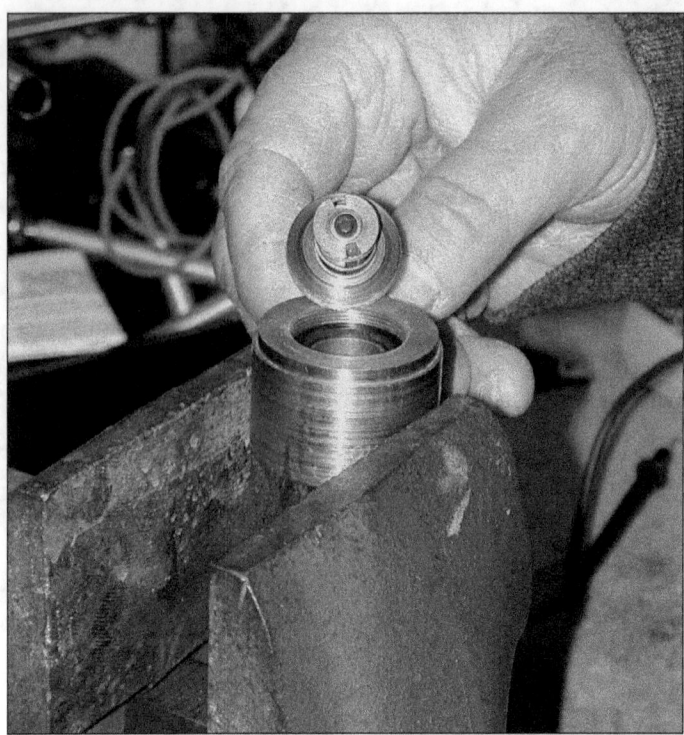
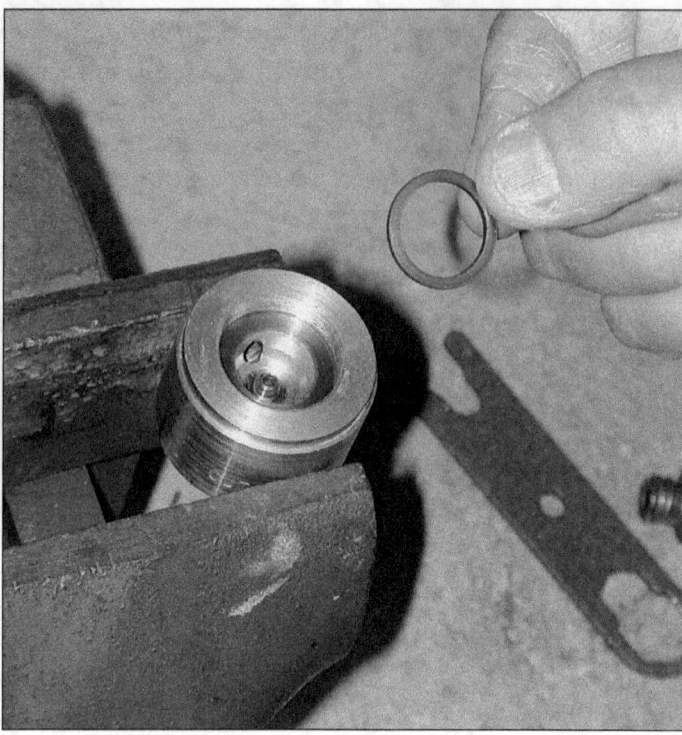

4 After the stem has been removed from the base, out comes the plunger with the internal seal or O-ring and return spring.

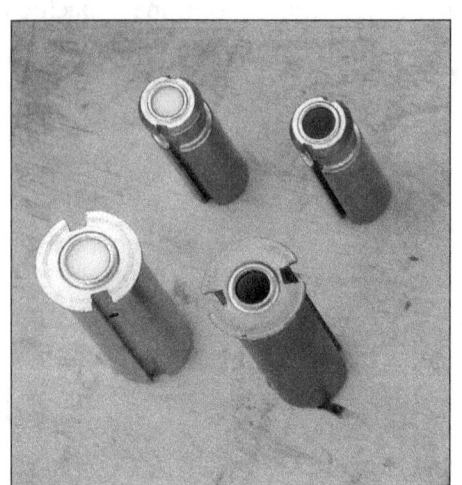

5 This comparison photo of N$_2$O and fuel plungers shows the difference between good-condition (left) and worn plungers (right). It's all in the seals.

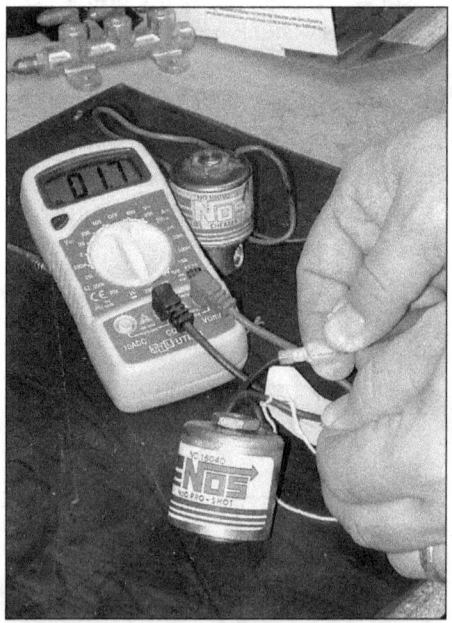

6 Use a Volt-O-Meter to check the voltage output of the nitrous coil, which in this case reads 1.7 ohms. If the coil is bad it either reads "0," signifying a dead short, or reads very high (around 22 ohms or more), signifying that the coil is stuck in the wide-open position.

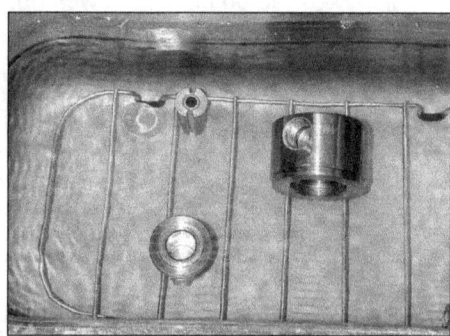

7 An ultra-sonic cleaner is used to clean the solenoid's internal components. If you don't happen to have one of these units, carburetor cleaner can also be used. The point is to get every component as clean as possible.

SINGLE-STAGE SINGLE-PLATE SYSTEMS

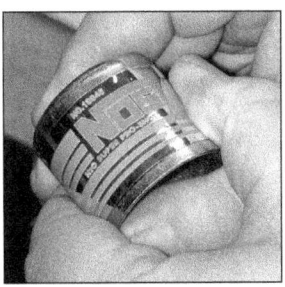

8 Begin by placing a new NOS sticker, provided in the Nitrous Solenoid Rebuild Kit, onto the nitrous coil housing.

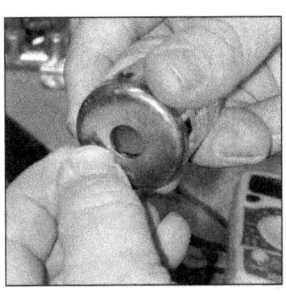

9 Install new rubber grommets on the solenoid housing.

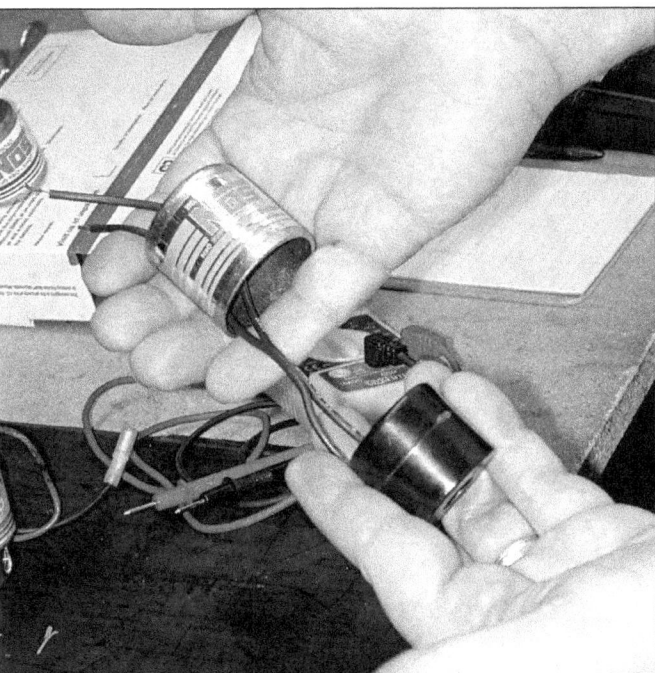

10 Route the coil wires through the rubber grommets. This completes rebuilding the nitrous solenoid coil and nitrous-solenoid coil housing assembly.

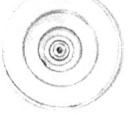 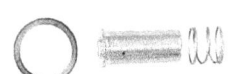 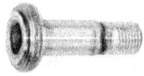 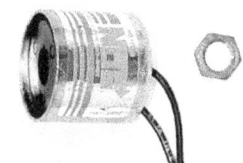

11 This exploded view clearly shows the coil and coil housing, stem, plunger, seal or O-ring, and solenoid body ready for re-assembly.

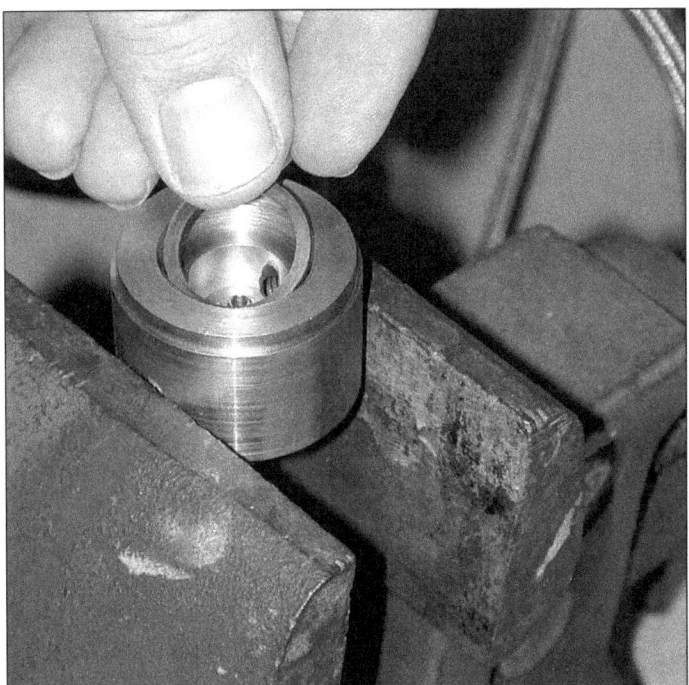

12 With the solenoid body back in the vice, install a brand-new O-ring.

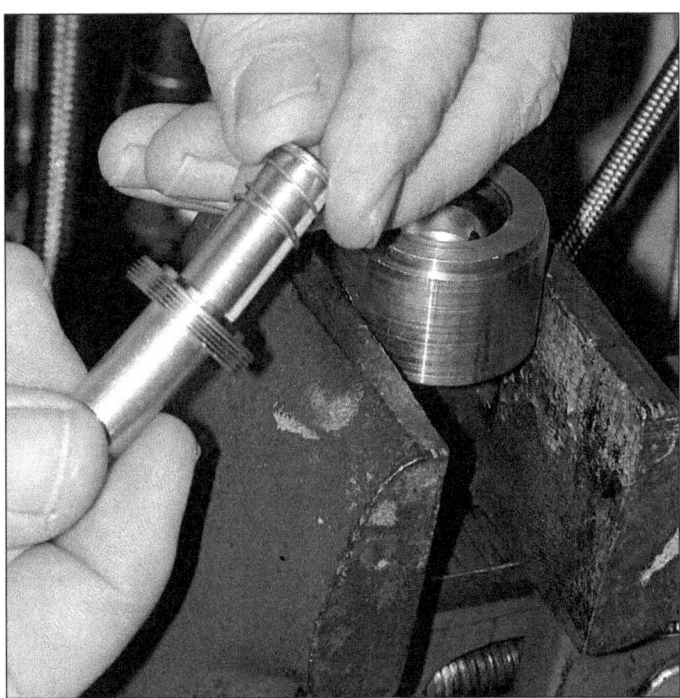

13 Install the plunger and spring onto the solenoid stem.

CHAPTER 1

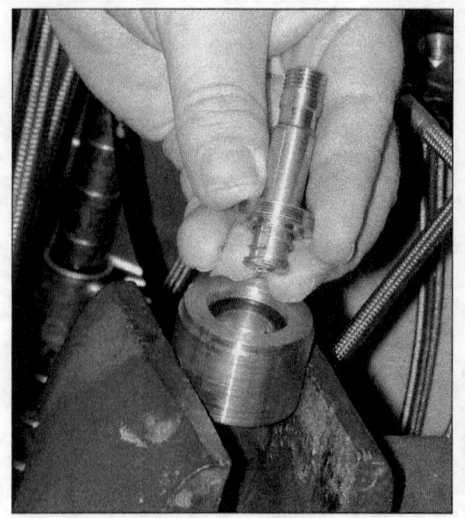

14 In goes the stem and plunder securely tightened, but not too tight, to avoid O-ring damage.

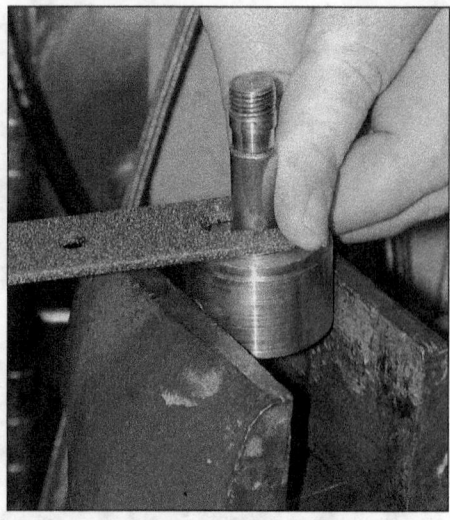

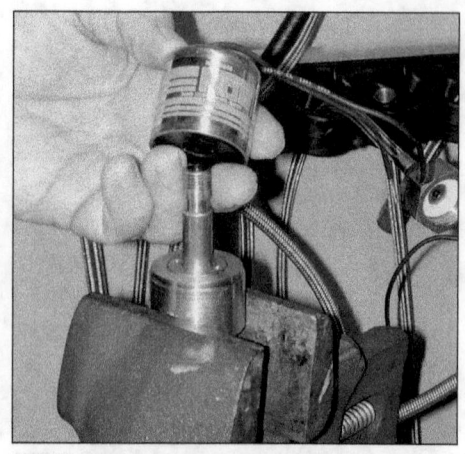

15 The coil and coil cover go on along with the retaining nut, and the N₂O solenoid rebuild is complete.

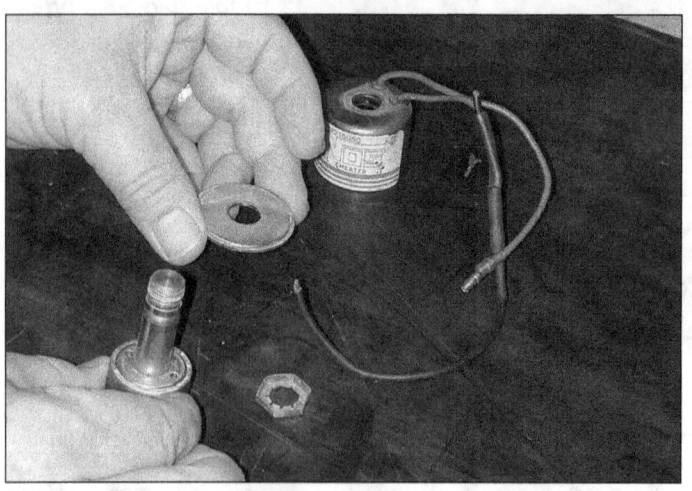

16 It's time to rebuild the NOS Fuel Cheater solenoid. Remove the retaining nut, the coil cover, and protective flux washer.

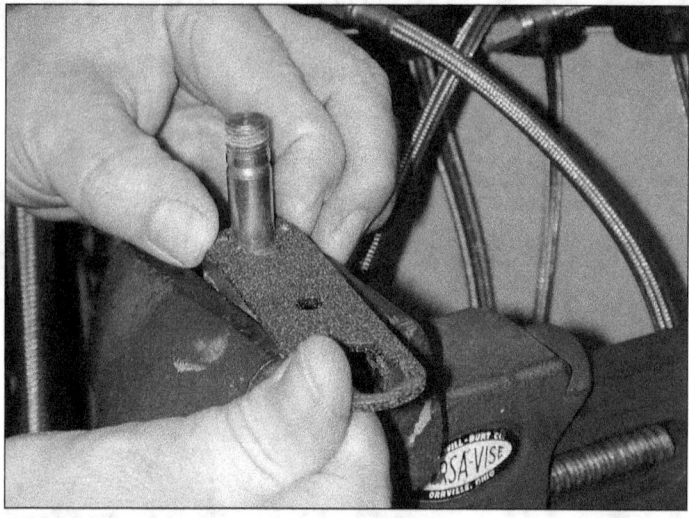

17 Remove the Fuel Cheater stem by using the spanner wrench available through Nitrous Supply.

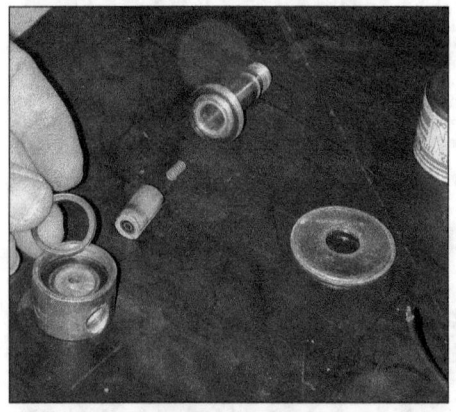

18 Here is the completely disassembled NOS Fuel Cheater solenoid ready for rebuilding.

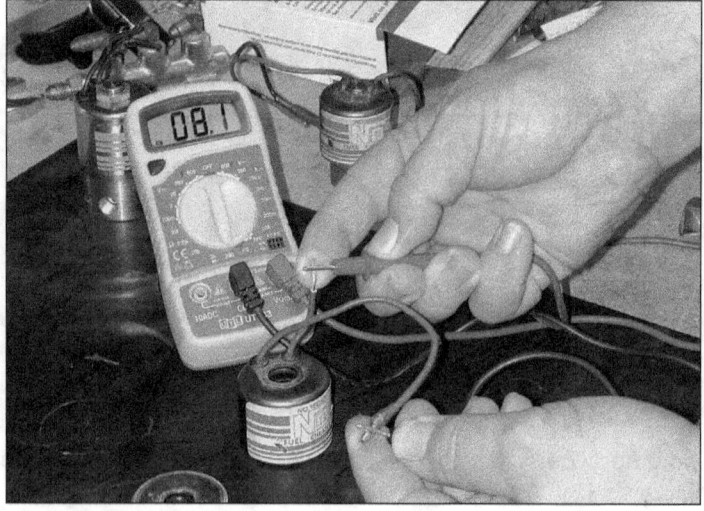

19 Check the voltage output on the NOS Fuel Cheater coil. This one comes up with an acceptable reading of 8 ohms.

HOW TO INSTALL AND TUNE NITROUS OXIDE SYSTEMS

SINGLE-STAGE SINGLE-PLATE SYSTEMS

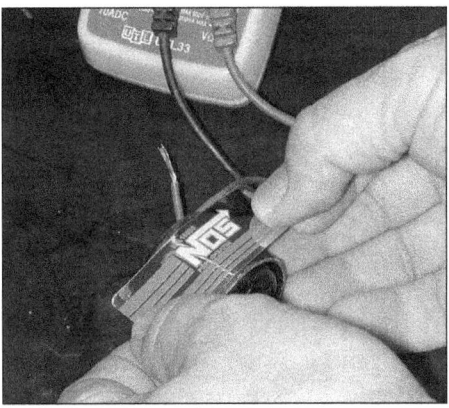

20 After the coil cover is fully reconditioned, install a new NOS Fuel Cheater sticker.

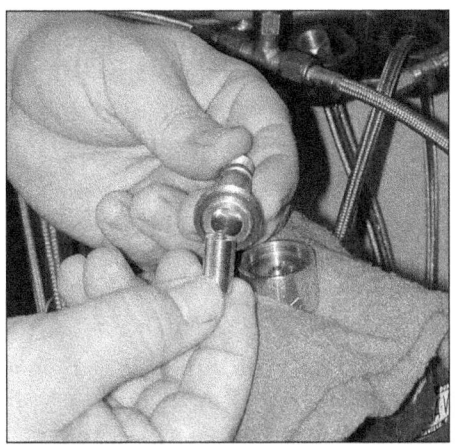

21 Install the plunger spring, which fits into a receiver hole on the plunger, and O-ring into the NOS Fuel Cheater base, or solenoid body.

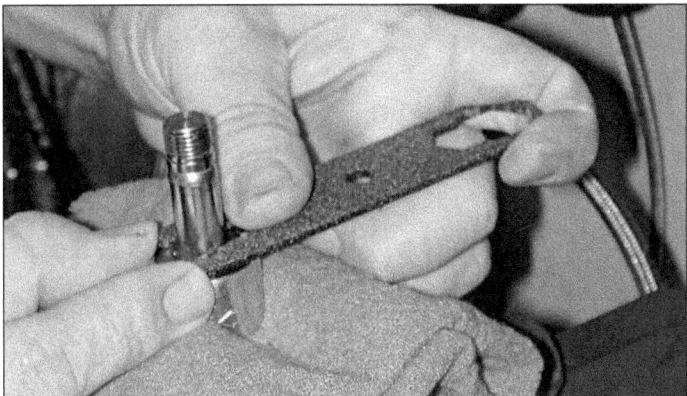

22 Tighten down the NOS Fuel Cheater solenoid stem (complete with flux washer) using a spanner wrench.

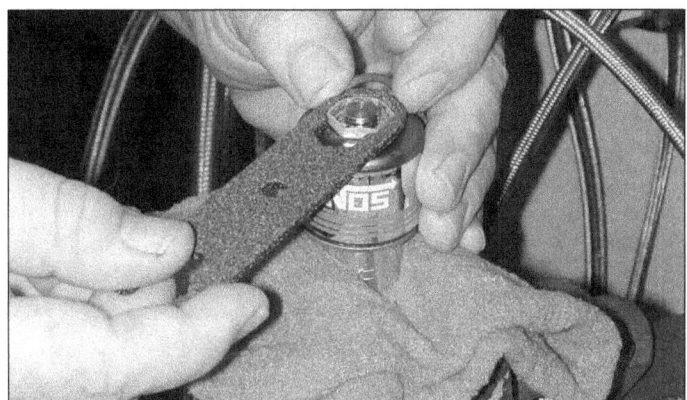

23 With the NOS fuel solenoid fully reconditioned, tighten the retaining nut that secures the fuel coil cover in place.

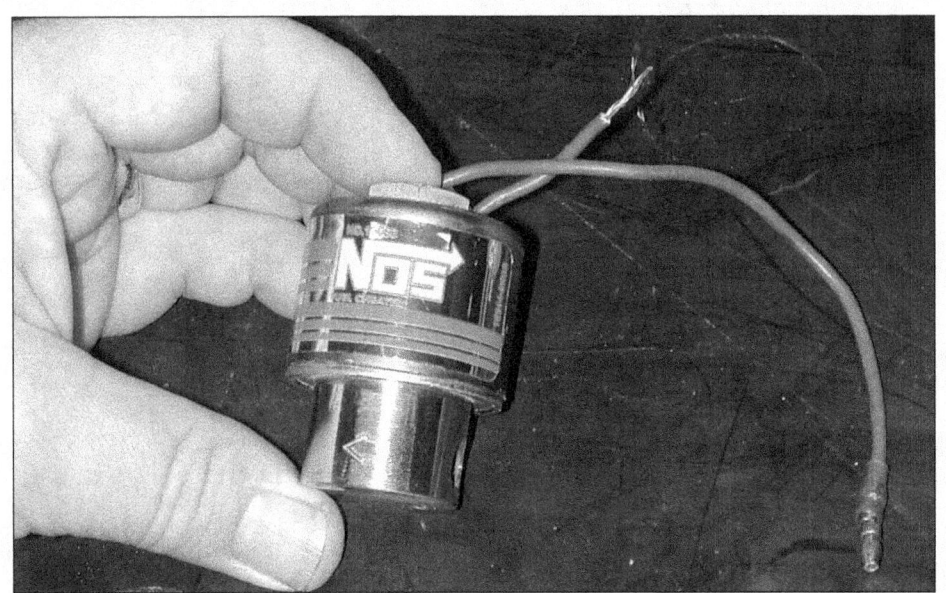

The fully rebuilt NOS Fuel Cheater solenoid.

CHAPTER 1

Nitrous Lines and Carburetor Supply Lines

When it comes to both 1/8-inch-diameter N_2O and fuel delivery lines going directly to the carburetor, user-friendly color coding of the accompanying fittings denotes the application. For example, the N_2O supply line features a blue fitting, while the fuel line fittings are red.

As far as the actual lines themselves, some kits such as Nitrous Supply's Powerstar Holley 350 Chevrolet single-stage nitrous kit, provide -4 AN-fitting-equipped, Teflon-lined flexible braided-stainless soft lines for fuel and nitrous carburetor supply. However, other manufacturers may choose to supply 1/8- to 3/16-inch-diameter hard lines, which feature a blue or red -4 AN fitting on one end and a yet-to-be-installed compression fitting on the other. These lines generally measure 8 to 10 inches in length. Here's a tip: Use an old coat hanger or discarded piece of welding rod to mock up these lines first before bending the actual hard lines. This saves you a lot of time and headaches. Then you can use a proper tube bender to complete the job.

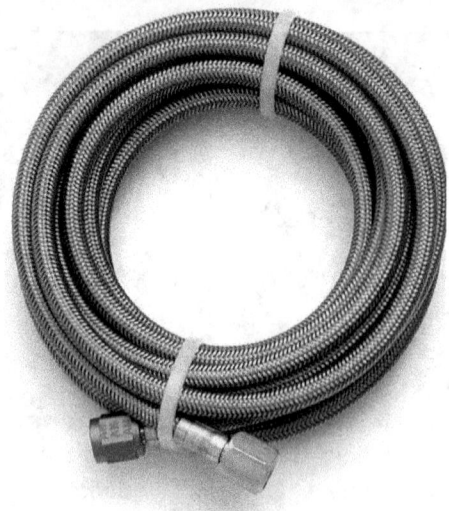

For safety reasons, N_2O delivery lines are comprised of a Teflon core encased in braided stainless steel. Inside-diameter size varies, but most single-stage single-plate carbureted street/strip N_2O kits use 1/8- to 3/16-inch-inside-diameter delivery line with a -4 AN fitting swaged on each end. Hose length also varies; most of these kits come with between 12 and 15 feet of it, depending on the particular application. Remember, braided stainless-steel lines may be flexible, impervious to the elements, and strong enough to ward off road debris, tars, and acid. Also, it cannot be kinked, or placed against sharp surfaces because then it frays, wears through, and ultimately fails.

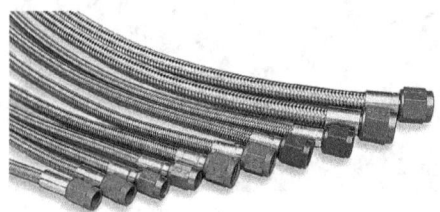

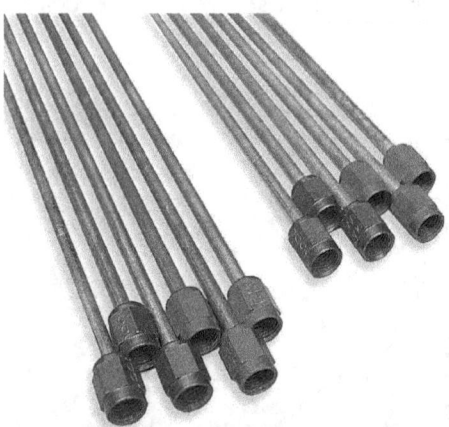

The N_2O and fuel delivery lines go directly to the carburetor (or carburetors) in single-stage dual-carbureted applications; the user-friendly color coding of the accompanying fitting denotes the application. For example, the N_2O supply line features a blue fitting while the fuel line fitting is red.

For safety reasons, nitrous oxide supply lines are comprised of a Teflon core encased in braided stainless steel. Inside-diameter size varies, but most single-stage, single-plate carbureted street/strip N_2O kits use 1/8-inch-inside-diameter delivery line with a -4 AN fitting swaged on each end. Hose length also varies; most single-stage carburetor plate kits give you between 12 and 15 feet of it depending on the particular application. The installer should always keep in mind that although a braided stainless-steel line may be flexible, is impervious to the elements, and is strong enough to ward off road debris, tars, and acid, it cannot be kinked or placed against sharp surfaces or it will fray, wear through, and ultimately fail. Most popular makes of cars feature pan rails, sub-frame connectors, factory-drilled holes, and pan plugs that can be used to safely route nitrous lines along the bottom of the chassis. Using rubber-encased crimp line connectors is another means of safely installing these lines.

Nitrous Oxide Filter

All single-stage carbureted nitrous oxide kits provide a nitrous oxide filter. If yours doesn't have one, perhaps you should consider installing one! The function of the filter in an N_2O kit is to trap any sediments and impurities in the nitrous line. Unlike an OE-type fuel filter, most of these inline N_2O filters are 100-percent serviceable.

Nitrous Oxide Bottles

Believe it or not, early nitrous oxide pioneers stored their N_2O in everything from scuba tanks to steel

SINGLE-STAGE SINGLE-PLATE SYSTEMS

acetylene bottles! That all changed in the late 1970s when Nitrous Oxide Systems founders Dale Vaznaian and Mike Thermos approached Luxfer Manufacturing Company (which specialized in the manufacture of lightweight fire-extinguisher bottles) and inquired if it was possible to manufacturer a 10-pound, 1,800-psi N_2O bottle out of lightweight aluminum rather than steel. Today, the Department of Transportation–certified, DOT-3AL-1800 10-pound aluminum N_2O bottle, which originally appeared in NOS blue, has become an industry standard. This bottle features a wall thickness of .0305 inch and weighs 14.2 pounds empty, and 24.2 pounds full. These bottles come equipped with a bottle valve, bottle valve adapter, and a pair of bottle brackets. Bottle mounting (particularly with a 10-pound bottle), because it features no internal siphon, should be done so the valve is elevated at a 15-degree angle to ensure optimum delivery of its contents. A nitrous filter should also be positioned in line with the remainder of the system to avoid any potential delivery issues.

Electrical Components

Wiring a single-stage carbureted nitrous-plate system is about as basic as it can get. You have an arming switch that consists of either a plastic or metal toggle switch. This arming switch connects to ground on one end, and the inline fuse link at the other end. Once activated, the micro switch is energized, which in turn activates the nitrous and fuel solenoids, which are also grounded. Pretty simple stuff!

Fuel Pumps and Fuel Pressure Regulators

High-pressure fuel pumps, like NOS' popular PN 15763NOS 110-gph Pump with Regulator (which is the same as a traditional Holley Blue Pump) are not usually provided with single-plate, single-stage carbureted N_2O kits; so why bring it up? Because most OE carbureted fuel pumps (mechanical or electric) function at a pre-determined output volume for stock engines. At three-quarter to wide open throttle, the OE fuel pump in your car is already operating near maximum capacity, so asking it to do any more than it was designed for is asking too much.

When purchasing a high-pressure carburetor-style supplementary fuel pump, there are four factors to consider:

1. The horsepower increase this supplementary pump must support.
2. The gallons per hour (GPH) required to support this increase in horsepower. (A common rule in determining the needed size of supplementary pumps is to multiply intended horsepower by .008 to .095 on a four-cycle engine like a Ford or Chevrolet small-block, or by .095 to .110 on a two-cycle engine like an ATV or motorcycle; and when it comes to alcohol, double these figures.)
3. You need to know the fuel pressure on which the engine operates. For carbureted engines like the aforementioned Ford and GM small-blocks, 6 to 10 psi is ideal.
4. The flow pressure of the pump under consideration. For example, the Holley/NOS pump is 110 gph, so your flow requirements should always be at or below the pump's maximum GPH rating.

When mounting a supplementary carburetor-style fuel pump, it's advisable to locate the pump as close to the fuel source as possible. Line size should be consistent with the remainder of the fuel system, and a high-quality fuel filter (preferably one that is serviceable) should be used.

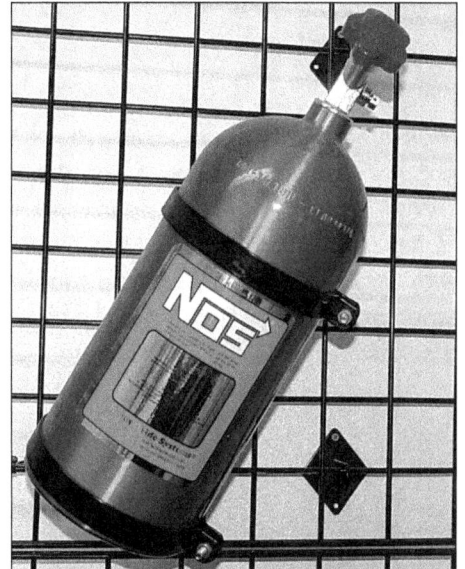

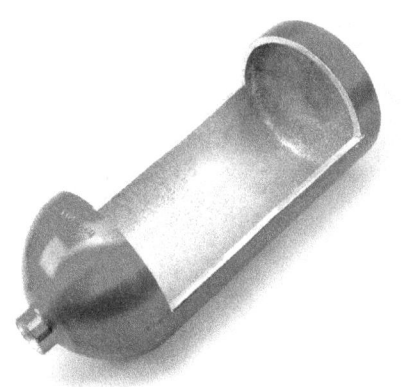

The 1,800-psi, 10-pound-aluminum N_2O bottle that originally appeared in NOS Blue has become a standard of the industry. This DOT certified (DOT-3AL-18000) bottle features a consistent minimum wall thickness of .0305 inch (shown in cutaway) and weighs 14.2 pounds empty, 24.2 pounds wet, and traditionally features no internal siphon.

Two types of fuel pressure regulators are available: deadhead or bypass. Regardless of which type of regulator you use, it is crucial that it is matched to the flow capacities of the fuel pump, or it could result in premature pump failure or burst fuel lines.

With a deadhead-style regulator, fuel pressure is controlled down to a set value using a diaphragm/spring arrangement that controls the fuel that passes into the engine. Once the system is disarmed or the engine shut off, fuel flow through the regulator ceases. If the pump is wired on a separate circuit, and remains on, line pressure climbs to the psi rating at which the pump stalls. This system is traditionally used on carbureted applications, so the previously mentioned Holley/NOS version is a good choice.

A bypass-style fuel pressure regulator controls fuel pressure by returning excessive fuel to the tank or back to the fuel line upstream of the pump. This particular loop approach reduces stress on the fuel pump by lowering the fuel pressure to the level at which the pump was designed to operate. Furthermore, fuel pressure is more constant with a bypassing regulator and the pulsing effect is eliminated. Bypassing regulator systems seem to work best with throttle-body injection (TBI) applications as well as sequential electronic fuel injection (SEFI) systems, which use either in-tank-mounted pumps, inline electric fuel pumps, or a combination of both.

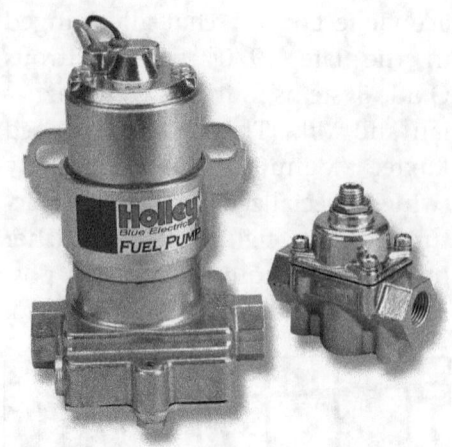

High-pressure fuel pumps, like the popular 110-gph Pump with Regulator (PN 15775NOS; the same as the Holley Blue Pump) are not provided with single-plate single-stage street/strip carbureted N_2O kits, but they are a necessity.

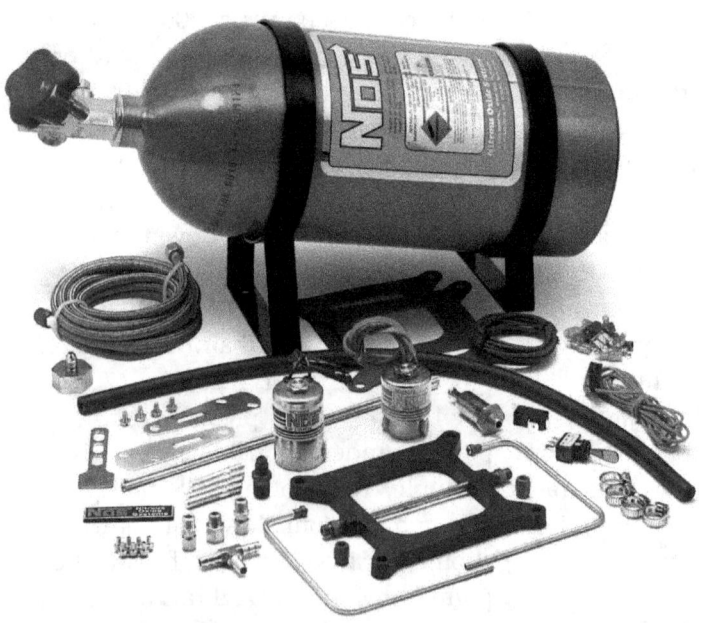

NOS 150- to 250-hp Cheater system contains 150-, 180-, 210-, and 250-hp levels. It boasts a total of six 4-barrel applications, including Holley 4-barrel/late-model Carter AFB (PN 02001NOS), Holley Dominator and Barry Grant King Demon-flange (PN 02002NOS), early-style Carter AFB (PN 02003NOS), spread-bore flange (PN 02004NOS), and Holley 2300 2-barrel application (PN 02005NOS).

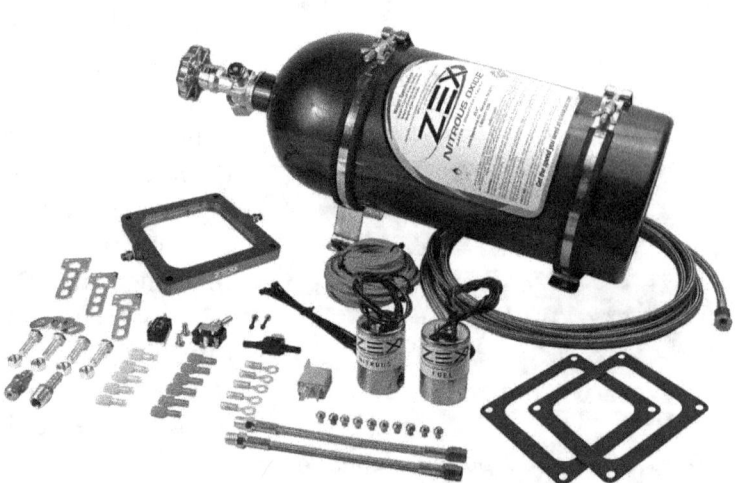

ZEX Nitrous Products bases its 4V single-stage single-plate N_2O kits around its Perimeter N_2O Plate, which features a series of finely drilled holes, referred to by the manufacturer as the Internal Delivery Channel. Horsepower increases of 100 to 300 hp can be achieved and ZEX markets kit applications in square-flange (PN 82040) and Dominator-flange (PN 82048) carburetor applications.

SINGLE-STAGE SINGLE-PLATE SYSTEMS

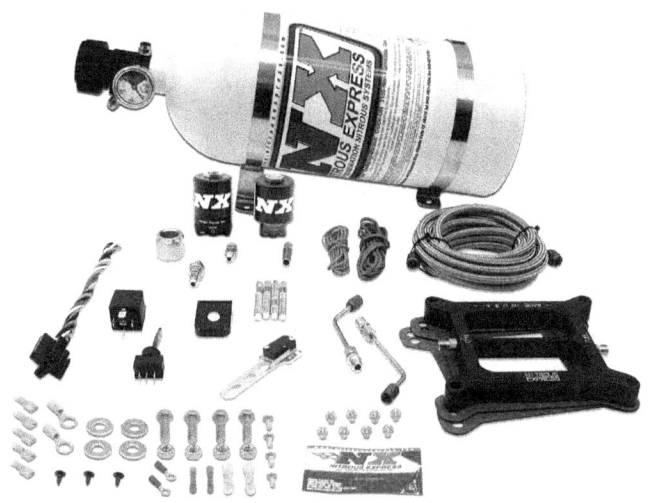

Nitrous Express entry-level single-stage, single-plate N_2O system goes by the name Phase 3 Conventional Plate System, and is capable of producing 50 to 500 hp (PN 30040-10).

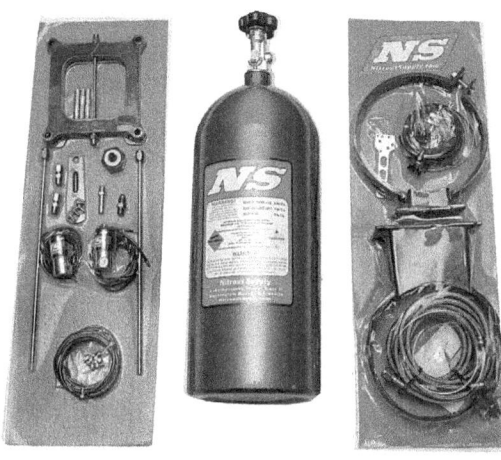

Nitrous Supply markets the NS Powerstar 8001 as an entry-level 4V, single-stage single-plate kit. NS' fully adjustable jet spray bar plate is capable of producing between 50 and 175 hp with advertised torque increases of up to 195 ft-lbs. It's a well-thought-out and well-designed kit.

Project: Nitrous Supply Powerstar 8001 for 350 Chevy Small-Block Installation

Nitrous Supply is one of the most recognized nitrous oxide systems and components parts houses in the industry. Founded by Mike Thermos, one of the original co-founders of Nitrous Oxide Systems, Inc., NS caters to hardcore nitrous racers and offers a huge inventory of nitrous system hard parts, ranging from maximum-power valves to lightweight composite nitrous bottles and trick nitrous solenoids. The company stocks myriad fogger-type nozzles, gauges, jets, braided nitrous line, and virtually anything needed to custom-build your own single- or multi-stage N_2O injection system.

NS also offers a modest line of street/strip nitrous kits geared toward the more common makes of engine, of which the small-block Chevrolet is the most popular. Not surprisingly, NS offers a 75- to 150-hp carbureted plate system for Holley-equipped small-block Chevrolet engines. (It's known as the NS Powerstar, listed under PN 8001.) The kit includes a 10-pound N_2O bottle/valve assembly, an N_2O bottle bracket set, nitrous valve/line adaptors, 14 feet of braided stainless steel

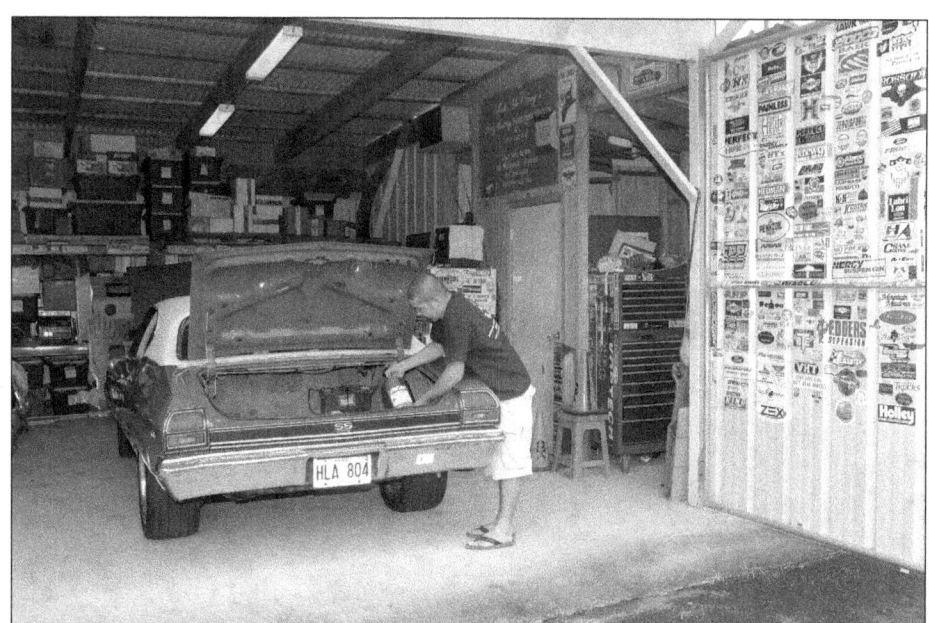

There's nothing like a shot of nitrous oxide to get a performance leg up on the other guy, and Nitrous Supply's Powerstar Single-Stage Carburetor Plate nitrous oxide kit (PN 8001) for the small-block Chevrolet V-8 safely delivers between 75 and 150 hp at the flick of a switch. Shown is Nicholas Morales' 1969 Chevelle SS 350 being trial fitted for an NS 10-pound bottle.

CHAPTER 1

nitrous feed line, nitrous and fuel solenoids, solenoid brackets, blue N_2O fuel filter fitting, gasoline filter fitting, blue N_2O feed tube, red gasoline feed tube, sprayer plate, a set of metering flare jets, carburetor plate gaskets, a carburetor stud kit, a gasoline hose T-fitting, nitrous micro switch and universal micro-switch bracket, nitrous arming switch, inline fuse wire and fuse, and a wiring and hardware pack. The retail price of this kit is $422, FOB from Huntington Beach, California.

The chosen recipient of an NS Powerstar 8001 kit was Nicholas and Charlene Morales' red 1969 Chevelle street machine. The car is powered by a 9.25:1 compression-ratio 1997 GM Vortec 350-ci crate engine. Nicholas' 350 also features a set of Dart Iron Eagle cylinder heads, an Edelbrock Air Gap RPM intake, a 750-cfm Holley carburetor, Hooker Shorty Headers, and a GM HEI ignition. The transmission is a Lokar-equipped GM TH350. This car is the perfect street candidate for a single-plate N_2O kit installation.

Installation time is quick (about six hours) and easy using a floor jack and common shop tools. Of course the proof is in the performance, so we strapped Morales' Chevelle onto Rob Gavel's Dyno Jet 248 portable chassis dyno. Nicholas' Chevelle recorded 278.50 hp at 5,275 rpm and 278.90 ft-lbs at 4,200 rpm as delivered. With the 100 N_2O jets installed and the nitrous switched on, the Chevelle cranked out 350.58 hp at 5,750 rpm and 341.43 ft-lbs at 5,000 rpm. When you take into consideration a parasitic loss of 20 to 22 percent at the flywheel, this old Chevelle is making some pretty good horsepower. See the dyno chart on page 38.

Our next stop was at Hilo Raceway Park, where the Chevelle clicked off 2.417-second 60-foot times and a best elapsed time of 14.029 seconds at 100.59 mph at sea level on the engine alone. With the NS Powerstar N_2O system activated, Morales' Chevelle cranked out a best of 2.227 seconds to 60 feet and registered a 13.281-second elapsed time with a terminal speed of 106.564 mph! Two weeks later, Nicholas and the Chevelle were back again at Hilo Raceway Park. With the Mickey Thompson tires thoroughly heated from the 30-plus-mile warm-weather drive, Morales lowered the tire pressure to 16 psi, and proceeded to crank off a 1.87-second 60-foot time and a 12.72-second pass at 105.99 mph! A couple of weeks later, Nick and his Chevelle made a return engagement and, with the 125 jets installed, the red-and-white Chevelle reeled off a best of 12.67 seconds at 108 mph!

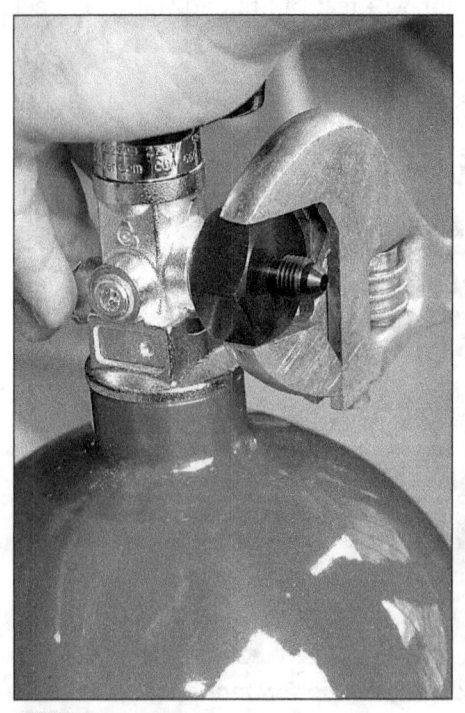

1 Begin the installation by attaching the nitrous and nitrous-valve-line adaptor snugly with a crescent wrench.

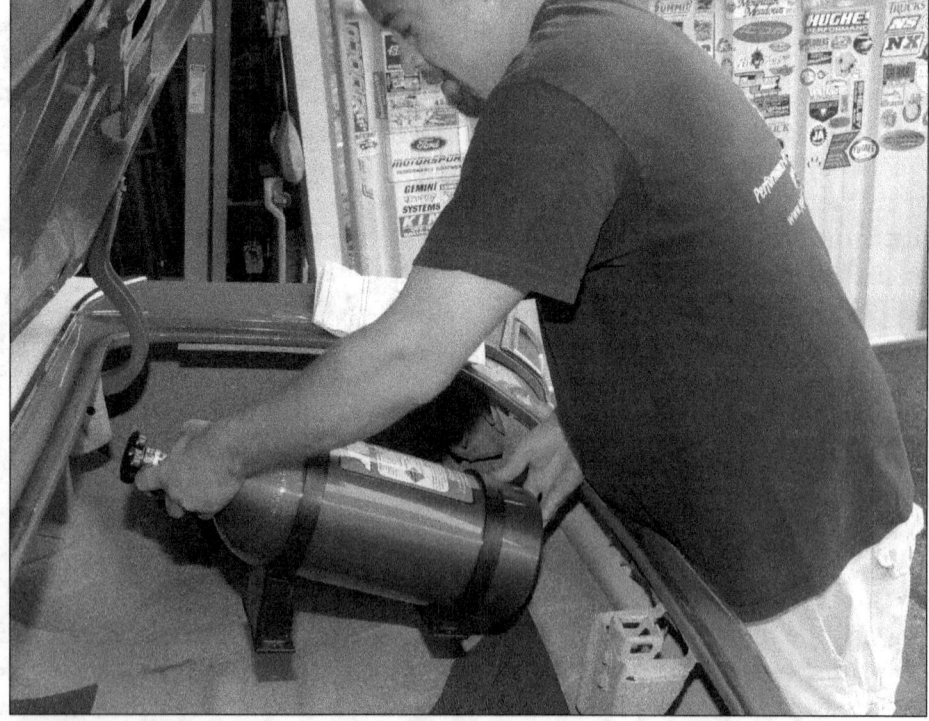

2 After installing the NS 10-pound bottle in the provided bottle brackets, spacing them approximately 10 to 12 inches apart, place the bottle inside the trunk on the passenger side with the bottle facing forward.

SINGLE-STAGE SINGLE-PLATE SYSTEMS

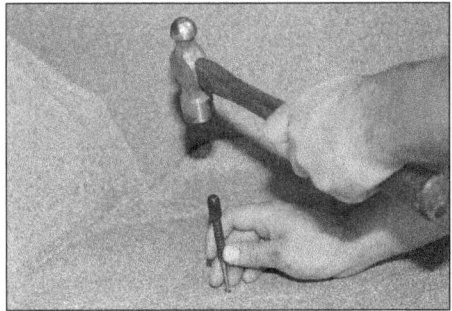

3 After choosing a suitable mounting location, use a marker to scribe the bottle bracket mounting hole, and then mark the trunk pan with a punch.

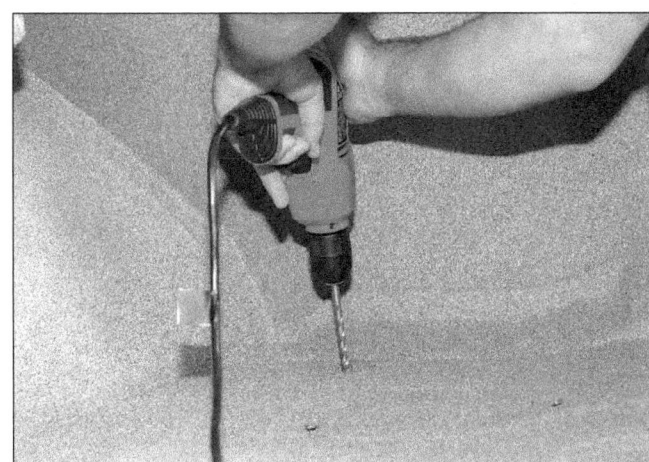

4 Drill four 5/16-inch holes.

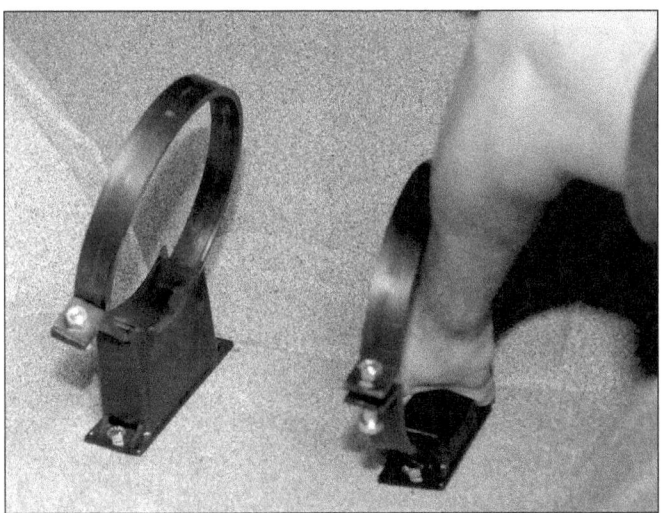

5 Install the NS bottle brackets, using the provided 5/16 x 1½-inch bolts.

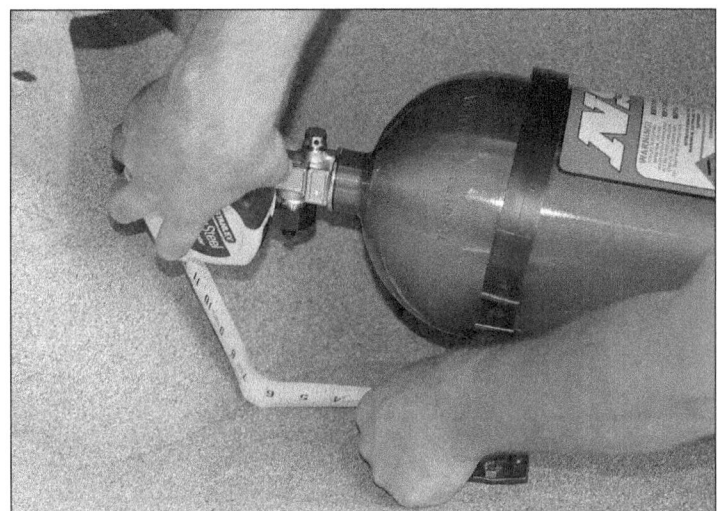

6 After strapping the 10-pound NS bottle into position, use a tape measure to indicate the proper spacing at approximately 4 inches from the front mounting bracket.

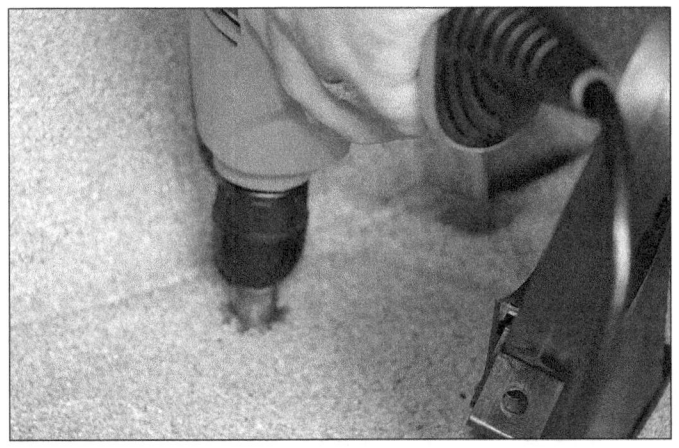

7 Use a step bit to create a 1/4-inch-diameter hole in the trunk pan for the braided stainless-steel N_2O delivery line.

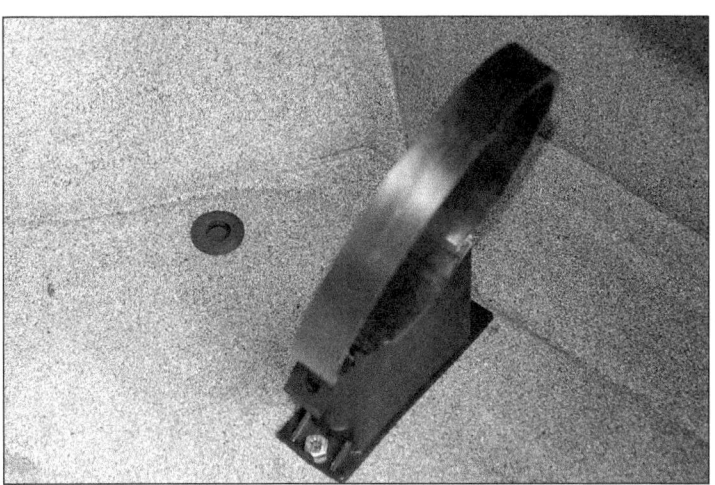

8 The finished hole, complete with protective rubber pan plug.

CHAPTER 1

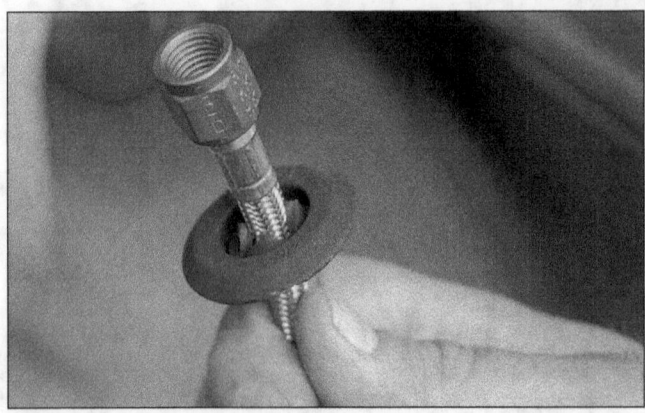

9 The center of the pan plug must be opened up to accept the actual nitrous feed line.

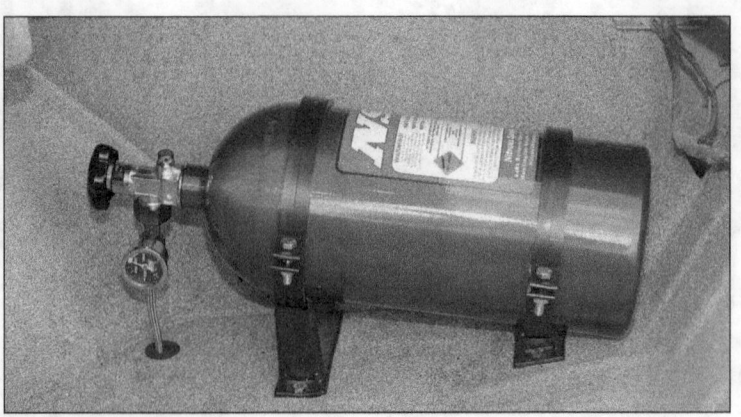

10 Fully attach the NS nitrous delivery line to the bottle and route it into the trunk pan. Note Nitrous Supply's optional 1,500-pound Gauge and Line Adaptor (PN 25910).

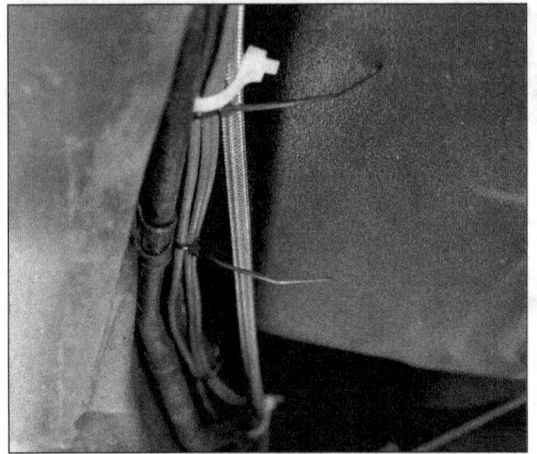

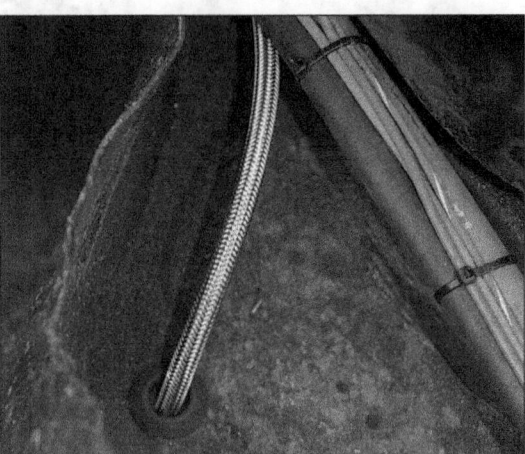

11 Route the nitrous supply line from the rear of the car to the engine compartment, using the front and rear sub-frames as anchoring points.

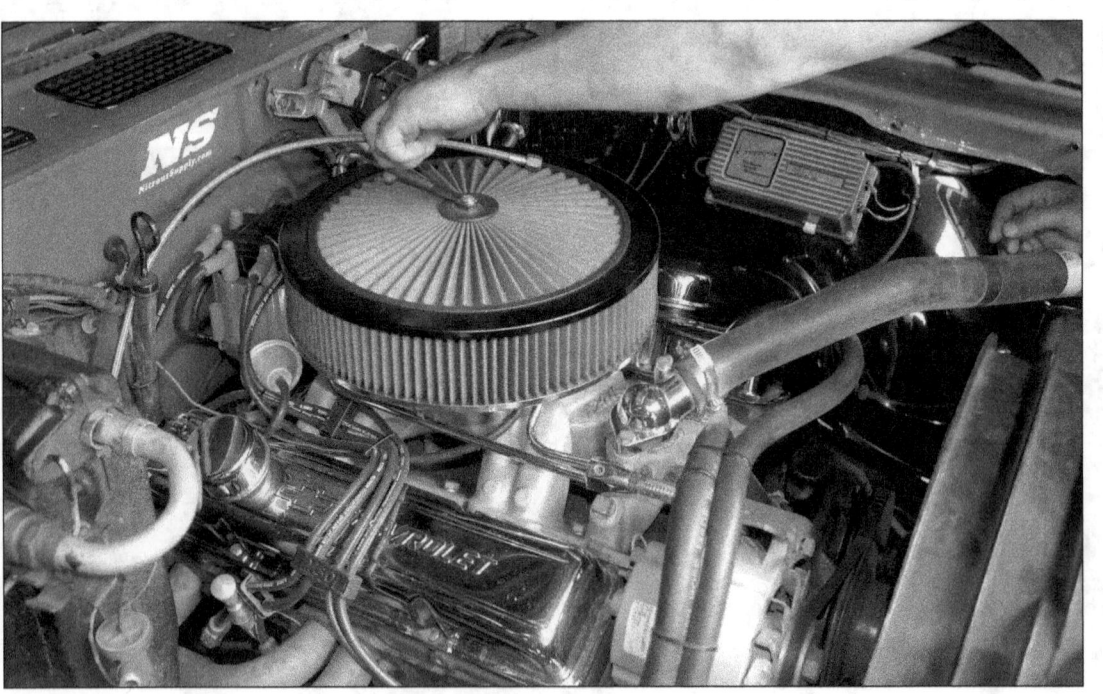

12 Next, route the nitrous supply line into the car's engine compartment between the passenger-side fender apron and air conditioning condenser, away from any heat.

HOW TO INSTALL AND TUNE NITROUS OXIDE SYSTEMS

SINGLE-STAGE SINGLE-PLATE SYSTEMS

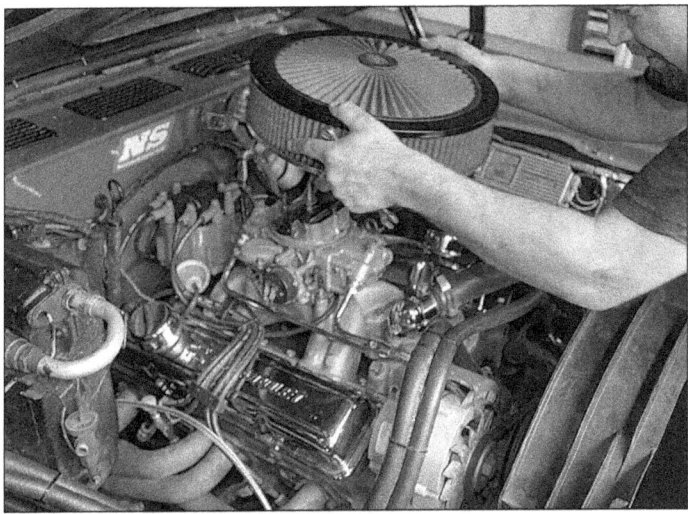

13 *Remove the Chevelle's K&N X-Stream Top High Performance Air Cleaner.*

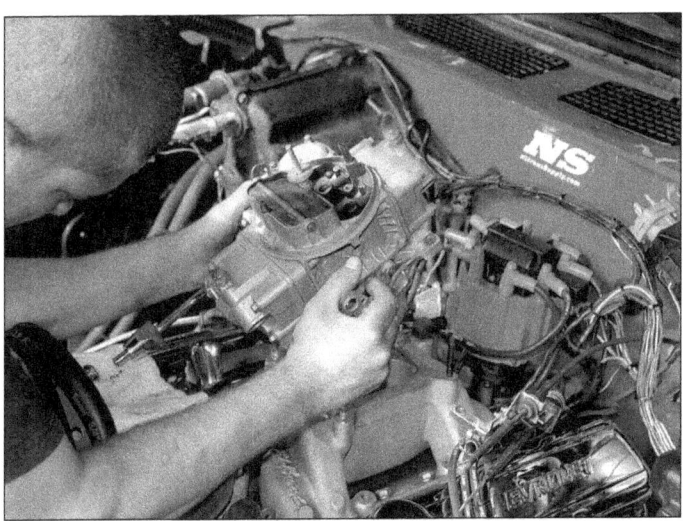

14 *Remove the carburetor from its intake. In this case it was a 750-cfm Holley.*

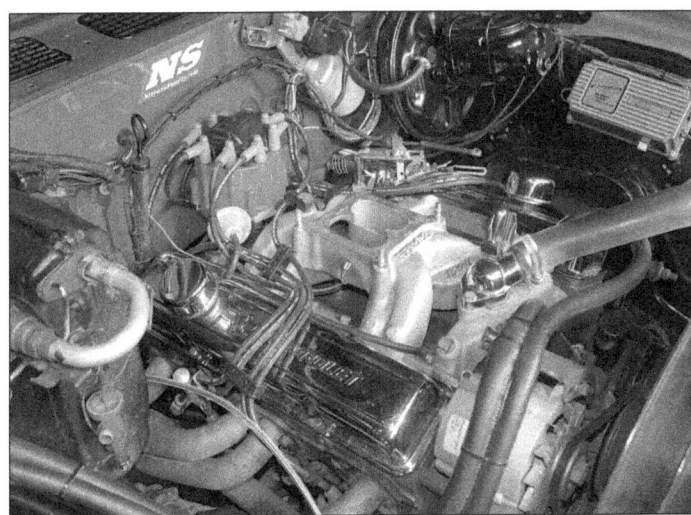

15 *With the carburetor removed, install the larger carburetor studs necessary to accommodate the 1/2-inch-thicker NS nitrous spay bar plate.*

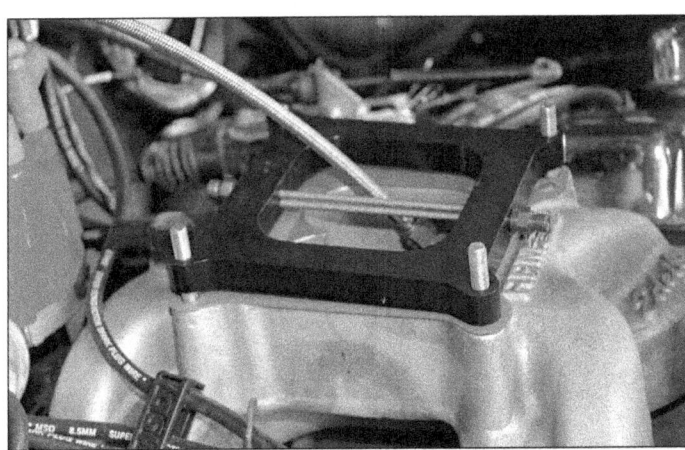

16 *Install the NS spray bar plate with the red fuel fitting facing forward.*

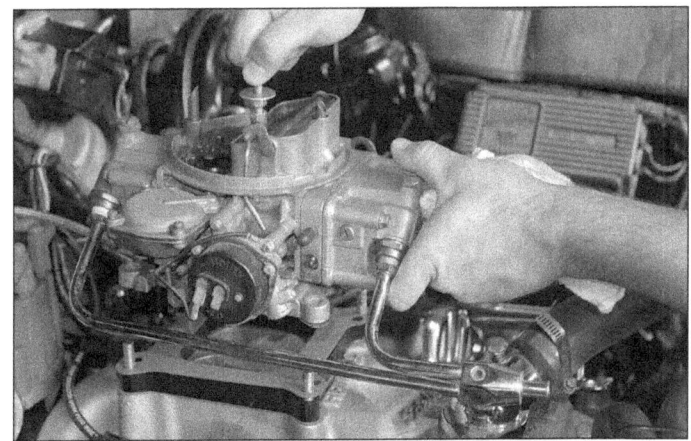

17 *With the NS spray bar in place, re-install the carburetor.*

HOW TO INSTALL AND TUNE NITROUS OXIDE SYSTEMS

CHAPTER 1

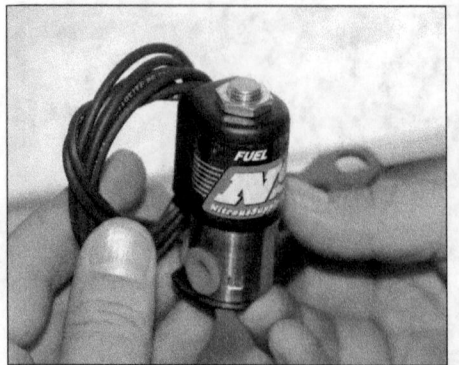

18 Set up the fuel solenoid on its corresponding mounting bracket, using the screws provided.

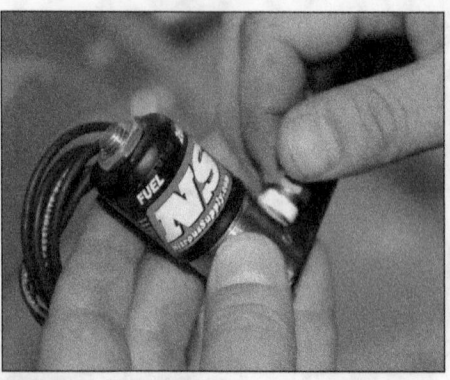

19 Use Teflon tape to secure the fuel line fitting to the fuel solenoid.

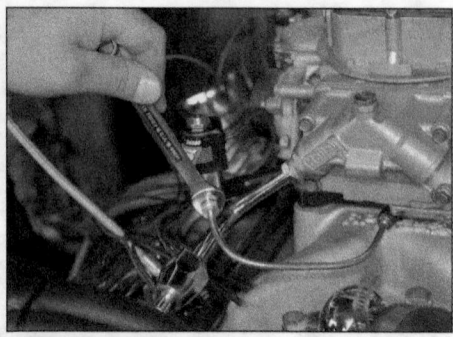

20 Install the fuel tag on the front carburetor onto the front carburetor stud on the passenger side of the engine.

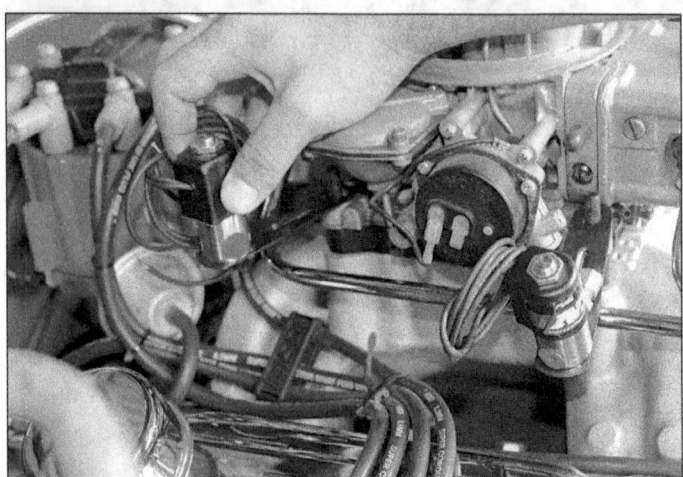
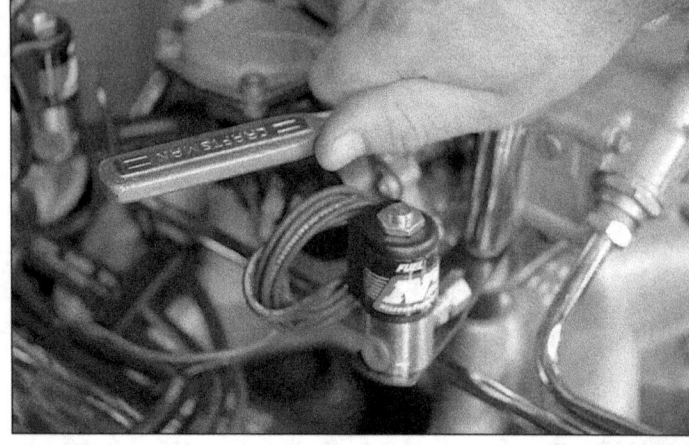

21 Next, place the N_2O solenoid onto the back stud of the carburetor.

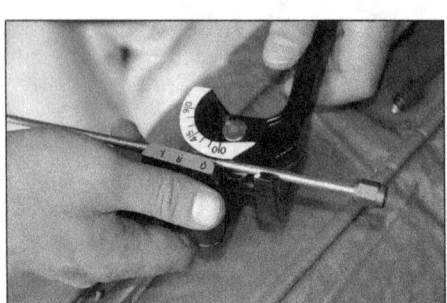

22 Bend the N_2O line extending from the N_2O solenoid to the carburetor plate.

23 Prior to hooking up the newly fabricated line, select a jet and insert it into the N_2O port at the rear of the spray bar. Then attach and tighten the nitrous line.

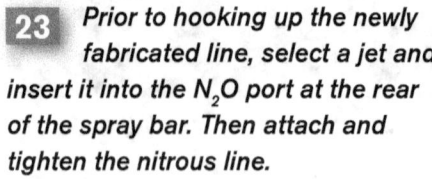
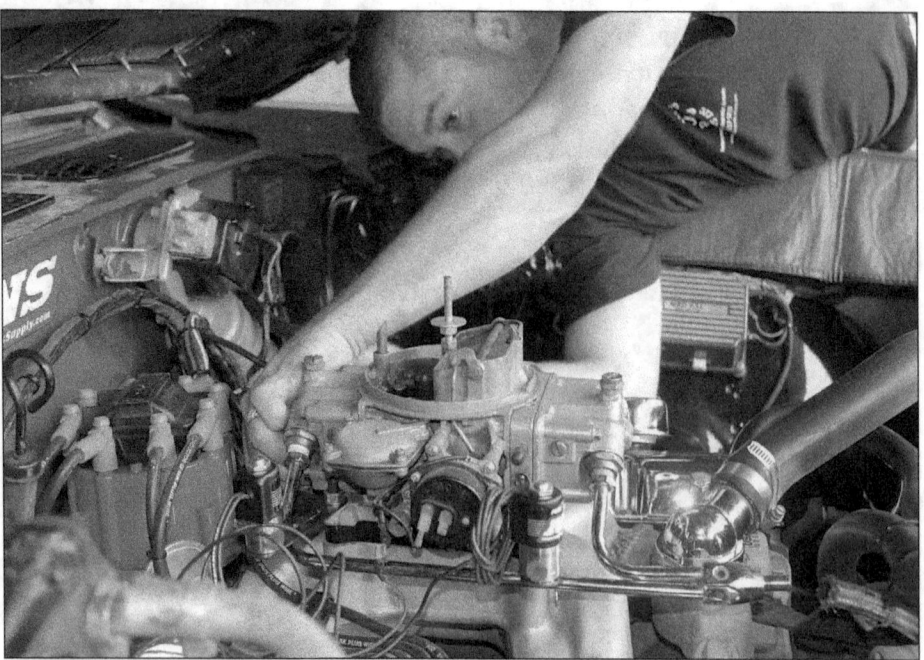

SINGLE-STAGE SINGLE-PLATE SYSTEMS

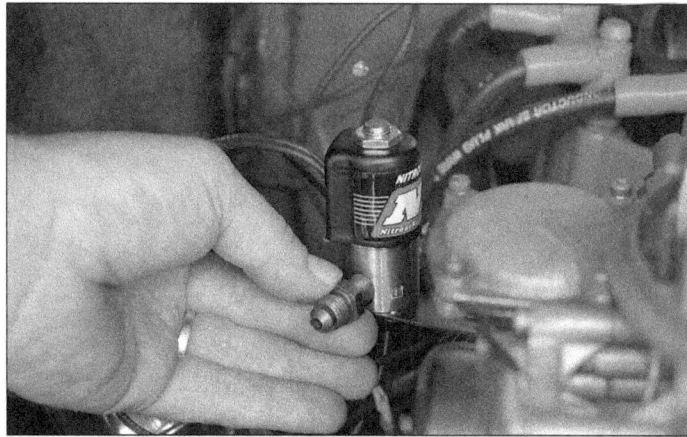

24 Fabricate and install the fuel line using the provided number-53 fuel jet. Then insert the fuel-filter fitting into the port of the N_2O solenoid.

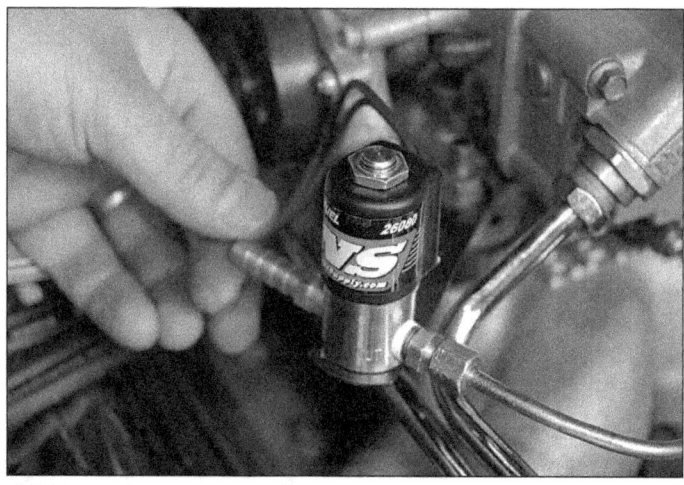

25 Install the barbed fuel-line fitting onto the fuel solenoid located at the front of the engine.

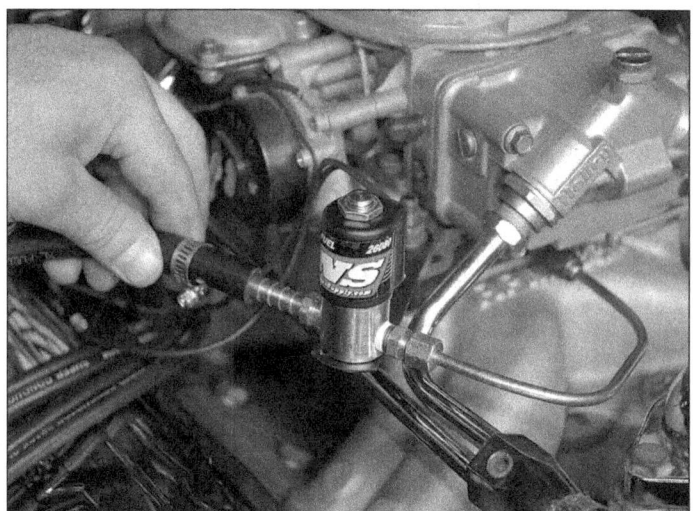

26 Install the fuel line.

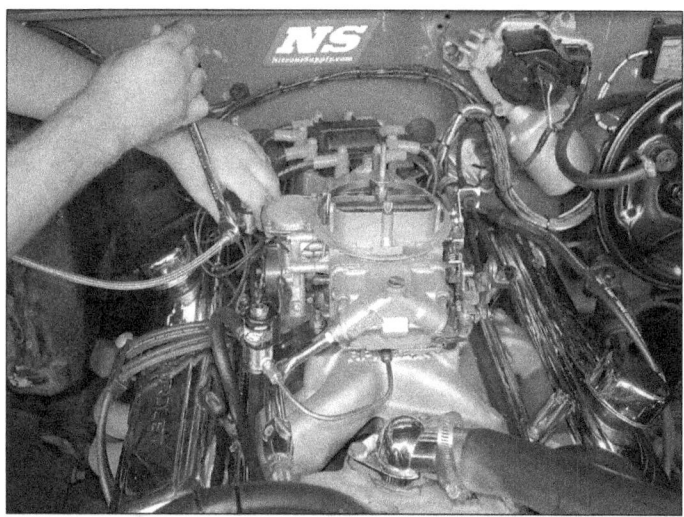

27 Install the nitrous supply line to the fitting located on the N_2O solenoid.

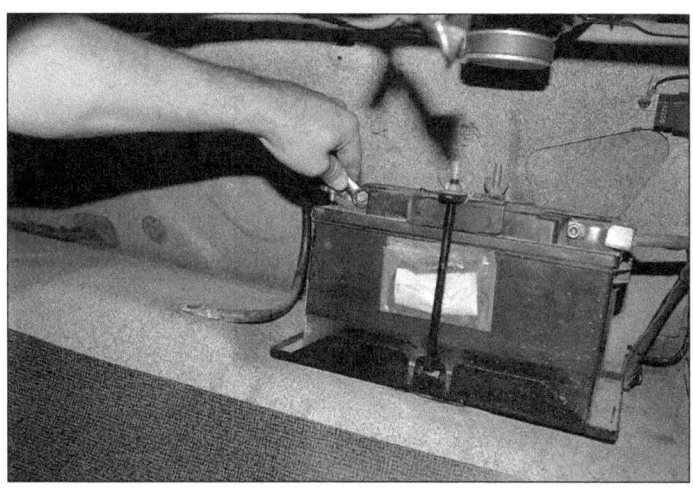

28 Prior to doing any electrical work, disconnect the battery.

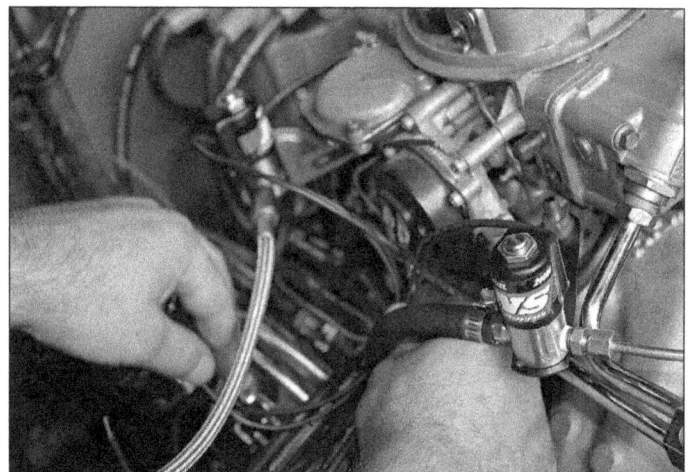

29 Wire the solenoids using the schematic in Nitrous Supply's Installation and Operation instructions.

CHAPTER 1

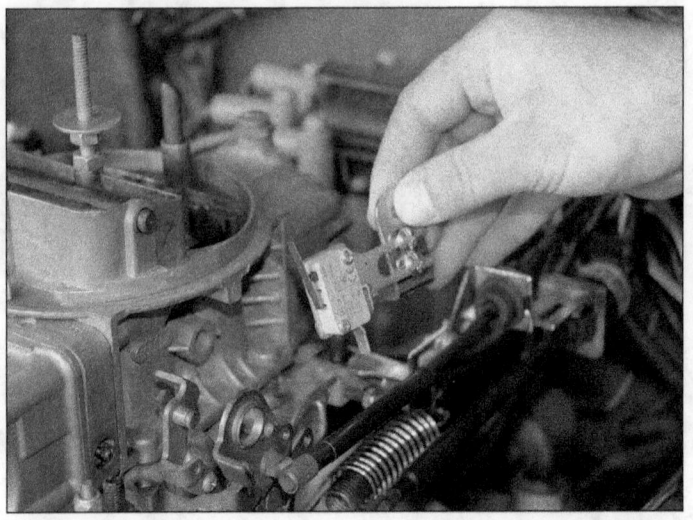

30 NS also supplies a micro switch and universal micro switch bracket, which can be activated at WOT, working off the Holley carburetor linkage.

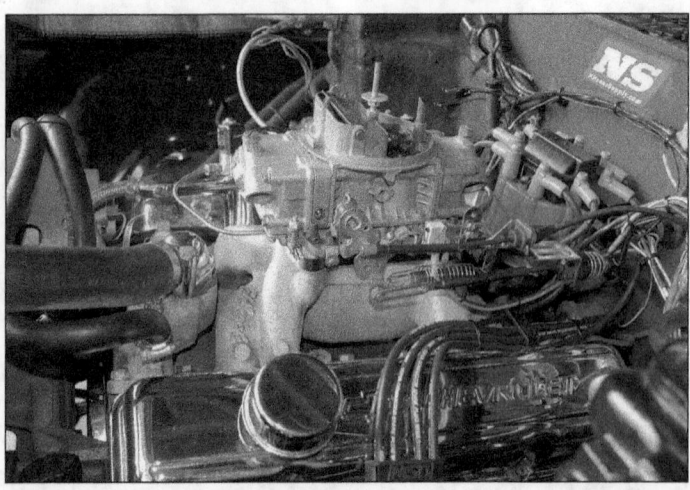

31 For this application, the installer chose to machine-screw this universal bracket to an old carburetor throttle bracket, which was simultaneously mounted to the rear stud of the carburetor. Simple!

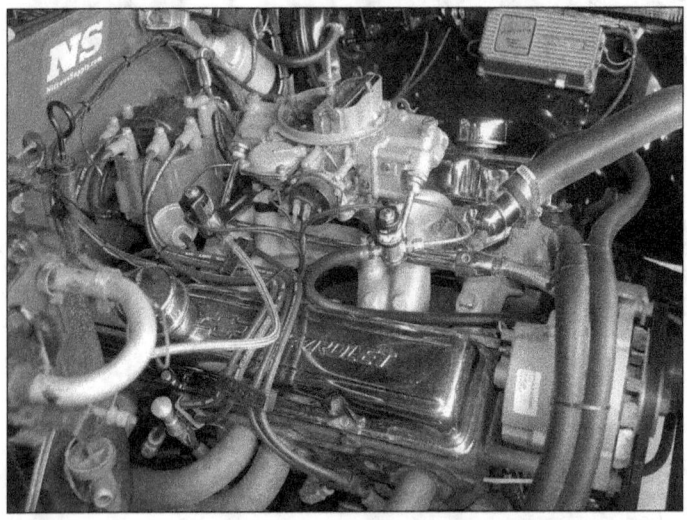

32 Here is the 350 small-block Chevrolet fully plumbed and ready to test.

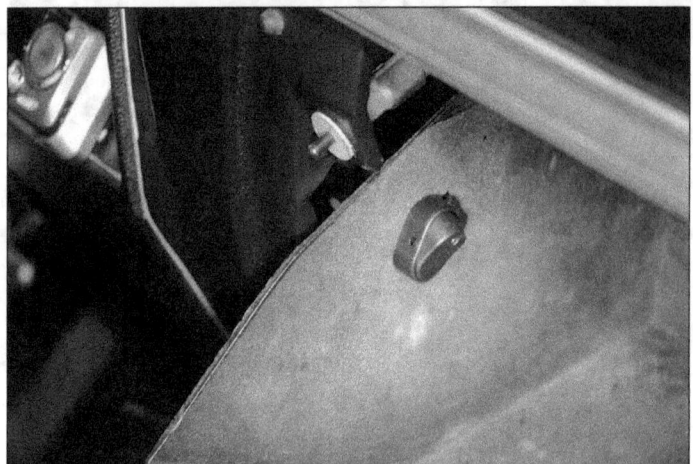

33 The last item of business; for safety reasons, the N_2O arming switch was located out of sight, inside the glove compartment.

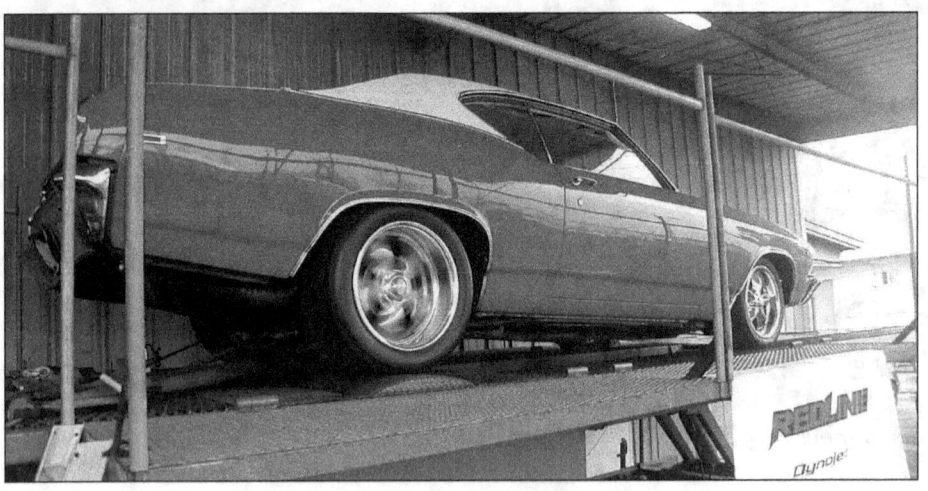

At Rob Gavel's dyno facility, the Chevelle cranked out 278.50 hp at 5,500 rpm on the engine.

SINGLE-STAGE SINGLE-PLATE SYSTEMS

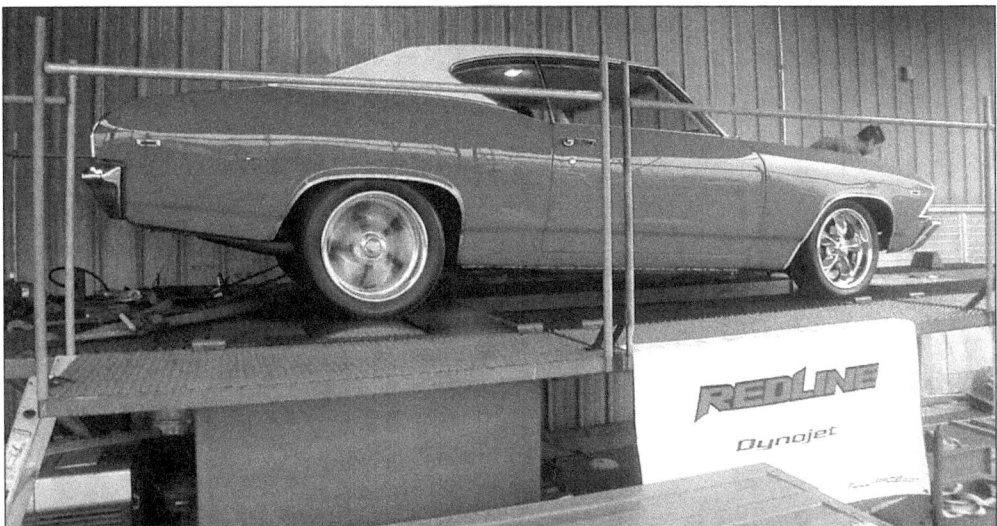

With the nitrous switched on, the red-and-white 1969 cranked out an incredible 350.58 hp at 5,750 rpm!

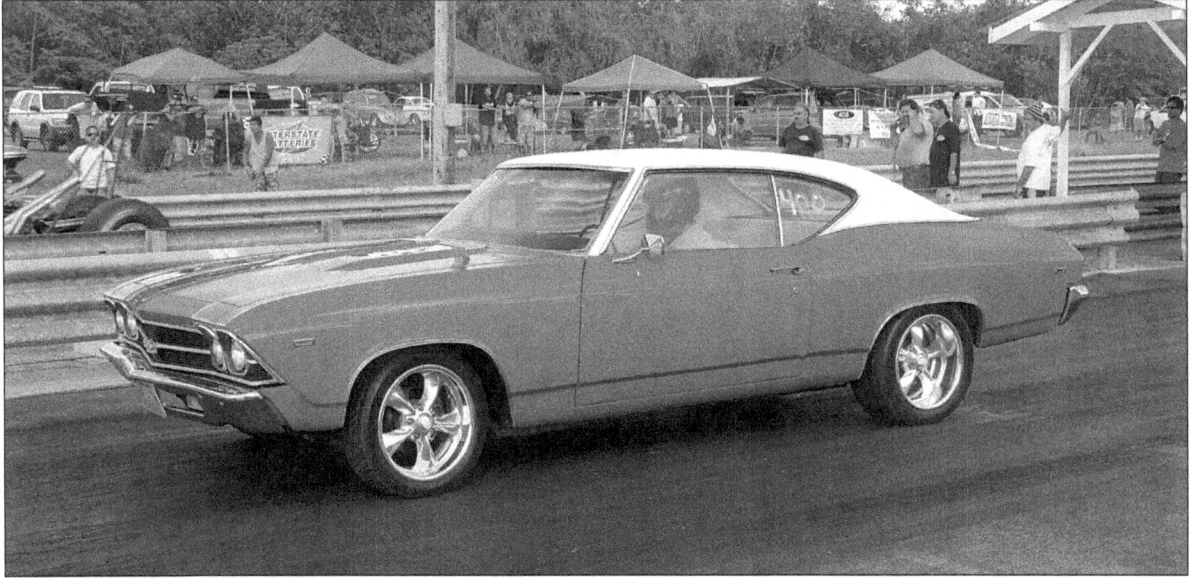

The owner stopped by Hilo Raceway Park where the Chevelle recorded a best of 2.417 seconds at 60 feet, with an ET of 14.029 seconds at 100.59 mph on the engine.

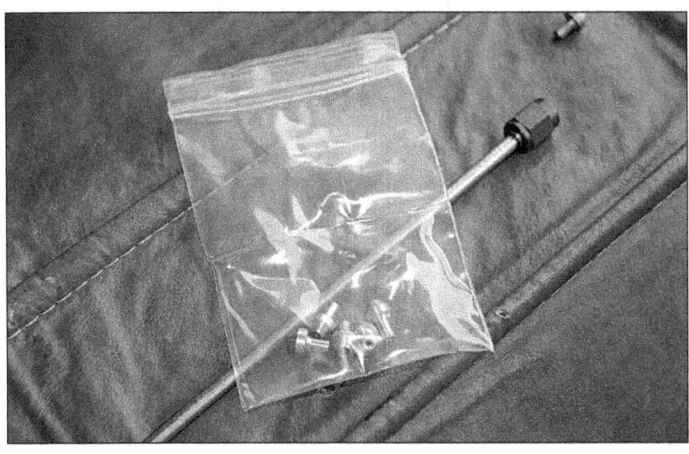
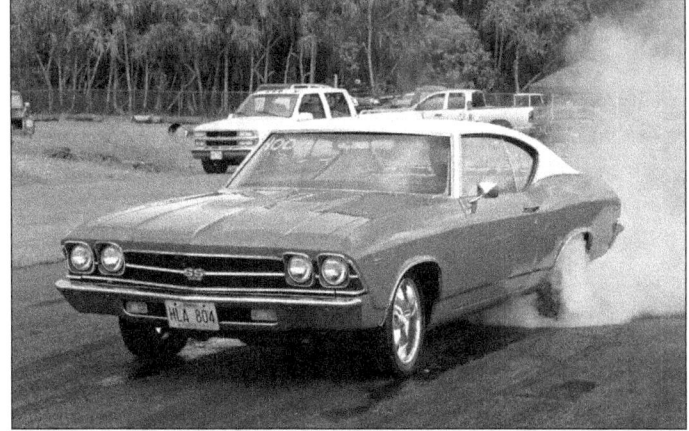

The Chevelle cranked off a respectable 60-foot time of 2.227 seconds while registering an elapsed time of 13.281 seconds at 106.54 mph at sea level. A few weeks later, the owner returned with the 125-hp jet installed and cranked out a best of 12.67 at 108 mph. Not too shabby!

Nitrous Oxide Safety Tips

"One of the things you learn when dealing with nitrous oxide is that it can either be a friend or foe," says N_2O pioneer Ron Hammel, whose 10,000 RPM Speed Equipment company pioneered user-friendly nitrous street/strip kits. "I've seen a lot of hoods blown off when a nitrous oxide system isn't installed correctly." Hammel continued.

"What I don't like about this industry is that a lot of people have jumped into the business thinking that they know all about the subject, but they really have no clue about what they're doing. If you incorrectly install N_2O in a car, it certainly runs faster than not having it at all, but you'll run lean, heat up pistons, backfire intake manifolds, and do all kinds of dangerous and expensive things to the engine!"

My first experience with nitrous oxide happened at the 1976 Car Craft Magazine Street Machine Nationals held in Indianapolis, Indiana. I was talking with my long-time friend (and early Funny Car pioneer) the late Richard Schroeder and former Keith Black Racing Engines technical representative Don Ewald. We were walking through the host hotel parking lot when we heard about a guy who just had his Don Hardy V-8 Kit Vega towed the last 126 miles to the event on the back of a tow truck after experiencing a horrendous engine fire!

We sought the owner out, and there sat the charred 1972 Chevrolet Vega, knee-deep in onlookers. The fiberglass hood was melted down around the 350 Chevrolet small-block engine so badly it looked like a huge potato chip. Its front fenders, windshield, and just about everything else in close proximity were severely warped from heat damage, and covered in soot! You could easily see that the owner and his two buddies were totally exhausted from this highly volatile and costly ordeal. When we asked one of them what had happened, he related that the trio had been up the entire week getting the Vega ready for the Nationals, and the nitrous system was a last-minute addition. He said they were about two hours outside of Indianapolis and everything seemed to be going fine until they decided to click on the nitrous.

Talk about complete and total humiliation! That became the catch-all phrase for the remainder of the weekend whenever our group of rag-tag journalists experienced any kind of SNAFU. But the grim reality is, when placed in inexperienced hands, nitrous oxide is no laughing matter!

The following is a list of safety/tech issues and pertinent advice, which, if considered and followed correctly, makes your N_2O experience a pleasant one:

Eye Safety First

When working with nitrous oxide, wearing eye protection is an absolute must. Nitrous oxide's release temperature is -127 degrees F. Permanent eye damage, perhaps even blindness, can occur if sprayed with nitrous oxide. Furthermore, hoses containing N_2O are not failsafe. Fittings can come loose, or hoses can rupture if they become kinked or frayed. Prior to running, always completely check your nitrous system for safety.

Transporting Nitrous Oxide

Never transport nitrous oxide cylinders loose in the back of a pickup truck where they can roll around and make contact with one another. Use only an approved bottle rack to store bottles standing up in a contained area, like those used by an oxygen, acetylene, or argon delivery truck. Never drill, machine, weld, deform, or modify an N_2O tank. Also never attempt to subject an N_2O tank to any type of plating process; this often affects the strength of the tank's material.

Battery Safety

Regardless of the amount of N_2O that an onboard cylinder contains, always disconnect the positive (+) side of the battery when working on any electrical components.

Manufacturer Guidelines

Most top-name N_2O manufacturers can provide some very valuable information concerning a particular engine application. Component strength and durability has also been taken into careful consideration to prevent damage to an engine. The kits and recommendations they offer are typically conservative and work effectively when installed and used as directed.

Not following the manufacturer's recommendations for the correct placement of system components and/or the correct way to plumb a system can cause major problems. Do not improvise! Follow the installation instructions—these kits have been expertly engineered, field tested, and dyno tested to maximize horsepower and to also maximize performance and reliability!

Engine Conditions

Before installing an N_2O system onto your engine, be certain that your engine is in good mechanical condition. The ignition system, carburetor, valvetrain, and other related components must be in top shape, because adding N_2O only accentuates existing problems. Furthermore, fluctuating fuel pressure, erratic nitrous cylinder temperatures, worn or sticky mechanical mechanisms, intermittent wiring problems, can all lead to erratic system performance and possible engine damage.

Restrictive Plumbing

The lack of space under the hood of some cars prompts people to use too many 45- and 90-degree fittings when installing an N_2O system. Nitrous oxide plumbing should be adequately matched to the powertrain, and as free-flowing as possible.

Safety Devices

Power relays, oil-pressure safety switches, wide-open-throttle switches, RPM-activated switches, and low-fuel-pressure safety switches and/ or warning lights or gauges are safety devices that can be installed within your N_2O system.

Safety Valves

Never disable the operation of the safety relief disk in the nitrous cylinder's valve. It's required by law and is there for your safety. Don't be foolish!

Fuel

Horsepower comes from the fuel, not the nitrous. N_2O is simply a fuel enhancer that allows you to adjust how much and how quickly an engine burns the fuel. If the fuel isn't there, the power won't be there either!

Detonation

Avoid detonation at all costs. Nitrous-enhanced detonation is even more damaging than naturally aspirated detonation due to the increased amount of fuel available and releasing energy. Using colder-range spark plugs or perhaps special nitrous-engineered spark plugs, such as those offered by ZEX Nitrous Products, helps reduce detonation. When checking spark plugs, be sure to check each one due to the potential variation of air/fuel mixture from cylinder to cylinder. Retarding the timing is also advised, and you should consult the particular kit manufacturer to learn how much. Get a nitrous-friendly high-performance aftermarket ignition system like those manufactured by MSD. Nitrous-specific computer chips, should the vehicle be electronically controlled, are available from companies like Diablo Sport Tuning.

Kit-Recommended Calibration

It is wise to begin with the lowest supplied level of calibration, or smallest N_2O and fuel jets when the system is initially installed and activated. After you've gained some confidence and experience with it, and the installation has proven to be trouble free, you can step up the size of the jets to deliver a higher level of power.

Nitrous Jet

At the first sign of detonation, backfire, or misfire, always first reduce the nitrous jet. The N_2O jet is an oxidizer, so the safest approach is to reduce the nitrous level first, identify the problem, and then proceed from there.

Filter Screens

Routine maintenance of fuel and nitrous filters pays off. Just like a standard carburetor, it doesn't take much to alter the calibration of an N_2O system. Even a miniscule piece of dirt can cause big problems!

Wrong Feel or Sound

If something doesn't sound quite right, shut it off! It's a lot cheaper to pull the system apart and diagnose the potential problem rather than just driving through it, and breaking expensive parts! Let the engine live to race another day.

CHAPTER 1

Project: Edelbrock Performer 70001 Big-Block Chevrolet Single-Plate Nitrous Kit Installation

Everyone knows the name Edelbrock as the recognized authority in high-performance automotive aftermarket induction systems, intake manifolds, carburetors, fuel injection, cylinder heads, cams and kits, etc. It's no surprise that Edelbrock Corporation is also involved in the N_2O induction systems aftermarket.

According to Edelbrock Corporation's latest catalog, the company's Single-Stage 50-75-85-100 Nitrous Plate System for the square-bore Holley-type carburetor, with silver-painted 10-pound bottle (PN 70001) or polished 10-pound bottle (PN 70031), was designed to be the best single-stage carburetor-plate N_2O kit available on the market. One of the reasons for this claim is that Edelbrock Corporation's N_2O kits use stainless steel CNC-machined precision jets, rather than the corrosive brass jets used by other kit manufacturers.

Also in this kit are a pair of Edelbrock precision-machined, flow-matched stainless steel nitrous and fuel solenoids with durable Teflon plungers. It also features: a high-quality, powdercoated or anodized aluminum nitrous plate featuring Edelbrock's patented stainless steel spray bar, which works on either single- or dual-plane intake manifolds; a pair of hinged, red-powdercoated steel nitrous bottle brackets equipped with rubber insulators to protect the N_2O bottle; an Edelbrock High-Flow bottle valve; the aforementioned nitrous bottle; 14 feet of braided stainless-steel nitrous feed line with AN fittings; extra-long carburetor studs; gaskets; a pre-terminated wiring harness; and some of the best detailed assembly instructions (which include Jet Map information) I've seen in an N_2O kit.

Edelbrock also offers single-stage, spread-bore/Quadra Jet-type Performer nitrous-plate systems as well. These are available through participating retailers (PN 70002 for silver-painted bottle, or PN 70032 for polished bottles). I was recently invited to follow along as Edelbrock technician, Mark Honsowetz, installed a Performer single-stage (50-75-85-100-hp) square-bore N_2O kit (PN 70001) on one of Edelbrock's test vehicles—a 454-ci TH400-equipped 1966 Chevrolet El Camino. This was followed by a four-phase dyno test using Edelbrock's Super Flow chassis dyno.

First, a baseline was established, then a 50-hp Performer N_2O jet was installed and the testing process repeated. This was followed with the installation and testing of a 75-hp Performer N_2O jet, and finally an 85-hp jet was tested. Testing parameters included the use of 92-octane Chevron Supreme unleaded fuel, a set of one-step-colder spark plugs (something in the 9 to 11 range), and

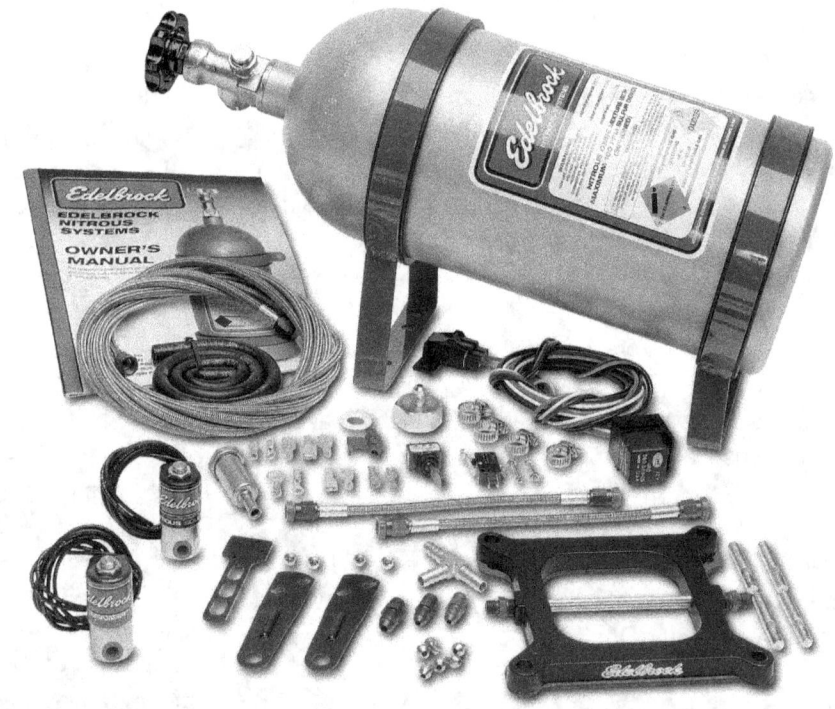

Chosen for this installation was the Edelbrock Nitrous single-stage 50- to 100-hp nitrous plate system (square-bore PN 70001; spread-bore PN 70002). This kit includes a selection of CNC-machined stainless-steel jets, a pair of precision-machined flow-matched stainless-steel fuel and N2O solenoids, micro-switches and mount brackets, anodized aluminum spray-bar plate, red bottle brackets, a silver painted or (optional) polished 10-pound nitrous bottle, a complete wiring harness, and fully detailed assembly instructions.

SINGLE-STAGE SINGLE-PLATE SYSTEMS

1 to 3 degrees of retard in the ignition advance as a starting point. Prior to hitting the squeeze, a baseline of 273.5 hp was achieved on the engine alone at 5,100 rpm. Stock torque numbers consisted of 296.2 ft-lbs at 4,400 to 4,500 rpm. However, after the nitrous system was activated, it was a whole 'nuther story!

The 50 Edelbrock Performer nitrous-jet data is interesting because horsepower at the flywheel and rear-wheel horsepower are near identical at 5,100 to 5,300 rpm. Call it the sweet spot, if you will. But maximum horsepower (323.6) peaks at 5,500 rpm, while rear-wheel horsepower comes in a little earlier (320.8) at 5,300 rpm.

Engine torque comes in between 4,600 and 4,700 rpm, 344.1/345.5 ft-lbs, while peak rear-wheel torque (388.4 ft-lbs) comes in at 4,700 rpm. The last thing you want is to dismiss that 50-shot jet as being inconsequential and toss it in the toolbox!

Tests conducted with Edelbrock's 75-hp Performer N_2O jet were likewise very productive. Engine horsepower using the 75-shot made 358.9 at 5,500 rpm, but remained consistently strong starting at 5,100 rpm. Rear-wheel horsepower was also quite close (351.8 at 5,500 rpm), making noticeable 6- to 7-hp jumps up the scale beginning at 4,900 rpm. The sweet spot was again at 4,600 rpm, where power jumps a full 33.3 hp. It also doubles and then some between 4,700 and 4,900 rpm.

Then there's torque. With the 75-hp jet installed, engine torque remains constant throughout the chart at 4,600 to 5,500 rpm, with a peak number of 361.5 ft-lbs at 4,700 rpm. Rear-wheel torque starts climbing at 4,700 rpm to 349.5 ft-lbs, and remains consistent up to 5,200 rpm, with the sweet spot being 354.4 at 5,100 rpm. After reading these charts, I instantly became a fan of the Edelbrock Performer 75-hp N_2O jet, but there was more!

With Edelbrock's 85-hp N_2O jet installed, engine horsepower peaked at 358.1 at 5,700 rpm, with an overall range of 262.6 at 4,600 to 358.1 at 5,700 rpm. Rear-wheel horsepower likewise remains consistent in the 358.1 to 358.2 range between 5,100 and 5,700 rpm.

Engine torque using the 85-shot N_2O Performer jet produced a best of 383.3 ft-lbs at 5,000 rpm. Optimum rear-wheel torque (375.9 ft-lbs) came in at 5,000 rpm!

So then, why not a 100-shot test? Because the 3,200-stall-speed torque converter in this particular test vehicle would be fine for the drag strip (as witnessed by the lower-RPM-torque numbers), but was basically played out at the higher horsepower and torque-RPM levels, and any performance gains were negligible at best.

"A 10-inch-diameter torque converter with either a 2,400 or 3,000 stall speed would have been a much better choice for this particular application," said James "Jimmy G" Galante from Racetrans.com. The main idea when running N_2O is your engine needs more torque, and more torque equals more stall speed. This is extremely crucial, as the exhaust valve needs more time to be able to effectively purge the combustion chamber of the engine. After all, when you don't have all that back pressure in the cylinder, you make more horsepower!

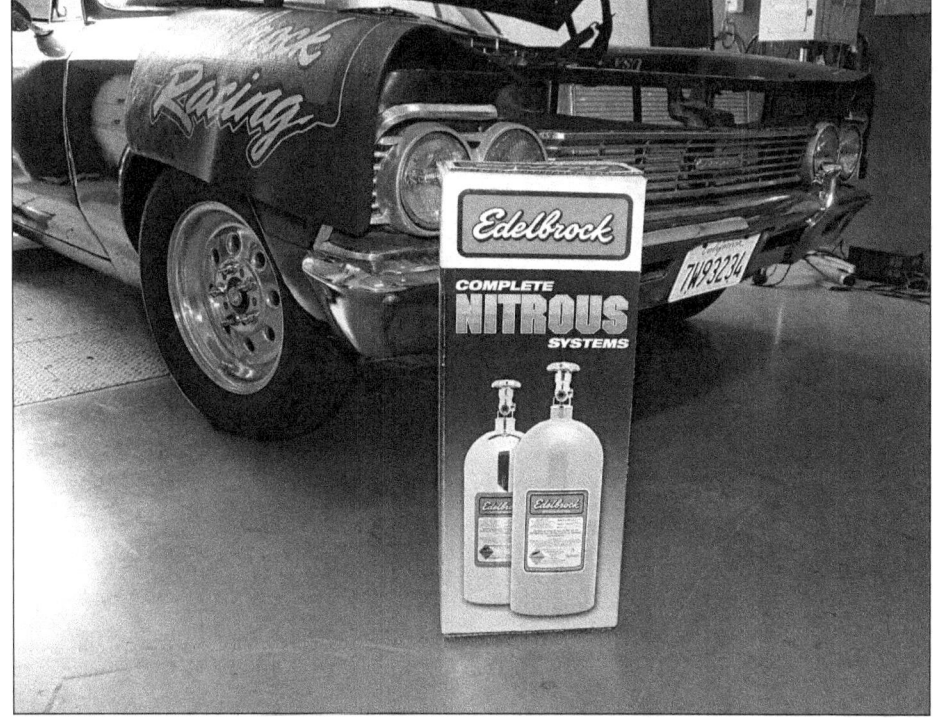

The complete Edelbrock Nitrous system (PN 70001) comes in a single box with everything needed to plumb a car equipped with a single 4-barrel carb with juice. This is exactly what we were looking for, and we'll have an additional 50-100 hp (depending upon which set of jets we choose to run) at the touch of a button.

CHAPTER 1

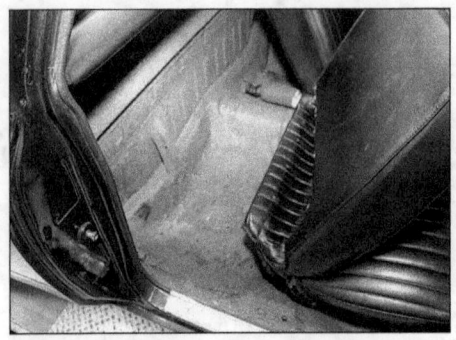

1 Traditionally, bottle placement on most cars is inside the trunk, but an El Camino is technically a truck and not a car; so the bottle needs to be mounted inside the passenger compartment. Here it's on the passenger side behind the seat because the spare tire is stored behind the driver.

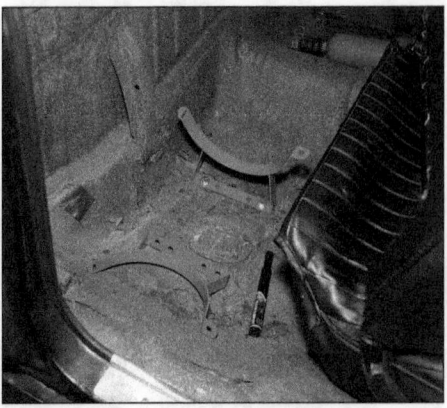

2 Edelbrock nitrous bottle brackets mount to the floorpan using a series of four 3/8-inch holes. The bottle brackets can be secured in place using the supplied hardware in the Edelbrock Nitrous Performer Single-Stage kit.

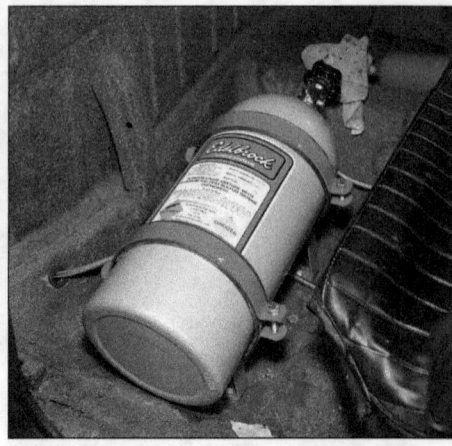

3 With limited space available, the 10-pound bottle mounts crossways behind the passenger seat, with the bottle valve and nozzle facing upward toward the transmission tunnel.

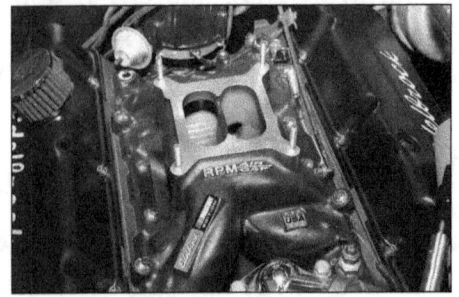

4 Moving on to the engine compartment, remove the carburetor and air cleaner. A new set of longer carburetor studs are provided with the Edelbrock Nitrous single-stage kit, to allow for the Performer N_2O square-flange plate.

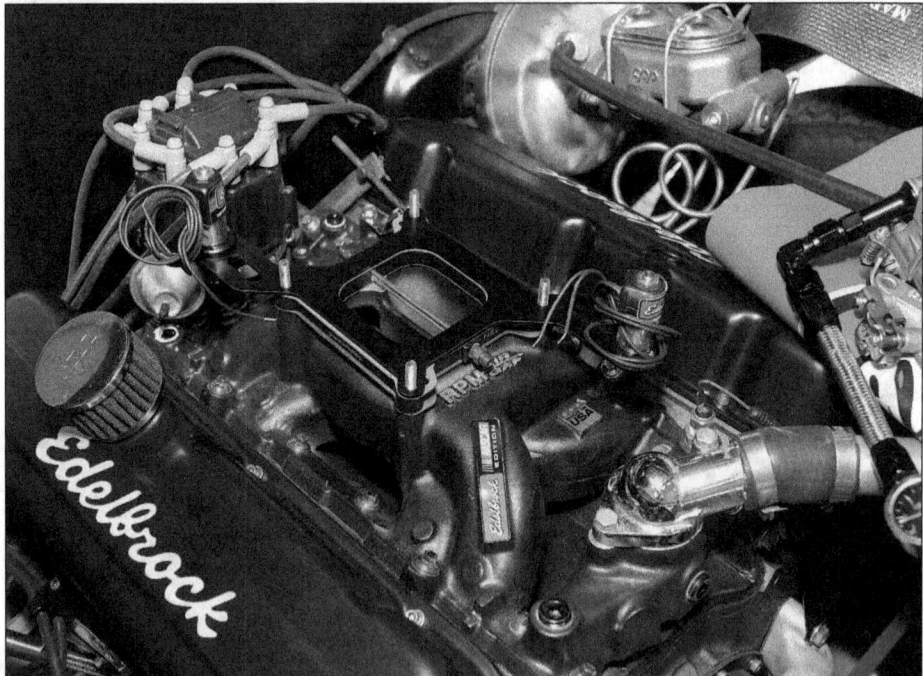

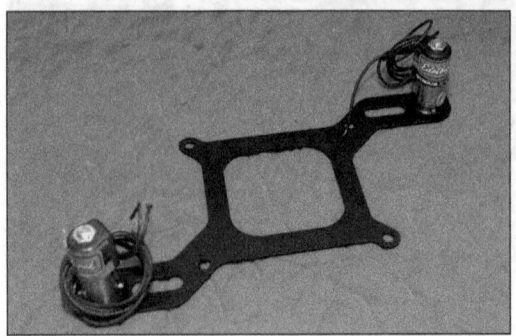

5 The setup after the CNC-machined N_2O plate, carburetor gasket, and extra-length carburetor studs have been installed. Note the red fuel AN fitting is facing forward.

6 The fully installed Edelbrock Performer solenoid plate. Remember, the red fitting hooks up to the fuel solenoid, and the blue fitting hooks up to the N_2O solenoid. Note that Edelbrock Nitrous cautions against using any sealant on these fittings.

SINGLE-STAGE SINGLE-PLATE SYSTEMS

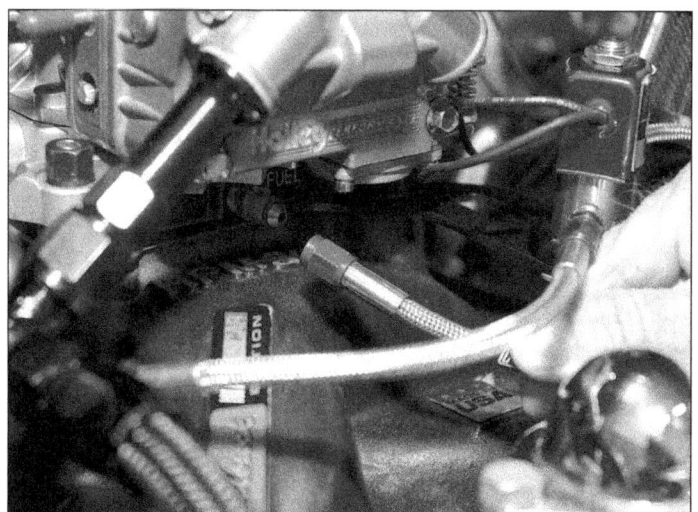
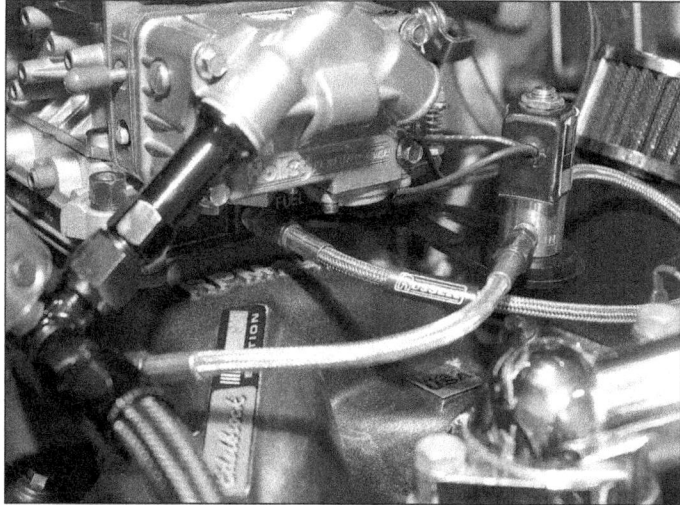

7 *Prior to installing the carburetor, the correct-size N₂O and fuel jets are installed into their ports, and the corresponding lines are snug but not over-tightened.*

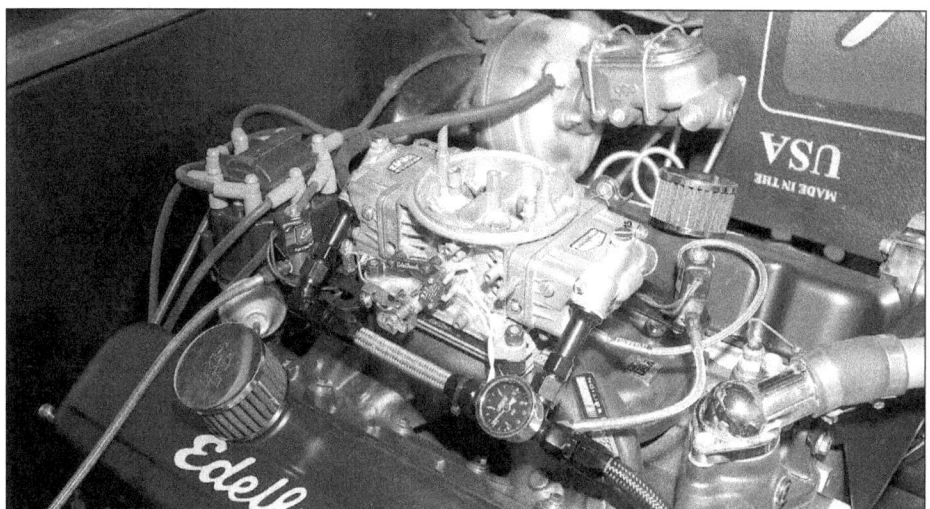

8 *Here is the El Camino 750-cfm Holley 4-barrel carburetor bolted back in place with all the corresponding nitrous supply and fuel lines hooked up.*

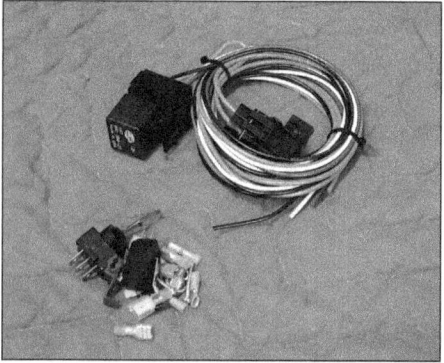

9 *The Edelbrock Nitrous Single-Stage Plate Kit's pre-terminated wiring harness, complete with relays and corrosion-resistant electrical fuse holder, electrical switch, and connectors.*

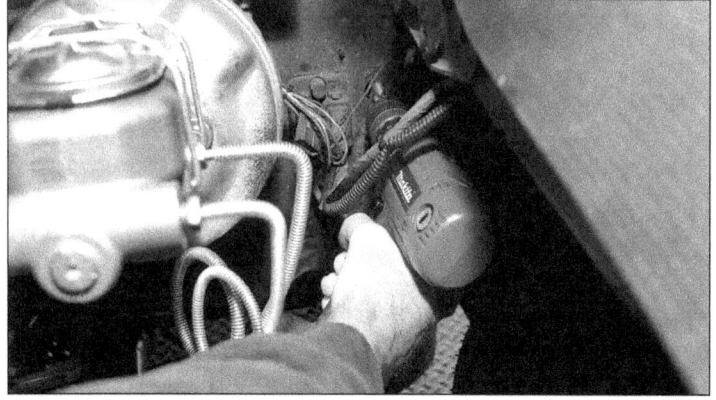

10 *If you can't locate a pre-drilled opening on the driver's side of the El Camino firewall, first drill a pilot hole, and then enlarge it to accommodate the wiring loom.*

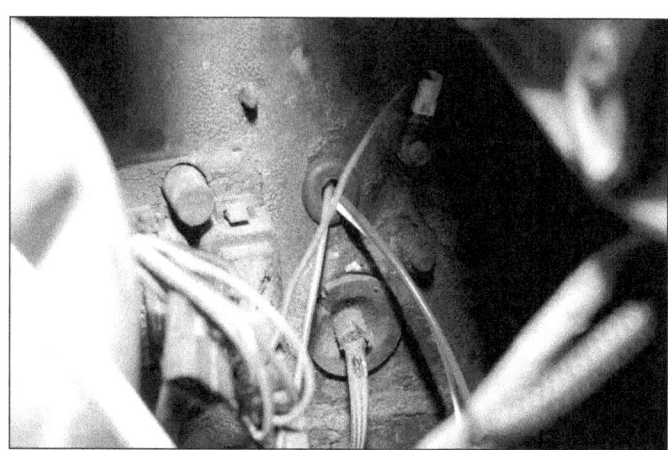

11 *The electrical wires for the solenoids route through the El Camino's firewall.*

CHAPTER 1

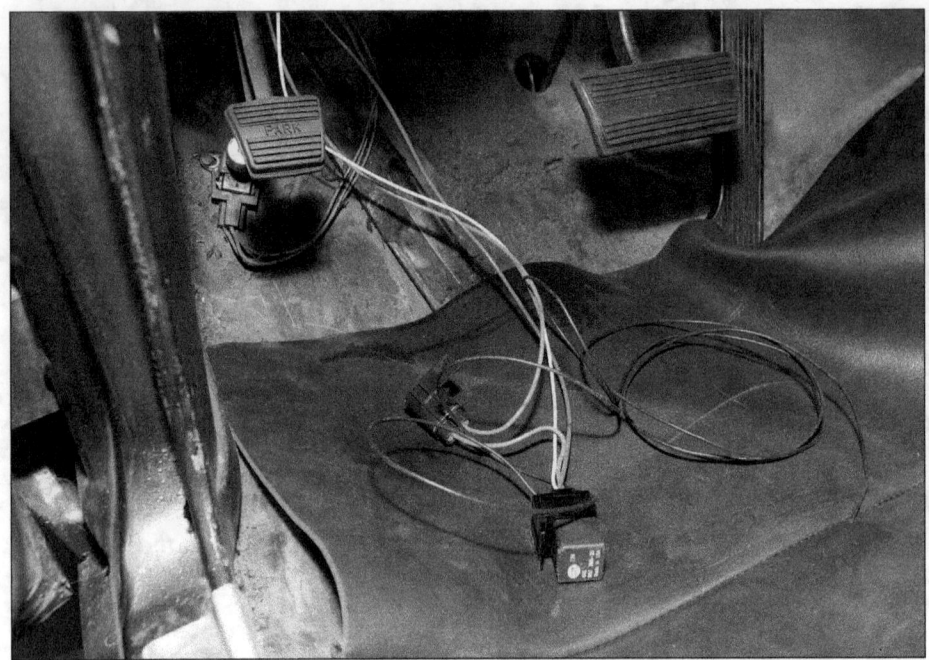

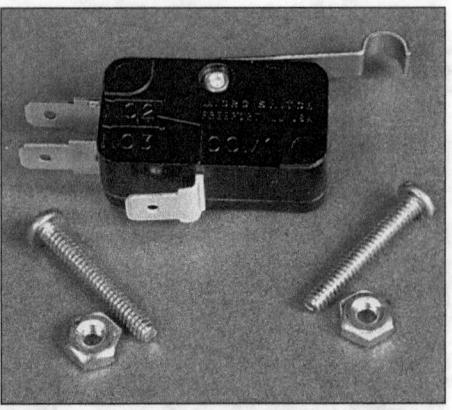

12 The pre-terminated electrical harness from the driver's compartment side. Proper wiring of the system is covered on page 16 of the Edelbrock Nitrous Installation manual (PN70001/70002).

13 Properly activating this system requires setting up the Throttle Linkage Micro Switch, which works with (yet does not interfere with) the OE carburetor-throttle linkage. Due to the micro-switch mounting bracket's flexibility, it can be set up to come on at half throttle, three-quarters throttle, or wide-open throttle at the operator's discretion.

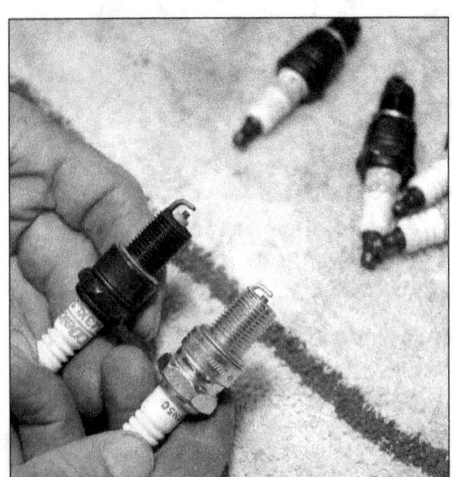

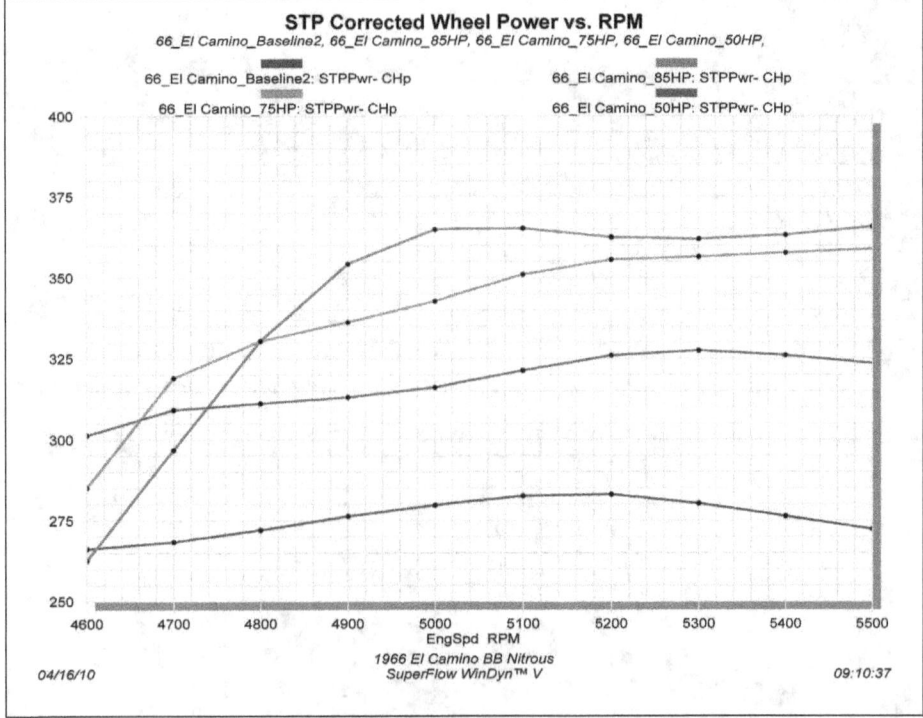

14 Because nitrous oxide creates a lot of cylinder pressure, and cylinder pressure creates excess heat, a colder-range spark plug helps avoid detonation.

This rear-wheel horsepower chart shows the effect of various nitrous oxide and fuel jets. The blue line represents the baseline, with no nitrous oxide being used. The purple line shows the horsepower produced with the 50-hp setup added. The green line represents the 75- jetting, The red line shows the results of the 85-hp package.

CHAPTER 2

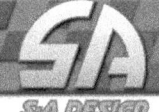

SINGLE-STAGE DUAL-PLATE CARBURETED SYSTEMS

Single-stage dual-plate (or 2x4) carbureted N_2O systems, and single-stage single-plate 4V N_2O systems pretty much share the same components, except the former uses two plates. The most commonly seen intakes are low-profile-intake-runner inline 2x4, medium-rise-intake-runner inline 2x4, and cross-ram 2x4 and tunnel-ram 2x4 dual-quad intake manifolds. On average, when equipped with a 2x4 standard-flange Holley, one of these systems can produce 50 to 250 hp. When equipped with a pair of Holley Dominator-style 4-barrel carburetors, one of these single-stage dual-plate setups can produce anywhere from 200 to 400 hp on a typically prepared small- or big-block engine, depending on tuning. For this type of nitrous setup, the following considerations apply:

- With 2x4 single-stage, dual-plate systems, carburetor jetting pretty much follows the same principle as with standard non-nitrous dual-quad setups. Namely, jetting differs (slightly) between front and rear carburetors based on the acceleration principle of dual carburetion.
- Carburetor plate positioning largely depends on the location of the throttle linkage, whether it is in-line, north/south, crossways, or east/west. Set your nitrous and fuel supply lines to follow suit.
- With some north/south throttle linkage systems, it's possible to

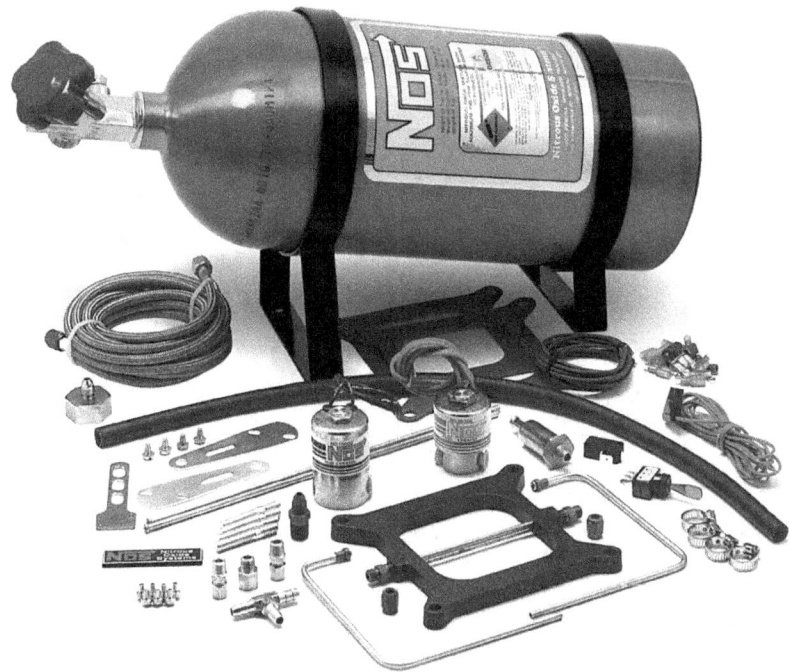

Nitrous Oxide Systems offers four 150- to 250-hp Cheater single-stage dual-plate systems. Applications include the 2x4 standard-flange late-Holley–style Carter AFB (PN 02010NOS), 2x4 Holley 4-barrel flange sideways mount (PN 020109NOS), 2x4 Holley Dominator flange (PN 02011NOS), 2x4 early Carter AFB flange (PN 02012NOS), and 3x2 Holley 2-barrel Tri-Power application (PN 02013NOS).

CHAPTER 2

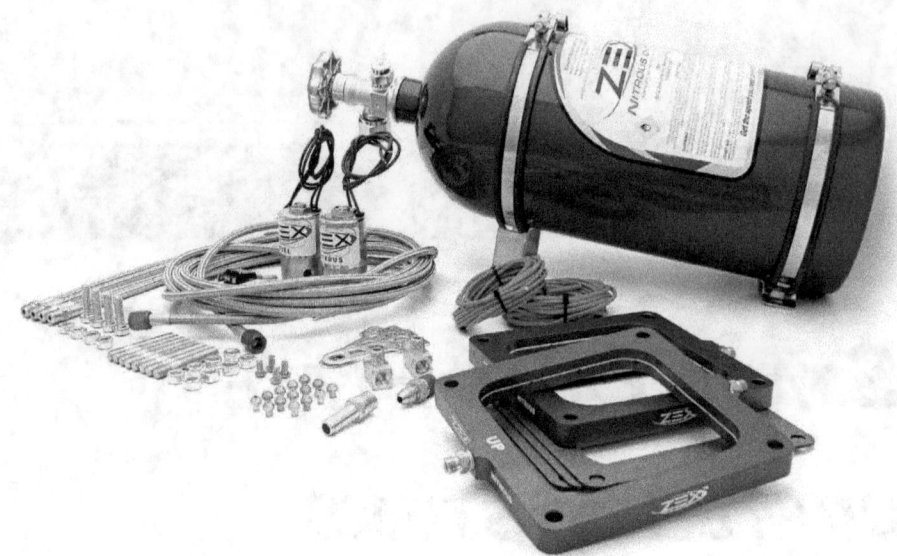

ZEX Nitrous Products' Dual Perimeter, Dual Plate nitrous systems are tunable from 100 to 300 hp. They fit square-flange Holley-style carburetors (PN 82185), and Holley/Barry Grant Dominator-style flanges (PN 82190).

- Fuel systems also have to be updated accordingly. Check with the manufacturer for recommendations.

Single-stage dual-plate street systems are becoming something of a dinosaur with the decline of pro/street and today's skyrocketing fuel prices. Many nitrous users feel you can produce just as much horsepower out of a large-CFM single 4-barrel carbureted N_2O system with less maintenance, cost, and hassles. But that is a matter of owner preference.

A number of companies manufacture single-stage dual-plate systems. For example, NOS lists four Cheater applications.

Nitrous Supply offers the 2x4 Sportstar Series N_2O system (PN 3010). It's designed to fit a standard Holley flange, on GM, Ford, or Mopar

set up the nitrous plates in tandem, linked together via a small line connector. However, this approach has problems with balancing out the two plates, making tuning quite problematic.
- On single-stage dual-late street/strips setups, like the 100- to 300-hp ZEX Nitrous Products dual-perimeter-plate nitrous system for either standard-flange Holleys (PN 82185), or Holley's Dominator dual-perimeter-plate nitrous system (PN 82190), individual nitrous and fuel solenoids are used, both of which flow more N_2O and fuel.
- You could assume that bottle size should be increased, due to twice the need for 2x4 single-plate systems. However, a 10-pound bottle is still the accepted size but you may have to refill it more frequently.

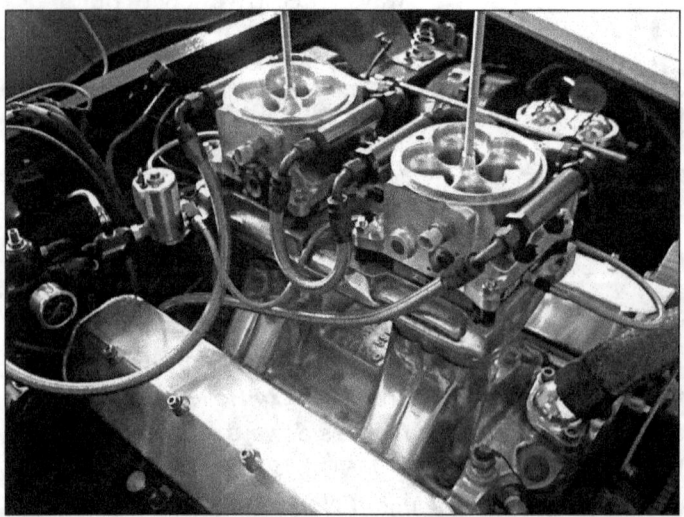
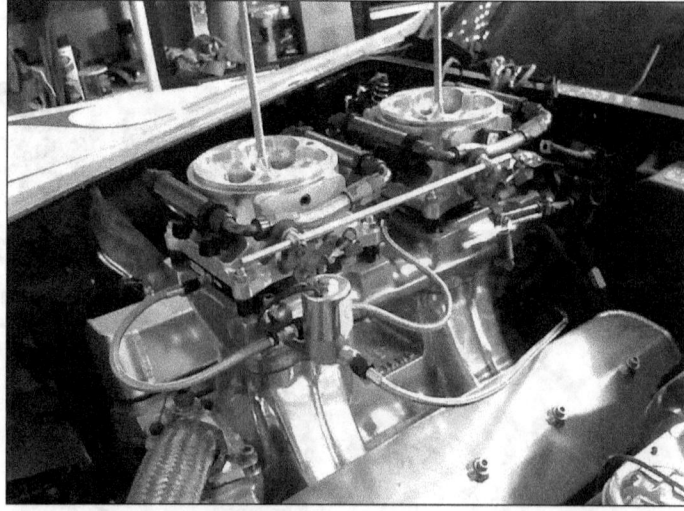

One of ZEX's Dual Perimeter Dual Plate 100- to 300-hp nitrous systems (PN 82185) installed on Ron Turnpaugh's 434-ci, RHS-headed small-block Chevy engine. Note the twin 785-cfm (1,530-cfm total) Holley throttle bodies instead of traditional carburetors.

SINGLE-STAGE DUAL-PLATE CARBURETED SYSTEMS

Nitrous Express' answer to a single-stage dual-plate 2x4 nitrous kit comes in two versions: PN 50040-00 (Pro Power Conventional Kit) for standard 2x4 Holley and PN 50270-NX for 2x4 Holley Dominator. These kits are power rated at an adjustable 50-100-150-200-250-300-hp capability!

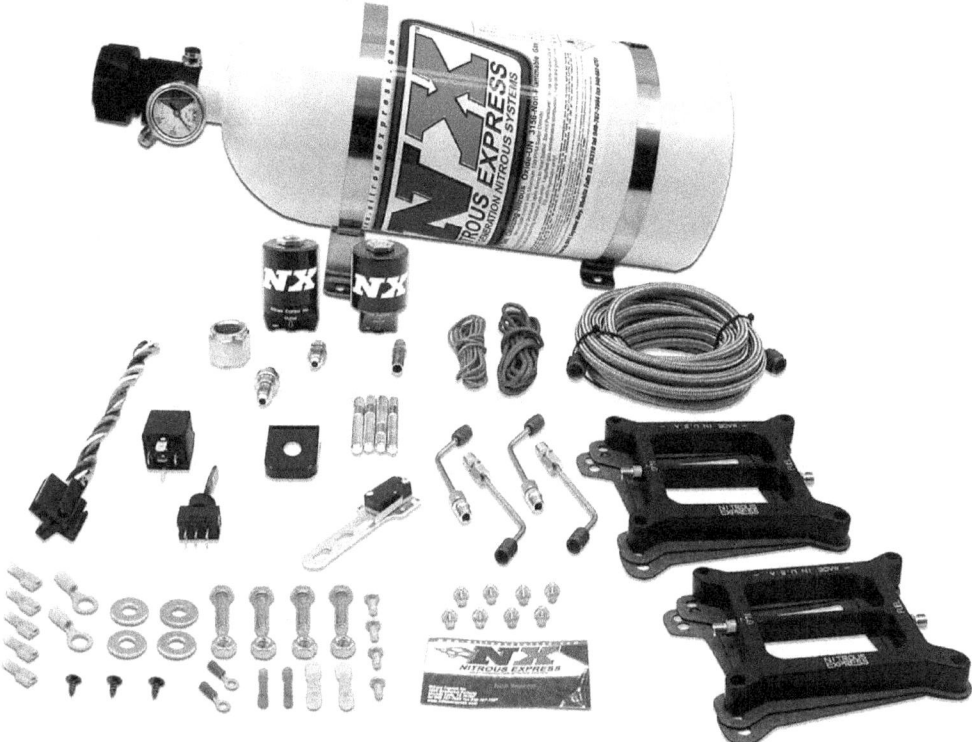

small-block setups and capable of delivering 50- to 250-hp increases. Nitrous Supply also offers a 2x4 single-plate system (PN 3011) for 50 to 250 hp in Dominator applications.

Nitrous Express offers the Gemini Twin Pro Power Plate Conversion Kit, or kits in this particular case for the Holley 4-barrel (PN NX614) or Holley Dominator flange (PN NX617).

Edelbrock Nitrous offers a 2x4 Performer RPM Dual Quad application, rated at 100 to 250, and Performer RPM II Dual Quad Application power rated at 100 to 400.

Remember that the single-stage dual-plate N_2O systems mentioned in this section are of the street/strip/sportsman variety. Hardcore 2x4 N_2O systems used in the Advanced Bracket classes, Top Sportsman, Pro Gas, and other forms of serious drag racing are usually dual-stage systems.

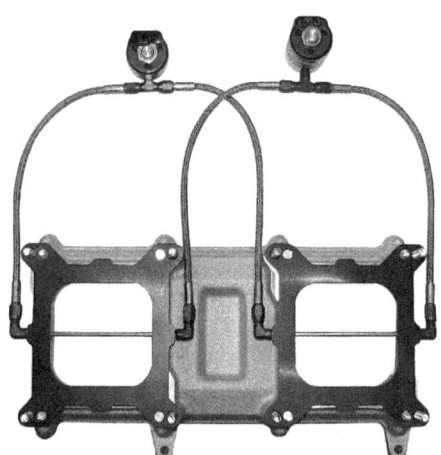

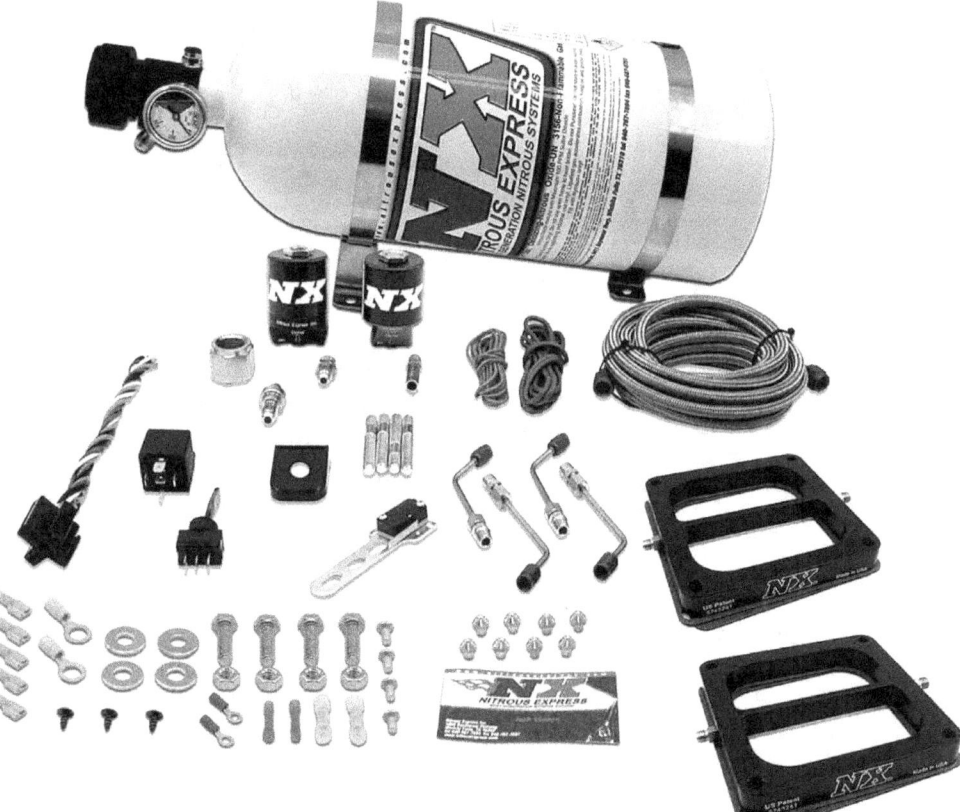

Edelbrock Nitrous offers a 100-150-200-250-hp 2x4 Performer RPM single-stage dual-plate application for either the square-bore or Holley-type 4500-series carburetors.

HOW TO INSTALL AND TUNE NITROUS OXIDE SYSTEMS

CHAPTER 3

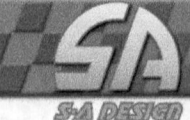

Two-Stage Single-Plate Systems

A single-plate system with two stages is commonly preferred by street enthusiasts and budget racers who need of plenty of power (200 to 400 hp) and who have an engine that can handle it, but not necessarily all at once. It is a less costly alternative to a more sophisticated, dual-stage dual-plate/nozzle-type system. A good example of a single-plate system is a standard-flange NOS Big Shot (PN 02401NOS) or Dominator-style Big Shot (PN 02402NOS), a TNW Billet Atomizer Dual-Stage Kit standard or Dominator/King Demon (PNs 12060 and 12070, respectively), or an Edelbrock Nitrous Performer RPM II (PN 70082 square bore, or PN 70083 4500 Series). All of these seem to work best on single-plane 4V or tunnel ram, and are traditionally controlled by two sets of nitrous and fuel solenoids and a jet-able block at the spray plate.

Basically, the first-stage solenoids are activated by a conventional

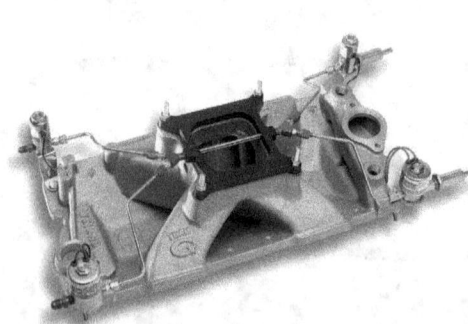

The NOS Dual Shot Cheater system Holley 4-barrel application (PN 02201NOS) or Dominator carburetor application (PN 02202NOS), can provide 100 to 250 hp, but in stages. The first stage is activated by a conventional carburetor throttle switch and, based on the size jet, can deliver anywhere from 100 to 150 hp. Once underway, you can activate the second stage, hence two sets of solenoids providing an additional 150 to 250 hp at the flick of a button. Or, you have the option to ramp up the nitrous in increments using one of NOS' optional Progressive Nitrous Controllers (PN 15974NOS).

TWO-STAGE SINGLE-PLATE SYSTEMS

throttle switch, while the second-stage solenoids are activated by pushing a button according to racer preference or by any one of a dozen brand-name progressive nitrous controllers on the market. Manufacturers like NOS, NX, NS, ZEX, etc., all offer dual-stage conversion kits and progressive nitrous oxide controllers.

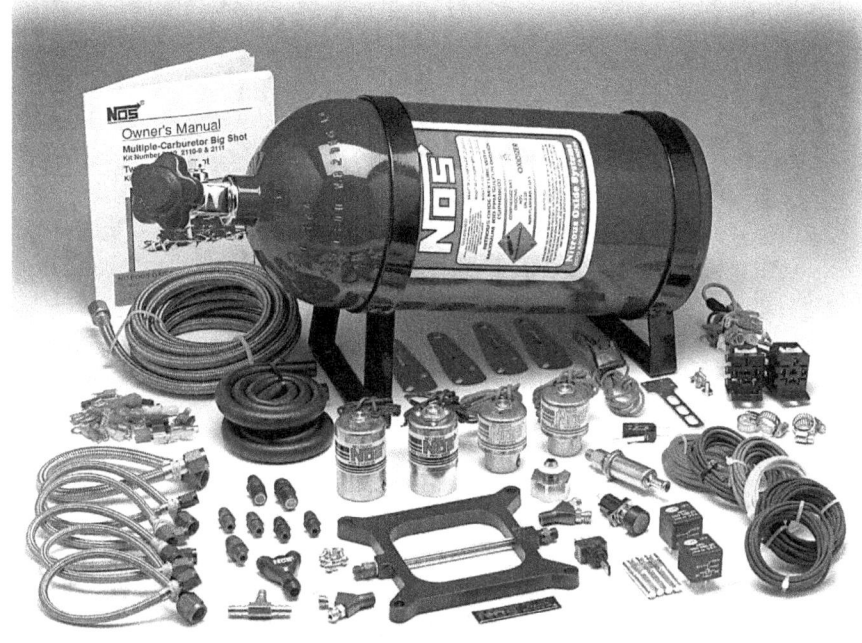

The NOS Big Shot Dual Stage system Holley 4-barrel (PN 02401NOS) or Dominator application (PN 02402NOS) provides an instant boost of 200 hp but provides a more gradual application of power so as not to shock the tires, and/or upset the chassis during critical launches. The first stage allows you to leave at a 200-hp shot. Once launched, Stage Two (200 more hp) can be activated by the flick of a button.

Nitrous Wagon

A practical application of a two-stage single-plate N_2O system in action is Nitrous Express Power's sports director Mike Golightly's well-weathered 1963 Plymouth Savoy four-door station wagon. This retired, 3,100-pound grocery getter has run a best of 6.255 seconds at 109.14 mph in the eighth-mile using an NX two-stage single-plate 250-shot system.

The engine is a .060-inch overbored 383-ci Mopar big-block. Now displacing 394 ci, the engine was prepared by Golightly and Dave Kleeman. Internally, it makes use of a knife-edged and micro-polished factory 383 Mopar crankshaft, a set of SCAT long connecting rods, Venolia forged-aluminum pistons with .900-inch wrist pins, and 11.0:1 compression. The cam is a Bullet-brand flat tappet with 268-degrees duration and .582 inch of lift. Other items include a Comp Cams multiple-index-roller timing chain, ARP engine fasteners, Comp Cams lifters, and an 8-quart Milodon oil pan and matching oil pump.

Bolted up top is a set of Golightly-prepared Chrysler 915-casting big-block cylinder heads equipped with 2.180-inch-diameter intake and 1.80-inch-diameter

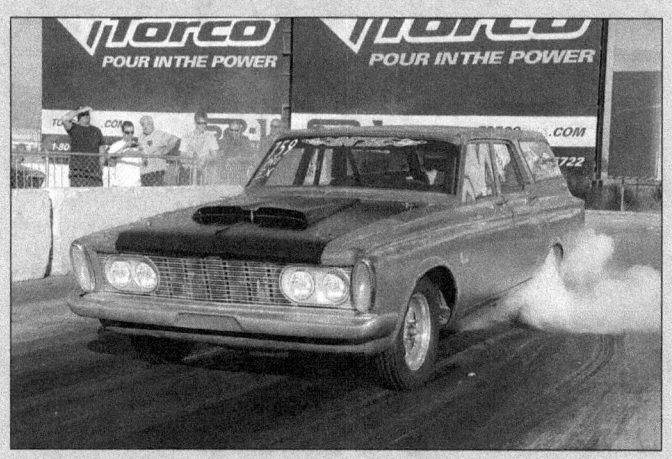

Nitrous Wagon CONTINUED

Mopar Performance exhaust valves, a set of 1.6:1 Harland Sharp intake and 1.5:1 exhaust rocker arms, and Smith Brothers pushrods. The ignition is a crank-triggered MSD setup with a 6AL box, while the exhaust system consists of Hooker Super Comp headers bolted to MagnaFlow mufflers. Backing things up is an owner-assembled Chrysler 727 Torqueflite using a TCI 3,500 stall-speed torque convertor, TCI manual valve-body shift kit, and B&M Bandit shifter.

When setting up the Savoy's chassis, Golightly equipped the wagon with a 4.88:1 Strange Engineering-geared and Strange billet-axle-equipped 8.75-inch Chrysler rear axle, riding on a set of Calvert Super Stock springs with Rancho Suspension shocks. CalTrac traction bars are also used. Getting the power to the pavement are a set of 15x10-inch Weld Racing Aluma-Star wheels riding on 30x10x15-inch Hoosier drag slicks. That's your basic package.

For the actual induction system, Golightly's Nitrous Wagon gets its oomph from a 250-hp Nitrous Express conventional plate system (PN 30040-10) equipped with a number-88 N_2O jet and a number-62 fuel jet. The plate is bolted to an Edelbrock 383 Victor intake manifold using a Pro Systems–prepared 750-cfm Holley carburetor. An NX Progressive Controller (PN 15835) allows the wagon to leave the starting line at 50 percent (125 shot) and ramp up to the full 250 horses in just .8 second. This system also makes use of an NX automatic bottle heater (PN 15940) and NX bottle jacket (PN 15945) to maintain consistent bottle pressure.

"She may be ugly, but she sure does run," says Mike. "You've just got to love it!"

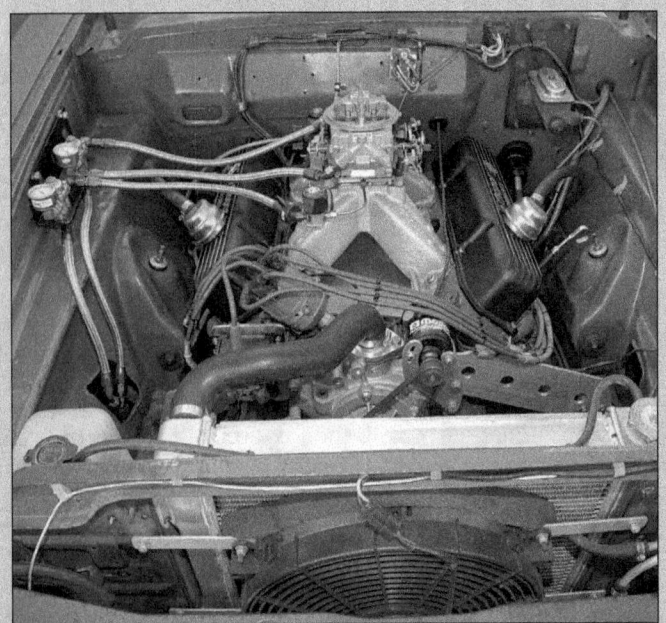 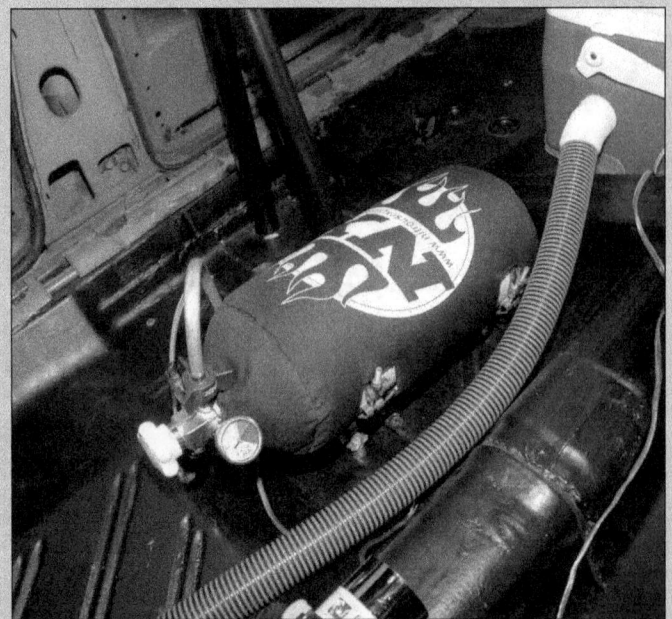

Nitrous Express Power's sports director Mike Golightly's well-weathered 1963 Plymouth Savoy four-door station wagon is a practical application of a two-stage single-plate N_2O system in action. It's a retired 3,100-pound grocery getter that runs a best of 6.255 seconds at 109.14 mph in the eighth-mile. The 383 block is punched out to 394 ci. A Nitrous Express Phase 3 two-stage single-plate 250-shot nitrous system (PN 30040-00) using a number-88 N_2O jet and number-62 fuel jet works in concert with a Pro Systems–prepared 750-cfm Holley and Edelbrock 383 Victor intake to get the job done. An NX Progressive Controller (PN 15835) allows Mike's wagon to leave the starting line at 50 percent (125 hp) and ramp up to the full 250 hp in just .8 second. This system also makes use of an NX automatic bottle heater (PN 15940) and NX bottle jacket (PN 15945) to maintain consistent bottle pressure.

CHAPTER 4

SINGLE-STAGE NITROUS SUPERCHARGER SYSTEMS

The granddaddy of the supercharged N₂O system was Ron Hammel, and his company, 10,000 RPM Speed Equipment, which developed an N₂O kit to interface with the GMC supercharger in 1962–1963. While superchargers and turbochargers are capable of producing significant gains in power, they also produce a great deal of heat. Because N₂O enters a system at -127 degrees F, and this is as much as a 750-degree drop in the intake charge temperature, frosted supercharger cases are a common sight. More importantly, useable horsepower gains and engine torque can increase as much as 40 percent.

For example there's Nitrous Supply's 175-hp stand-alone 16-nozzle supercharger plate kit. It's designed to fit GMC and aftermarket 6-71 to 8-71 superchargers and available in unassembled steel line (PN 3520) or unassembled stainless-steel line (PN 3521).

Nitrous Oxide Systems' 175, a 16-nozzle application for the 6-71/8-71 GMC supercharger (PN 02520NOS) comes pre-assembled, and includes a tank, solenoids, wiring, hose, etc. Also available is NOS' Blower System Show Kit, listed under PN 02520-CNOS. It should also be noted that Weiand, another division of Holley Performance Products, works hand-in-hand with NOS not only on traditional 6-71/8-71 street superchargers, it also markets individual plate systems for smaller street superchargers applications. Consult the manufacturer.

So what about supercharger houses like Blower Drive Service

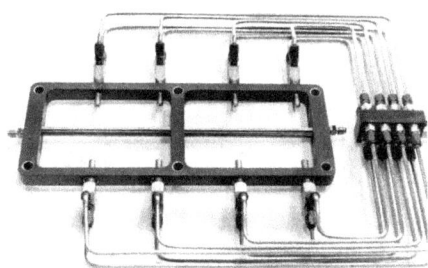

Ron Hammel and his company, 10,000 RPM Speed Equipment, pioneered the first nitrous oxide supercharger system as far back as 1962, when he bolted a kit on the Top Hat Special AA/FD. Hammel and AA/Dale Armstrong also tried N₂O on a Chrysler-powered, steel-bodied 1963 Chevy Nova called The Kanuk in the earliest days of the sport, with moderate success.

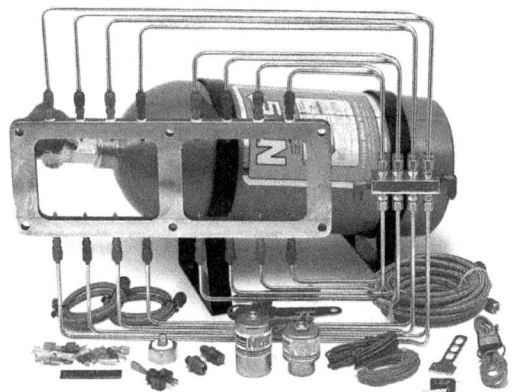

Shown is NOS 16-nozzle application for the GMC 6.71 and 8.71 supercharger, as well as aftermarket variants like Wieand, BDS, Dyers, Littlefield, the Blower Shop, etc. This plate can be mounted either way to clear the distributor and carburetor linkage, and to optimize solenoid placement. It comes pre-assembled and includes stainless-steel pre-bent lines with 175 hp jets, tank, solenoid hoses and lines, wiring, and installation hardware pack. It is listed under PN 02520NOS. A polished Show Kit is also listed under PN 02520-CNOS.

CHAPTER 4

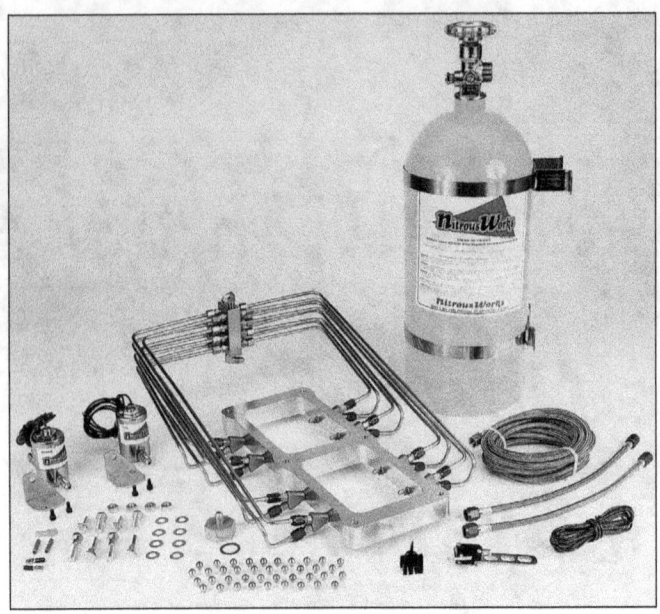

The Nitrous Works approach to bolt-on nitrous blower power consists of a plate system (PN 14060) based around eight TNW Power Wing nitrous-port nozzles that accept 250-300-350-hp N_2O and fuel jets. This system also comes pre-assembled and ready to go with tank, solenoids, hose, brackets, wiring, and jets.

(BDS), The Blower Shop (TBS), Littlefield Blowers, Mooneyham Superchargers? Do they offer kits?

"We don't sell nitrous kits," says BDS CEO Craig Railsback. "All a customer has to do is tell us what particular nitrous manufacturer he intends to use and we set up our blowers for that particular application."

And finally, what about centrifugal superchargers like ATI, Paxton, Vortech, etc., or screw blowers like Edelbrock E-Force, Kenne-Bell, and Whipple? Companies like Nitrous Supply and others offer custom systems for these superchargers and turbochargers.

Project: Nitrous Supply/Weiand 6-71 Supercharger Kit Installation

Nitrous Supply manufactures a 1/2-inch-thick, 16-port, dual-carburetor plate application for the Roots-type GMC 6-71 and 8-71 supercharger, as well as all of the aftermarket GMC/Roots-type variants. These plates arrive at your door drilled and pre-tapped, and ready to accept NS port-design, blue (N_2O) and red (fuel) jet spray nozzles. Of course, jet size determines the amount of horsepower generated. According to NS, performance gains of up to 300- to 450-hp are realistic when counting in the intercooling effect from the nitrous.

Two applications are available: PN 3520 (which consists of unassembled steel lines, carburetor plate, and nozzles and jets) and PN 3521 (the unassembled stainless-steel version). NS can provide solenoids, in this case a set of PN 26045 for N_2O and PN 26050 for fuel. The bottle, one of NOS' 10-pound units, is listed under PN 24745. The bottle adaptor is catalogued under PN 262230. Shown here is one of Nitrous Supply's PN 3521 plates being installed on Thomas White's 1962 Ford Falcon, powered by a Holley-Weiand 6-71 supercharged 350-ci Chevrolet.

Nitrous Supply's 1/2-inch-thick, 16-port-nozzle, dual-carbureted, supercharger-plate application for the GMC Roots-type 6-71/8-71 blower (PN 3520 unassembled steel line, PN 3521 unassembled stainless-steel Show Kit) also fits all aftermarket GMC/Roots-type variants, such as Weiand, BDS, Mooneyham, Littlefield, and The Blower Shop blowers. These plates arrive at your door drilled and pre-tapped and ready to accept NS blue (nitrous) and red (fuel) Jet Spray Nozzles. Of course, jet size determines the amount of horsepower generated. According to NS, performance gains of up to 300 to 450 hp are realistic when taking into consideration the cooling effect from the nitrous. When ordering, specify the type of carburetors being used.

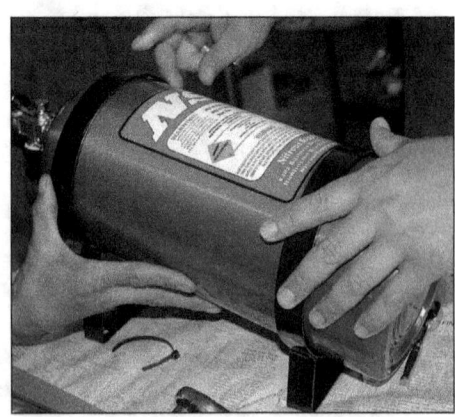

1 *Begin the installation by loosely attaching the NS bottle brackets to the 10-pound NS bottle for positioning in the car.*

SINGLE-STAGE NITROUS SUPERCHARGER SYSTEMS

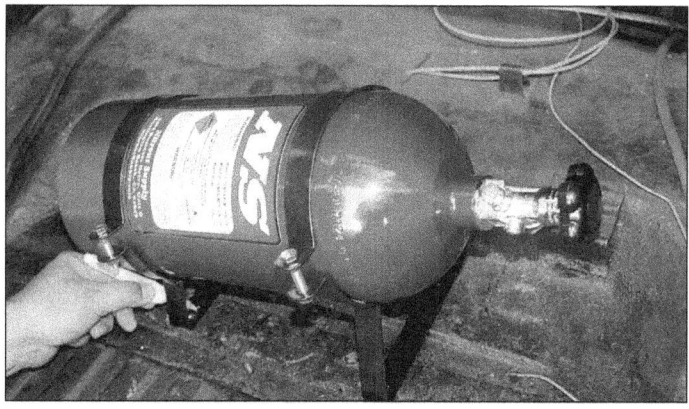

2 If you have a battery and fuel tank to contend with, you can mount the new bottle sideways in the trunk. The floorpan of Thomas W. White's blown Chevrolet-powered 1962 Ford Falcon street machine is marked for drilling.

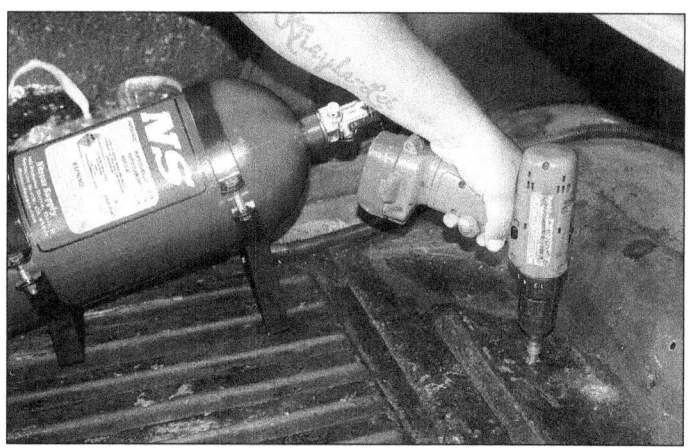

3 Drill the necessary pilot holes in the floorpan and and then use a 3/8-inch drill bit to achieve the correct size.

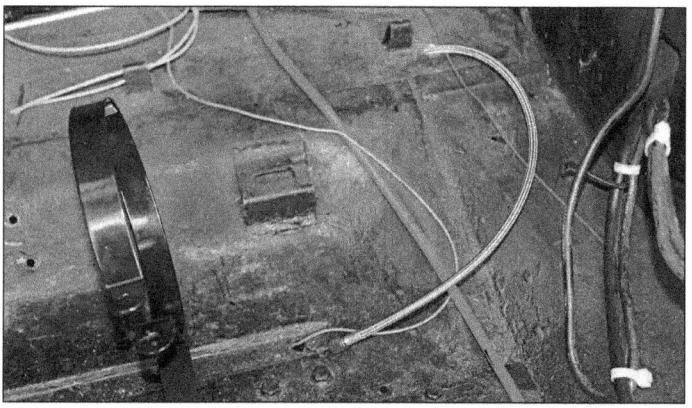

4 Next, route the -4 AN nitrous oxide supply line from the trunk to the car's engine compartment. Here, the line is attached to the Falcon's floorpan using rubber-isolated clamps held in place by machine screws.

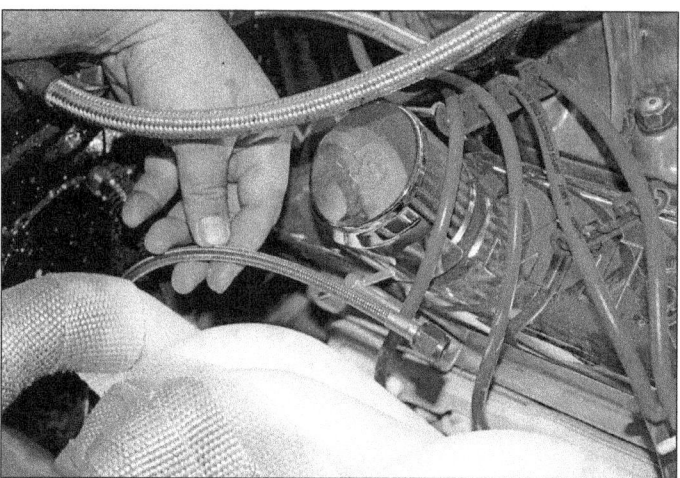

5 This is where the nitrous feed line enters the engine compartment.

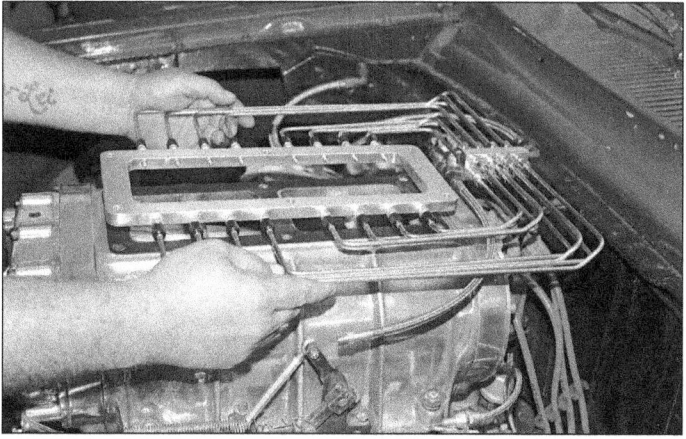

6 On goes the 1/2-inch-thick universal NS Supercharger Show Kit plate. It's a real looker with its polished-aluminum, stainless-steel lines, and red and blue annodized nozzles.

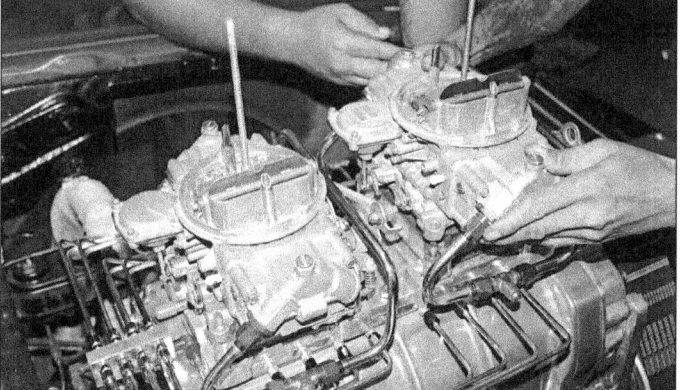

7 After installing the NS supercharger plate, Sensano re-installs the Weiand dual 4-barrel carburetor adaptor plate that originally came with the blower. This is followed with the installation of the dual 750-cfm Holley carburetors, and everything is looking good.

HOW TO INSTALL AND TUNE NITROUS OXIDE SYSTEMS

CHAPTER 4

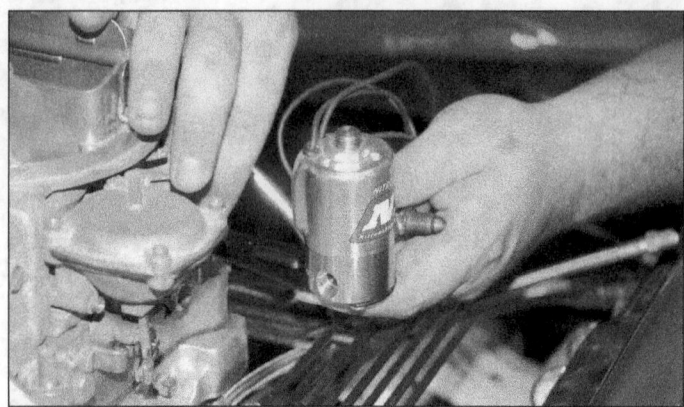 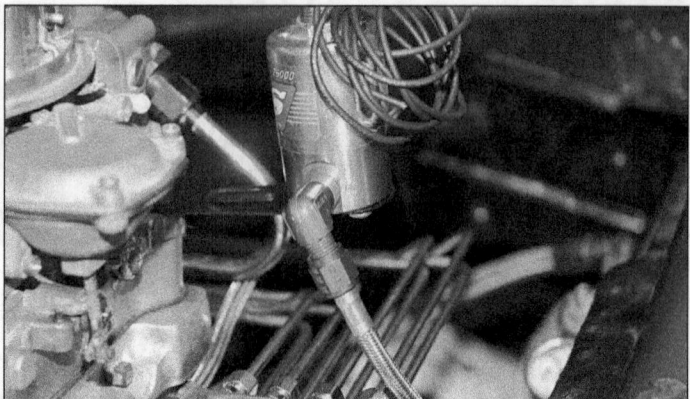

8 Installing the NS N20 solenoid comes next, followed with the attachment of the -4 AN blue-nipple nitrous supply line.

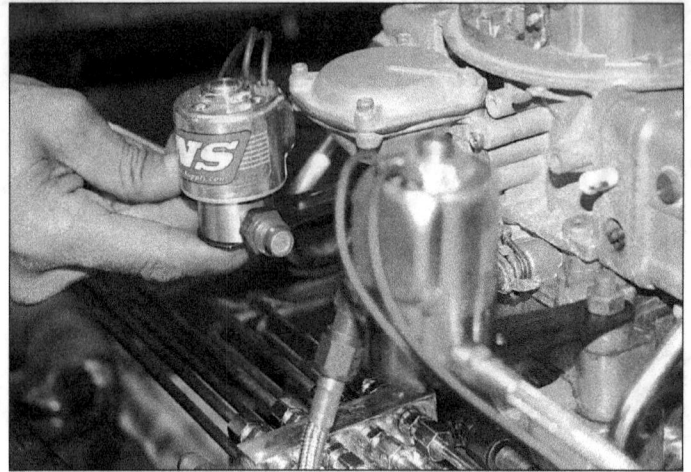 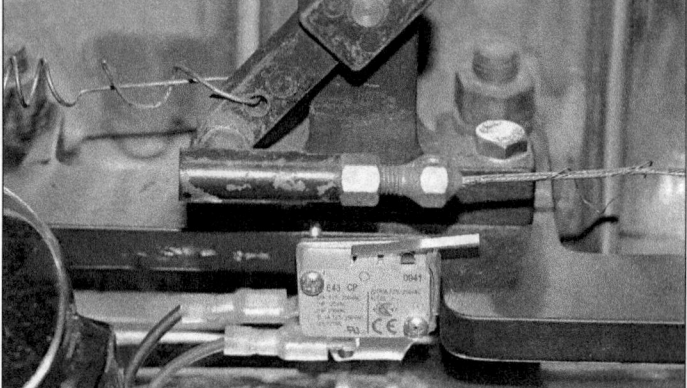

9 A T-fitting is used to tap into the existing fuel line in order to be able to supply gasoline to the NS fuel solenoid.

10 Wiring the throttle position sensor micro-switch comes next, using the provided bracket. Once a suitable hot-wire lead is located it is wired to the arming switch located inside the car and the system is sufficiently grounded.

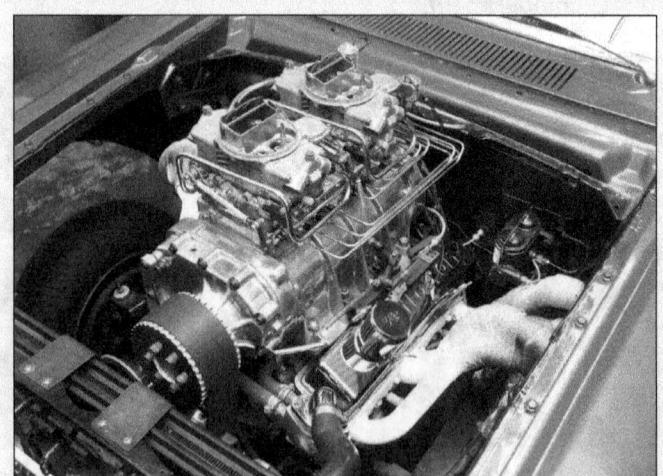 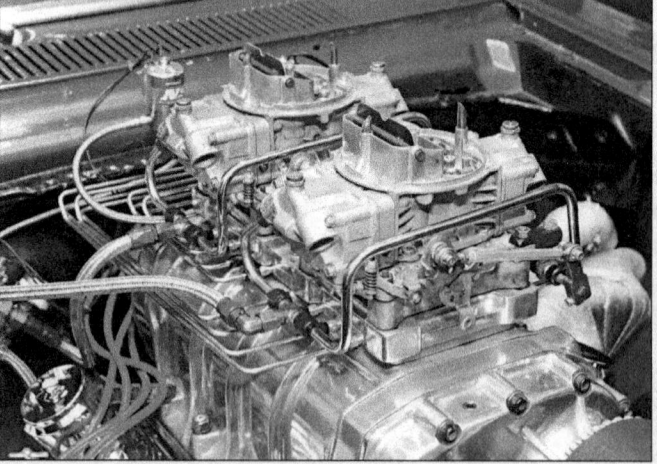

With the system fully plumbed and wired, this is what it should look like. It should also be noted that with this application, an auxiliary fuel pump capable of supporting 400 to 500 hp at 5 to 10 psi is required if you don't already have one like those manufactured by either Holley or Magna Fuel.

CHAPTER 5

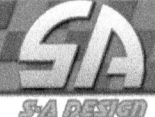

HIDDEN SINGLE-STAGE SYSTEMS: TOP SHOT AND FRIENDS

One of the big advantages of nitrous oxide systems are their ability to be concealed. This was much more important when use of nitrous oxide was relatively new and popular with the street racing crowd. When big money was bet on clandestine backstreet races, hiding the potential within your car (or motorcycle) was a big deal. Today, nitrous oxide is relatively common, and hiding it is much less of a concern. But, for those who still enjoy the lure of a "sleeper," here are some setups that work great, but remain out of sight.

Top Shot

The term "Top Shot" was originally branded by Nitrous Oxide Systems in the mid 1980s, and the principle behind the product is fairly self explanatory. The Top Shot system uses the carburetor as a mixer with a cylindrical injector module attached to the carburetor/air filter-cover stud. It comes complete with a thermal safety switch (TSS) in case of carburetor backfire. The Top Shot is totally hidden and utilizes N_2O and fuel flare jets to produce 75 to 150 hp on stock engines, and 100 to 150 hp on modified engines.

However, NOS wasn't the first N_2O manufacturing company to come up with the hidden system. That was Ron Hammel from 10,000 RPM Speed Equipment, one of the original developers of street/strip automotive N_2O systems. Hammel's invention, however, didn't employ the actual Top Shot sprayer-solenoid principle. True, his High-Speed RPM Power Ring also went on top of the carburetor as a mixer, but was not attached to the air cleaner stud like the Top Shot.

When attached to one of 10,000 RPM's 4-barrel carburetor plates, it was still a one-stage system, but looked and acted like a two-stage system. Tests indicated a gain up to 50 hp when used with the aforementioned carburetor plate. One of Hammel's fuel pressure regulators was also required to increase pressure because you were adding .5 psi per horsepower per hour. Also recommended for use with this application was 10,000 RPM's Stage-V nitrous solenoid valve. Although the company no longer actively promotes the High-Speed RPM Power Ring, it is still available.

Street Heat

A similar product is the 20- to 100-hp Street Heat portable N_2O system being marketed by Compucar Nitrous. This system (which is contained in a gym bag) can be installed

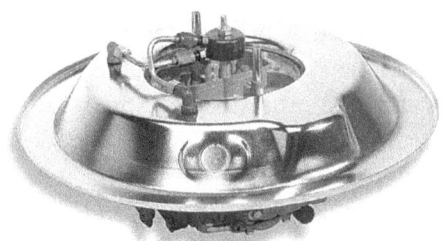

NOS' Top Shot is a cylindrical injector module that uses the carburetor as the mixer and uses adjustable flare jets. The Top Shot is mounted to the air cleaner stud and is totally hidden. Nitrous oxide is fed to the Top Shot from a well hidden line located at the rear of the intake manifold, and the unit touts a Thermal Safety Switch in the event of a carburetor backfire. Horsepower increases of 75 to 150 hp on stock engines and 100 to 150 hp on modified engines are possible.

CHAPTER 5

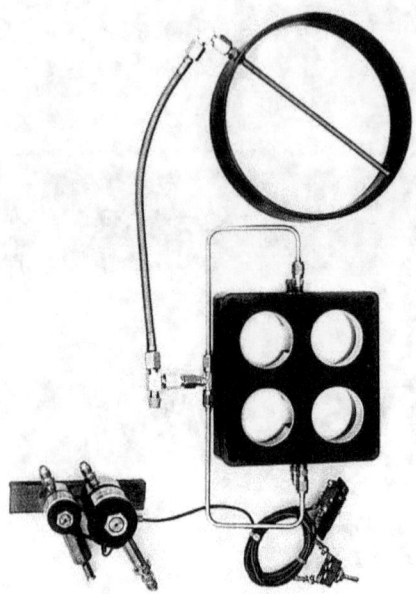

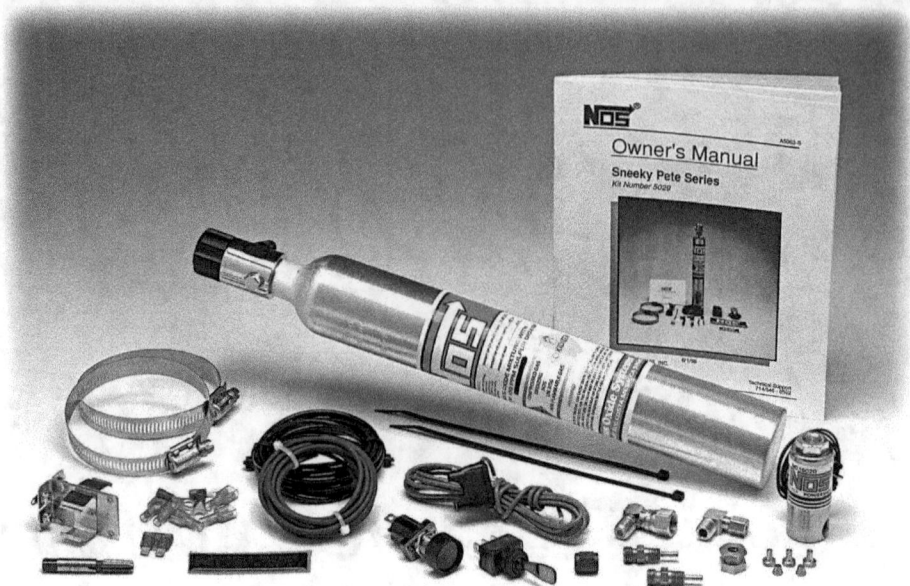

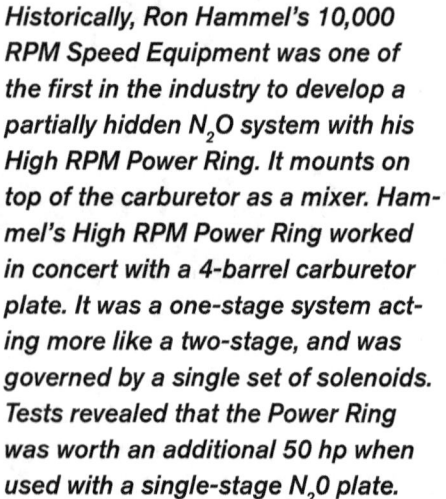

Historically, Ron Hammel's 10,000 RPM Speed Equipment was one of the first in the industry to develop a partially hidden N_2O system with his High RPM Power Ring. It mounts on top of the carburetor as a mixer. Hammel's High RPM Power Ring worked in concert with a 4-barrel carburetor plate. It was a one-stage system acting more like a two-stage, and was governed by a single set of solenoids. Tests revealed that the Power Ring was worth an additional 50 hp when used with a single-stage N_2O plate.

The NOS Sneaky Pete was designed to obtain an extra tenth of a second and an extra 15 to 25 hp without being obvious.

on any motor vehicle in 10 minutes or less, typically through the air intake tube of a late-model EFI car or through the carburetor lid of a traditionally carbureted car. It draws its electrical power from the cigarette lighter or power port. (For more information on the Street Heat system, contact the manufacturer.)

Also available on the market is a series of compact, easy-to-install nitrous kits capable of being used on applications from Harley-Davidson to ATV/ Jet Ski to most popular makes of carbureted and EFI-controlled light-duty cars and trucks. Of course, horsepower is limited by jetting and the amount of fuel available. Since these kits typically rely on a 10-ounce bottle of nitrous, they can't be expected to produce much power for very long. With these systems, it is also necessary to richen the jet on the carburetor to compensate for the extra shot of nitrous, since no additional fuel source is being utilized.

Sneaky Pete

The NOS Sneaky Pete is a portable cheater system. It was designed for the operator to obtain an extra tenth of a second with the additional 15 to 25 or so horses, without being obvious. This kit (PN 05090NOS) comes complete with a compact, easy-to-conceal 10-ounce N_2O bottle, a single N_2O solenoid, nylon nitrous supply line, wiring, a 9-volt tandem battery pack, and an assortment of jets.

The NS version is known as Little Sneaky (PN 06090NS). It also offers performance gains of 15 to 25 hp, and this system also operates on two 9-volt batteries wired in parallel.

The Stealth Nozzle

The Stealth Nozzle, designed and created by Scott Vander Schoor from Nightmare Motorsports, is considered a breakthrough product in single-stage N_2O kits. The Stealth Nozzle is mounted in the base of a single-plane, or Air Gap-type 4-barrel intake manifold, where Stealth's 360-degree nozzle (machined out of 6061 T6 aluminum) delivers a precise and direct shot of N_2O and fuel to each intake runner. With the carburetor bolted on, this 75- to 250-hp wet nozzle is 100 percent out of sight. The N_2O and fuel lines are routed to the bottom of the nozzle, where they are also accordingly jetted. This single nozzle effectively acts more like a direct-port nitrous delivery system rather than a fogger setup. At this writing, the list of single-plane Air Gap applications is growing, including all Edelbrock Victor, Edelbrock Victor Jr. and Holley/Weiand raised-floor intakes.

Also note that each nozzle has a different spray pattern based on the application, such as both small-block and big-block Fords and Chevrolets, with the latter including the popular LSX- and LM-Series engines. Available as a kit, all Stealth applications include single-stage Stealth Nozzles, N_2O and fuel solenoids and supply lines, a 10-pound nitrous bottle, and all the wiring and hardware necessary to complete the installation. Heck, Nightmare Motorsports even includes a blocking plate, should you ever wish to remove the system and return to stock.

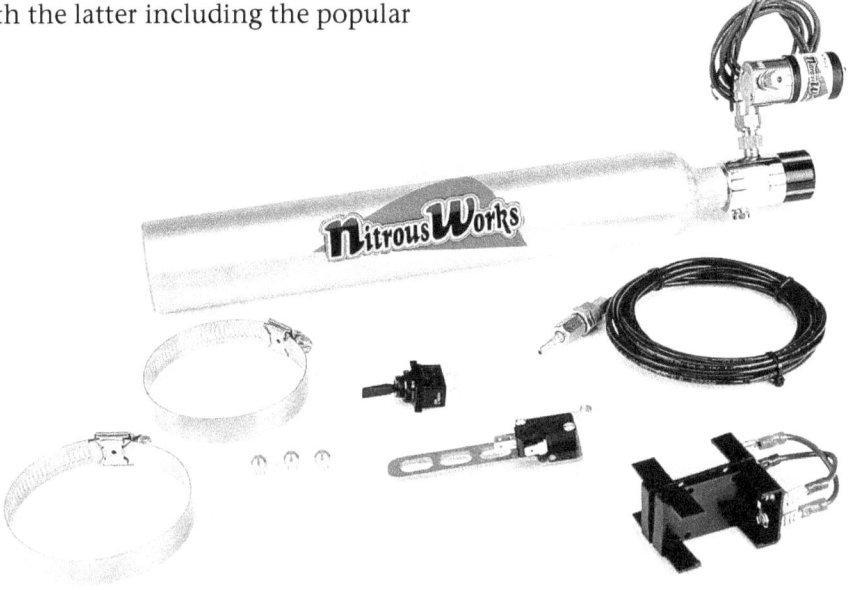

The NitrousWorks manufactures an easy-to-install, hideaway N_2O system, similar to the Sneaky Pete, called Mr. Mister (PN 15100), complete with 10-ounce Skinny-Minny N_2O bottle capable of delivering 15 to 25 hp. This fully adjustable 18-VDC kit also uses twin 9-volt batteries and is perfect for on-the-fly carbureted or EFI applications.

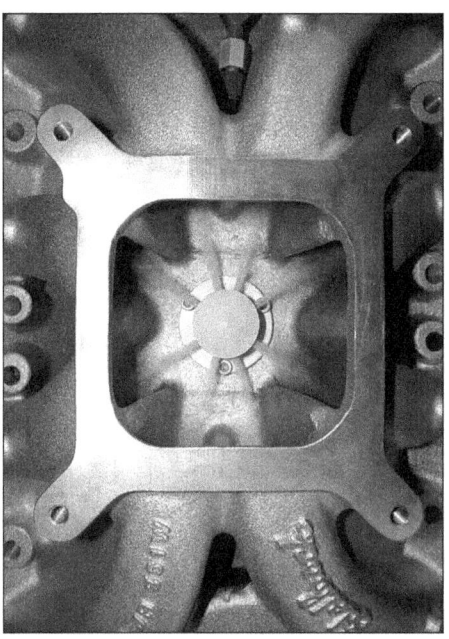

Judging from its spray pattern, Nightmare Motorsports' Stealth Nozzle acts more like a direct-port N_2O system, with its 360-degree nozzle that mounts dead center on the floor of an intake.

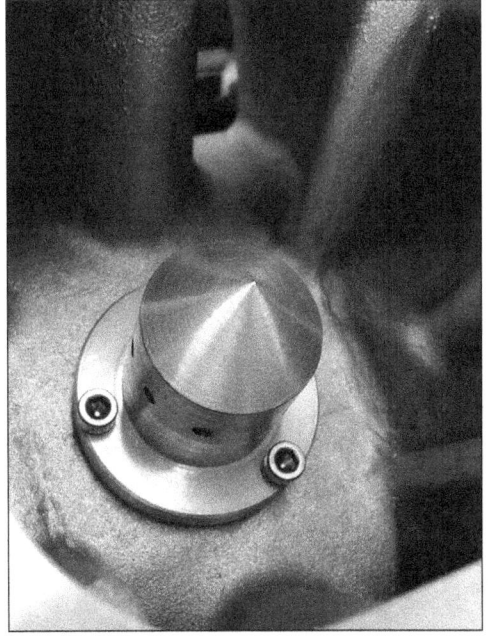 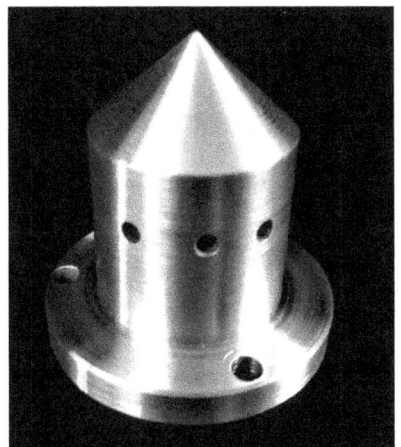

The Stealth works with any single-plane intake, such as a conventional Edelbrock Victor, Offenhauser Equipment Company, Blue Thunder, or Edelbrock Victor Jr. 4V intake, or an air–gap-design 4V intake like a Holley-Weiand or Edelbrock. Stealth's 360-degree, 6061 T-6 aluminum nozzle delivers a precise, direct shot of N_2O and fuel to each individual intake runner. With the carburetor bolted in place, Stealth's fully adjustable 75- to 250-hp wet nozzle is visibly un-detectable. The N_2O and fuel lines are routed to the bottom of the nozzle, where they are accordingly jetted. Stealth's nitrous and fuel solenoids are likewise hidden from sight. Different nozzle patterns are available for different applications. Nightmare Motorsports even provides a block-off plate, should you want to remove your Stealth N_2O system and use it on a different application.

CHAPTER 6

NITROUS FOGGER

Originally invented and patented in the early 1980s by Nitrous Oxide Systems, the term/name "Fogger" not only describes a particular means or process of introducing N_2O into an engine, it is also a name trademarked by NOS, now a Division of Holley Performance Products, Inc.

"The first nitrous oxide systems were obviously the plates," says nitrous industry pioneer Mike Thermos. "However, as horsepower requirements went up, the plate design became limited because of distribution issues. NOS engineers knew they had to individually spray into each port, and that's when the Fogger concept was designed."

The Fogger is a jet-based nozzle-type system that gives you the option to change both the N_2O side and the fuel side of the nozzle, which allows you to crank up the power and affords the option to either richen or lean-out either side of the nozzle, thereby allowing the tuning of the system runner-to-runner. Simply said, the

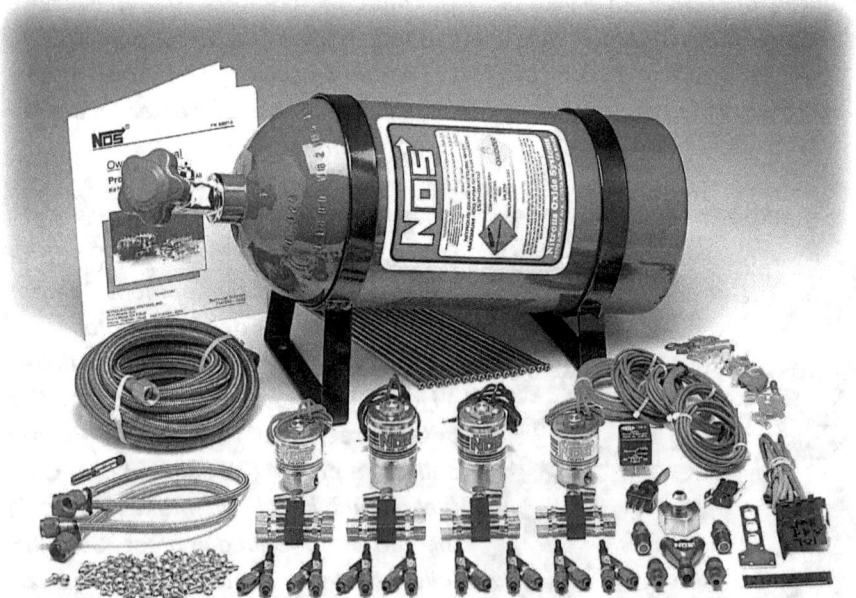
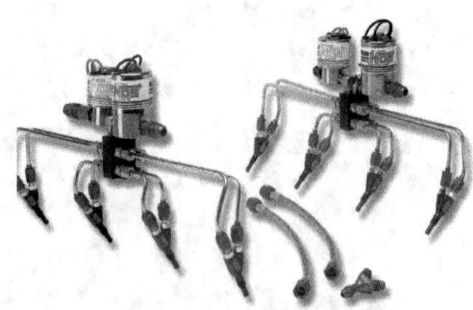

Originally patented in the early 1980s by Nitrous Oxide Systems, a Division of Holley Performance Products, Inc., the term Fogger not only describes a particular means or process of introducing N_2O into an engine, it is also a trademarked name. The Fogger is a jet-able nozzle-type system, and it gives you the option to change both the N_2O side and the fuel side of the nozzle, which allows you to not only crank up the power, it affords the option to either richen or lean either side of the nozzle, thereby allowing runner-to-intake-runner tuning of the system. The Fogger simply gives you a much better point of N_2O and fuel distribution.

NITROUS FOGGER

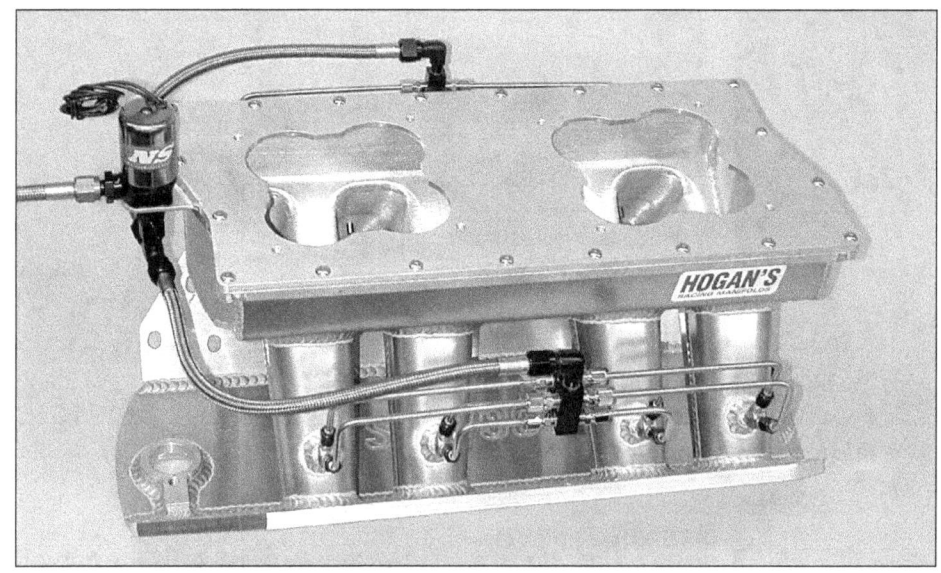

This Nitrous Supply–prepared single-stage system was installed on a Hogan Manifolds Dominator-style 2x4 sheet-metal intake, and uses a set of NS Mutha Fogga 360-degree nozzles.

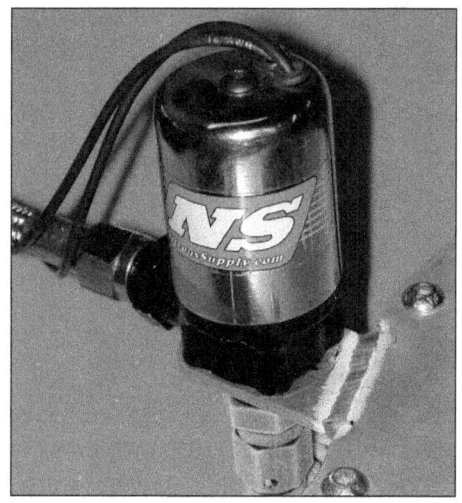

Another integral component in this system is one of NS Slayer high-yield N_2O solenoids, which features a huge .250-inch orifice.

Fogger gives you a much better point of N_2O and fuel distribution.

Foggers can be used on all types of intake manifolds/engines ranging from a conventional individual-runner, single 4-barrel-carbureted intake, to a dual-runner tunnel-ram 2x4 intake manifold, in both single-stage (Street Fogger and Sportsman Fogger) and dual-stage applications such as Pro Shot Fogger, Pro Shot Twin Fogger, etc.

EFI Fogger applications can include something as simple as a single fogger nozzle (inserted into the air intake tube of a computer-governed late-model EFI engine) or an eight-nozzle system hidden in the underside of an EFI intake (see "Bullit Reloaded" on page 101 in Chapter 9).

The heart of the Fogger concept is the nozzle. NOS sticks by its tried-and-true original pattern, the dual-jet Fogger- and Fogger2-brand nozzles, which continue to be the best sellers on the street/strip market. For high-horsepower/racing applications there's NOS' single-function Annular Discharge Fogger nozzle. Conversely, NOS also markets the Soft Plume 90-degree Fogger nozzle specifically designed for EFI applications.

Nitrous Supply's version of the fogger is the 90-degree Fine Plume 1, which works best with EFI applications, and produces a homogenized air/fuel mixture.

The company's competition-use High-Flow fogger nozzle pretty much

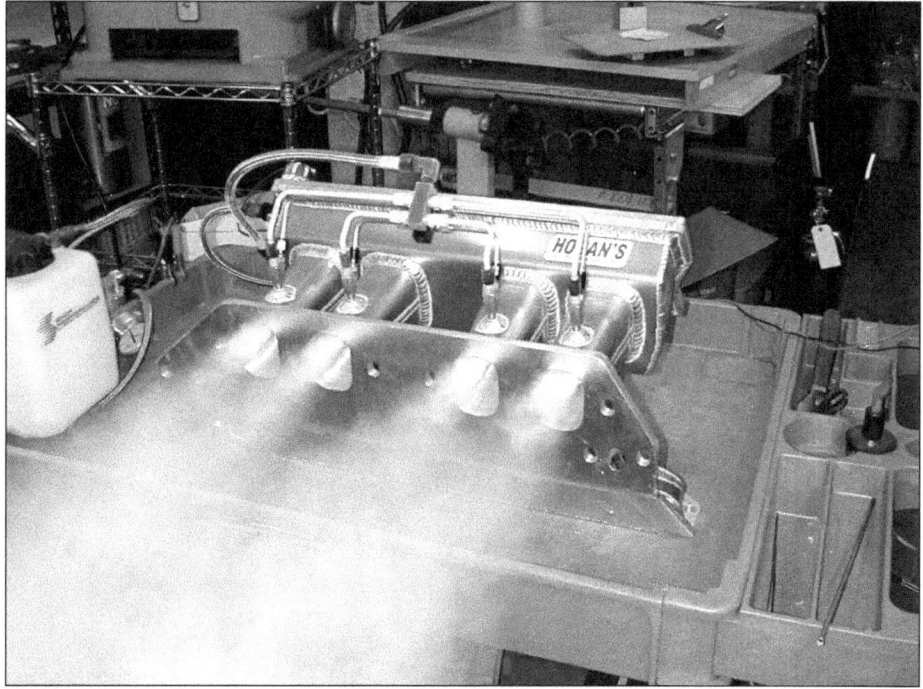

To ensure proper operation and nozzle orientation, a test firing is done once all of the components are installed. As you can see, each plume of nitrous is similarly sized and flowing nicely. This installation is ready for action!

CHAPTER 6

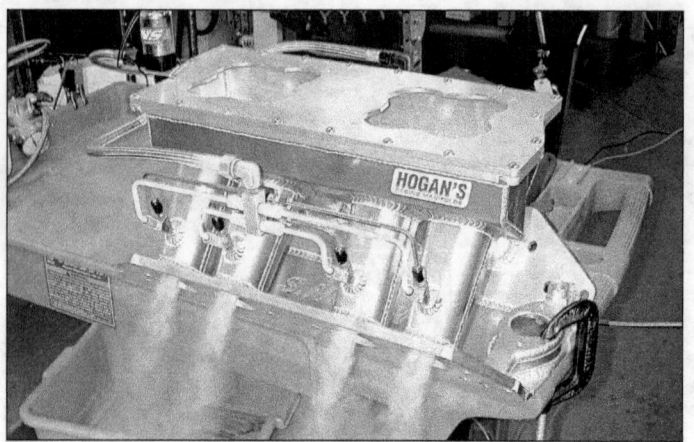
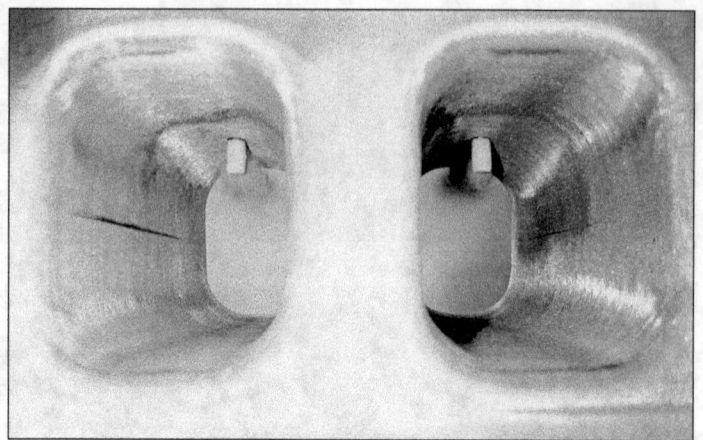

Nitrous Supply's CEO Mike Thermos test-fires this fogger-equipped, large-volume-solenoid Hogan Manifolds 2x4 sheet-metal intake—man, is that sheer volume or what?

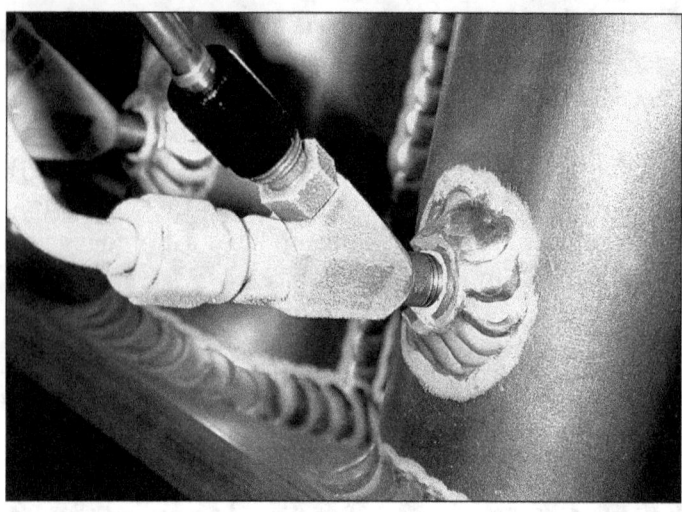

Injected into the ports of an engine at -127 degrees F, it's easy to understand why these nozzles frost up, especially when equipped with a big jet backed up by a large-volume nitrous solenoid.

speaks for itself. NS 90-degree Fang, is the next step up. The Fang is a higher-level competition-style nozzle with fuel outlets on either side of the N_2O plume. The ultimate is the full 360-degree Mutha Fogga, a high-density nozzle that actually injects droplets of fuel and N_2O into the cylinders of an engine, all geared for serious high-horsepower usage.

Nitrous Express calls its top-of-the-line fogger nozzles the Vortech, the Piranha, the Shark, and the SX2. The company also markets a GM NXL fogger-nozzle application to fit the LS- and LM-series GM EFI engines.

ZEX refers to its product as the 90-degree Power Advantage 1 & 2. And finally, Edelbrock Nitrous refers to its fogger nozzles as the 90-degree E1 & E2, while the competition-version E3 Series is a straight-shot fogger nozzle doing exactly what its name implies. When it comes to putting the nitrous where you need it, the fogger style (in its various brand names and incarnations) is one of the best and most effective N_2O systems on the market.

CHAPTER 7

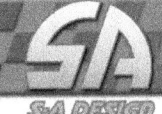

MULTI-STAGE SYSTEMS

Multiple-stage N₂O systems are intended for hardcore racing applications. They cover the full range, from the ultimate street racer and advanced bracket classes to Sportsman class racing, where you're going to need a lot of horsepower to cross the finish line first. A number of multi-stage N₂O kits are commercially available: NOS Pro Shot Twin Fogger and Pro Race Fogger, NS Racestar Pro, and Nitrous Express Shark Direct Port and SX2 Direct Port systems. They all work great with either single 4-barrel intakes like an Edelbrock Victor, 2x4 intakes like an Edelbrock or Weiand tunnel ram, or single 4-barrel or 2x4 sheet-metal-type intakes like those manufactured by Hogan's Racing Manifolds. These systems are capable of producing between 600 and 1,200 hp, depending on the tune-up and the engine. Now let's take a closer look at their physical makeup.

All multi-stage systems basically operate on the concept of two fully adjustable fogger-type N₂O and fuel solenoids operating separately, albeit in tandem, per bank of cylinders. The idea is to deliver as much nitrous as possible to the engine via a series of eight fogger-type nozzles (one per intake runner) for the ultimate in fuel/nitrous atomization and distribution. All these systems require plumbing the intake

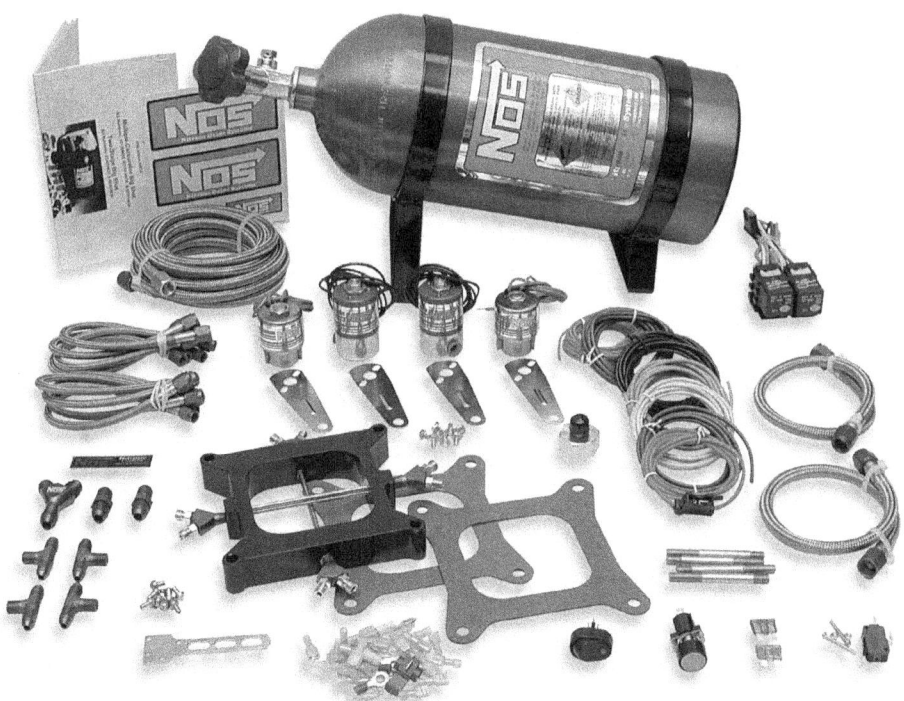

Billed as the World's Most Sophisticated Plate Systems, NOS Double Cross and Pro Two-Stage Plate Kits are available in either standard Holley (PN 02321NOS), or Dominator (PN 02322NOS) flange. The 90-degree-crossbar-angle Double Cross is most effective when used with complex intake manifold designs and/or deep-runner intakes like Pro-Stock/Pro-Mod/Top Sportsman intake manifolds, where maximum coverage is critical. The Two-Stage Double Cross kit provides anywhere from 250 to 500 adjustable horsepower.

Joe and Michelle Barry's

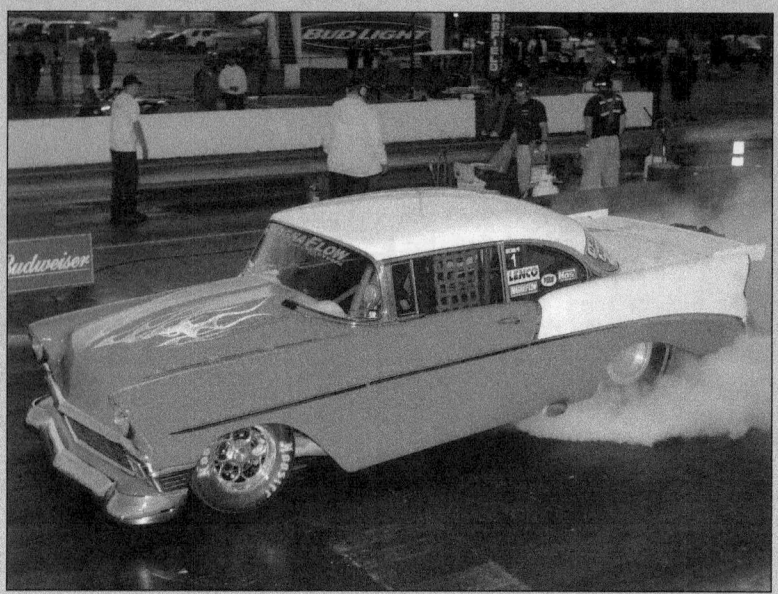

When it came to building a Pacific Street Car Association (PSCA) Heavy Street class entry, Colorado Springs, Colorado, racer Joe Barry could have chosen any kind of car he wanted. Not surprisingly, he chose a 1956 Chevrolet Bel Air.

"It takes real talent to build a successful heads-up Heavy Street car out of one of these old tanks," says Joe, who has run a best of 7.33 seconds at 189 mph using an NOS dual-fogger setup on his Mike Blackstone/Watson Racing Engines 632-ci Dart/Chevrolet big-block. The foundation for Joe's incredibly quick Nitrous 1956 is a Jerry Bickel Race Cars' (JBRC) 115-inch-wheelbase Pro Mod–style chassis. It features a Mark Williams 4.29:1-geared 9-inch Ford axle. The axle is suspended by Hyper Coil springs and Koni shocks.

Powering Joe's 7-second door slammer is the aforementioned 632-ci Dart Industries big-block, equipped with a Winberg forged-steel crank riding on Federal Mogul Performance engine bearings, ARP engine fasteners, a set of GRP connecting rods, and Ackerly-Childs–equipped 14.5:1-compression Ross forged-aluminum pistons. Also on board are a Lunati Cams roller cam, Jesel lifters, and Manton pushrods. Cam timing is handled by a Jesel belt drive, while lubrication comes from a Johnson four-stage dry sump system. A Stewart high-flow aluminum water pump and a Modine aluminum radiator handle engine cooling. Bolted up top is a set of Jones Racing–prepared Dart Big Chief's big-valve aluminum cylinder heads sporting ARP, Manley, and Jesel valvetrain hardware.

Another key player in this equation is a Dart Big Chief 2x4 intake outfitted with dual NOS Fogger plates and a pair of 1,050-cfm Braswell-prepared Holley Dominator carburetors. The crank-trigger ignition system on Barry's 1956 comes from the nice folks at MSD, firing a set of Autolite spark plugs through a set of MSD spark plug wires. A set of Hooker stepped headers with a 5-inch collector dumps into a 5-inch exhaust system equipped with a set of Flowmaster racing mufflers.

Like most shoe box racers, Barry's 1956 features removable steel front fenders, one-piece fiberglass front bumper, and a Glass Tech scooped fiberglass hood. Credit for the paint and body work goes to "Denver Dave" Hildebrand, who painted the car two-tone Hugger Orange

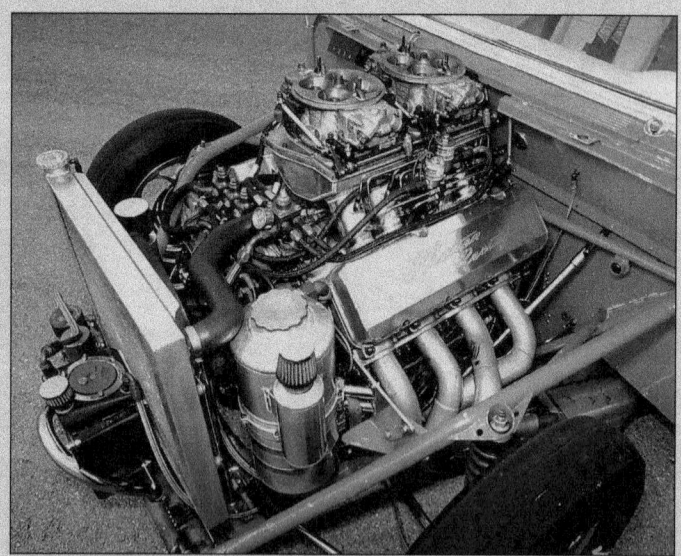

A Mike Blackstone/Watson Racing Engineering 632-ci Dart Industries big-block powers Barry's shoe box, which gets its oomph from a Nitrous Oxide Systems Dual Fogger Dart-Braswell/Holley Dominator induction system.

MULTI-STAGE SYSTEMS

Heavy Street Nitrous 1956 Shoe Box

and Vanilla Milkshake. Big Joe's 1956 also features Danchuk trim, GM factory window glass, and a Mark Lynn rear-deck-wing parachute brace for the twin Stroud Safety parachutes.

Housed inside the trunk is a JAZ fuel cell and twin Optima batteries. Joe's 1956 features carbon-fiber door panels equipped with Billet Specialties door handles, JBRC aluminum trim, twin carbon-fiber Auto Weave–upholstered bucket seats, Stroud Safety harnesses, Pete's Billet 1956 Chevy dash, Auto Meter instruments, and let's not forget those twin 15-pound polished NOS bottles!

Weighing 3,640 pounds, Joe and Michelle Barry's 1956 Chevrolet Bel Air 210 may be the bain of its competitor's existence, but the fans absolutely love the car. Says Joe with a huge grin, "That run of 7.33 seconds just so happens to be a tad quicker than the PSCA's 7.50-second NHRA class certification and we've been accused of killing the class. Hell, all I'm doing is making it all the more interesting, but it looks like the old Chevy's going to get itself re-factored."

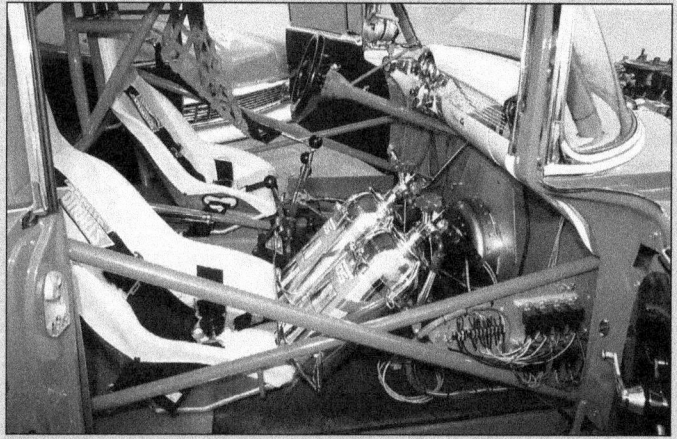

Inside, Joe's 1956 uses JBRC aluminum, a pair of twin carbon-fiber Auto Weave–upholstered fiberglass bucket seats, and Stroud Safety Equipment. There is also a JBRC steering column and pedal assembly, a Pete's Billet/Auto Meter–equipped dash, and those polished 15-pound NOS bottles.

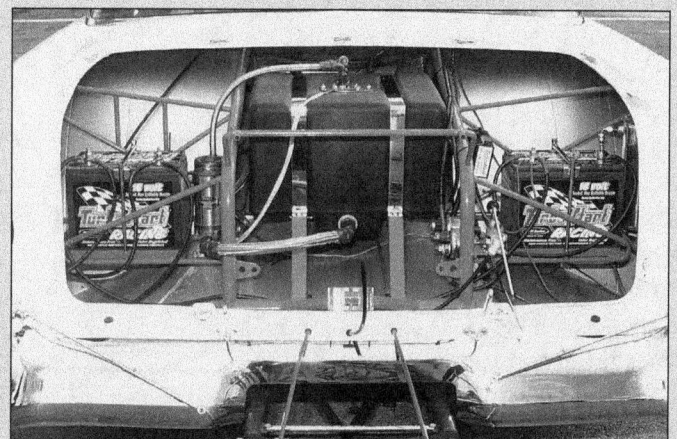

Housed inside the removable trunk lid are twin Turbo Start gel-cell batteries, Magna-Fuel twin fuel pumps, and a JAZ fuel cell. Nothing but the best!

manifold, which any competent machine shop or N_2O specialty house can do. They utilize a single 15-pound, siphon-type Super High Flow N_2O bottle, although it has become standard practice with serious racers to use one nitrous bottle per side. These setups also require a fuel system (or systems with twin bottles) capable of delivering 5 to 10 psi per side with a flow rate of at least 0.1 gph at 6 psi. Holley, NOS, NX, Nitrous Supply, etc., offer pumps and matched regulators for these applications. Typically, a good nitrous controller for an application like this is a Fuel Air Spark Technologies (FAST) XFI NOS Programmable Nitrous Controller, an Edelbrock Progressive Nitrous Controller, or similar.

With higher-horsepower applications like in NHRA/IHRA Top Sportsman and Pro Mod, 1,500- to 2,000-plus-hp multiple-stage setups (as many as six) are quite normal. However, you won't be finding them in an off-the-shelf kit, although all of the necessary components can be purchased in parts for any brand-name N_2O manufacturer. These kinds of systems are usually best handled by a specialist like Jeff Prock's Applied Nitrous Technologies, Wilson Manifolds & Nitrous Pro-Flow, Steve Johnson's Induction Solutions, etc.

CHAPTER 7

Project: Nitrous Supply Two-Stage Nitrous 2x4 Intake Buildup

The most popular intake system for serious all-out drag racing is the Holley Dominator/2x4 sheet-metal tunnel-ram intake like those built by Hogan's Racing Manifolds. The company's tall-runner big-block Chevrolet 2x4 intake lends itself quite nicely for custom-fabricated, two-stage N_2O applications. Shown here is pioneer AA/Fuel Altered drag racer and Nitrous Supply resident machinist Bill Thurman setting up one of these systems. When installed on a nitrous-specific Chevy big-block engine, this two-stage nitrous intake produces 1,000-plus hp.

Stage 1 makes use of a set of eight NS Fine Plume 1 90-degree fogger nozzles (PN 23716), which, for the sake of setup, initially employ a number-26 nitrous jet and a number-22 fuel jet.

Stage 2 features a set of eight NS Fang style 90-degree nozzles (PN 23712), which, again for the sake of the initial tune-up, features a number-24 nitrous jet and a number-18 fuel jet. A set of two NS .0015-inch-orifice N_2O solenoids (PN 26048), and two .187-inch-orifice fuel solenoids (PN 26050) are also integral components of this take-no-prisoners two-stage N_2O system, and simultaneously flow up to 125 psi!

Nitrous Supply's CEO Mike Thermos says, "You can set this thing up to come in 1 plus 1, the stages can be sandwiched, or set up 1-3 using something as simple as a Digi-Set controller (PN 25835), or any of a number of different N_2O controllers on the market." Of course, with a controller, you not only time the stages, you can also adjust the fuel curve and leanness!

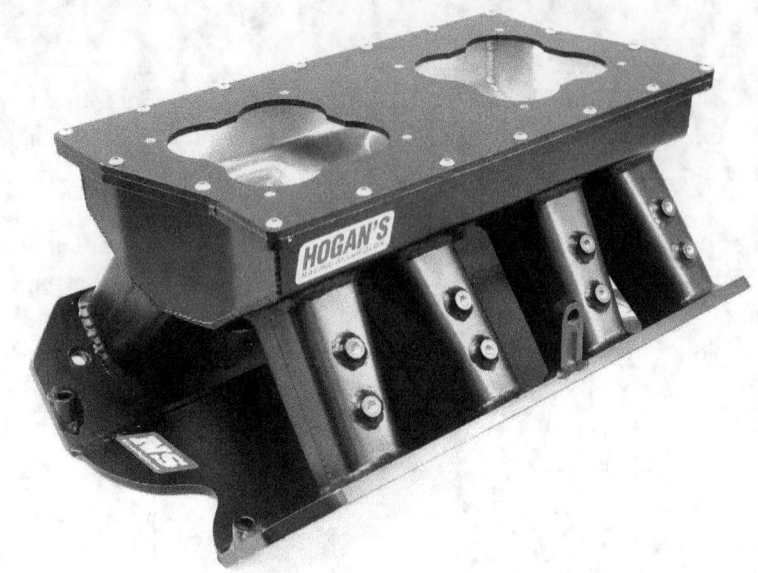

A Hogan's Racing Manifolds 2x4 tunnel ram for the big-block Chevrolet. In its various forms of preparation, this manifold has become a mainstay with bracket racers to Pro Gas and Top Sportsman racers.

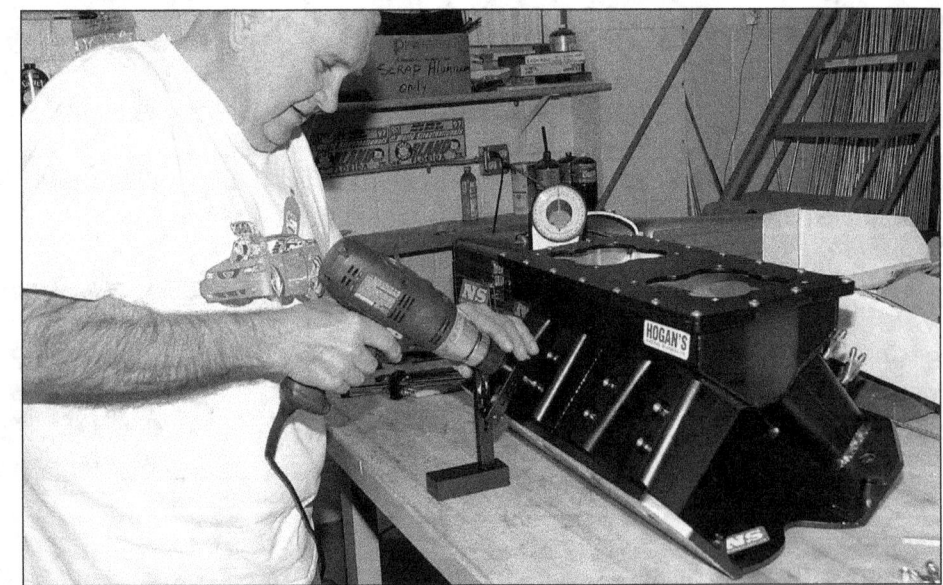

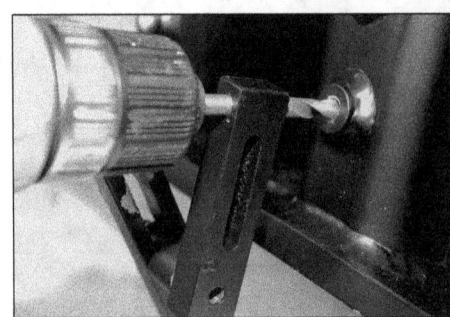

1 *Set up a fixture to align the top-most set of N_2O port nozzles for this two-stage tunnel ram setup. Use this fixture to drill the holes and mount nozzles straight and true using a 1/16-inch drill. Then tap the holes and chase the threads using a 1/6-inch NPT tap.*

MULTI-STAGE SYSTEMS

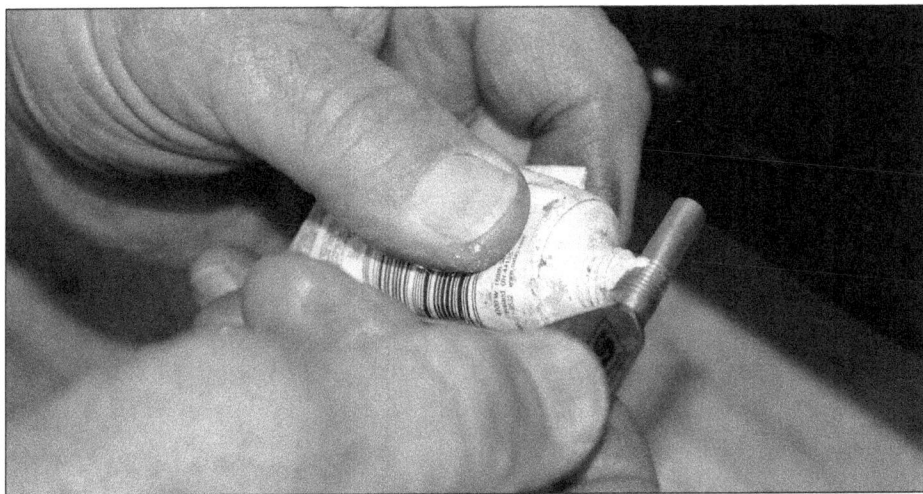

2 With nozzle ports set and ready, apply a dab of anti-seize to the threads of the nozzles and begin installation with NS Fine Plume nozzles installed in the top row, and NS Fang nozzles installed in the bottom row.

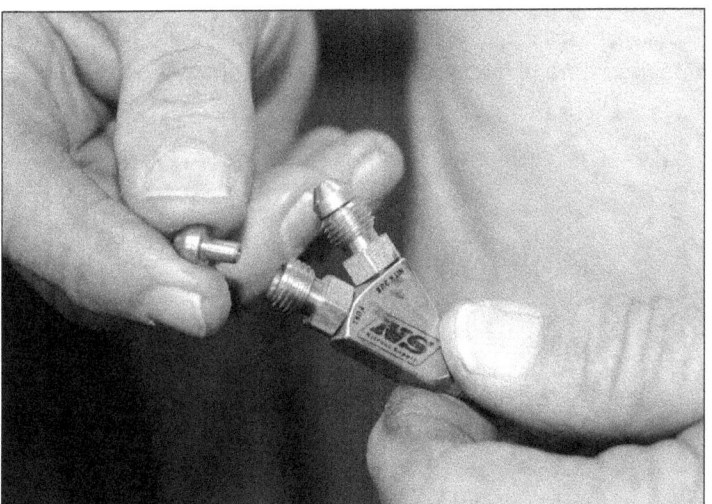
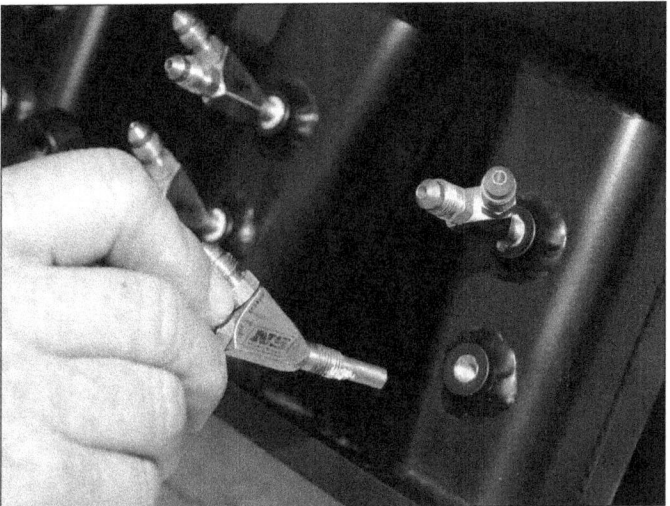

3 Install the nitrous jets into the nozzles, making sure that the business end of the 90-degree sprayer is facing downward.

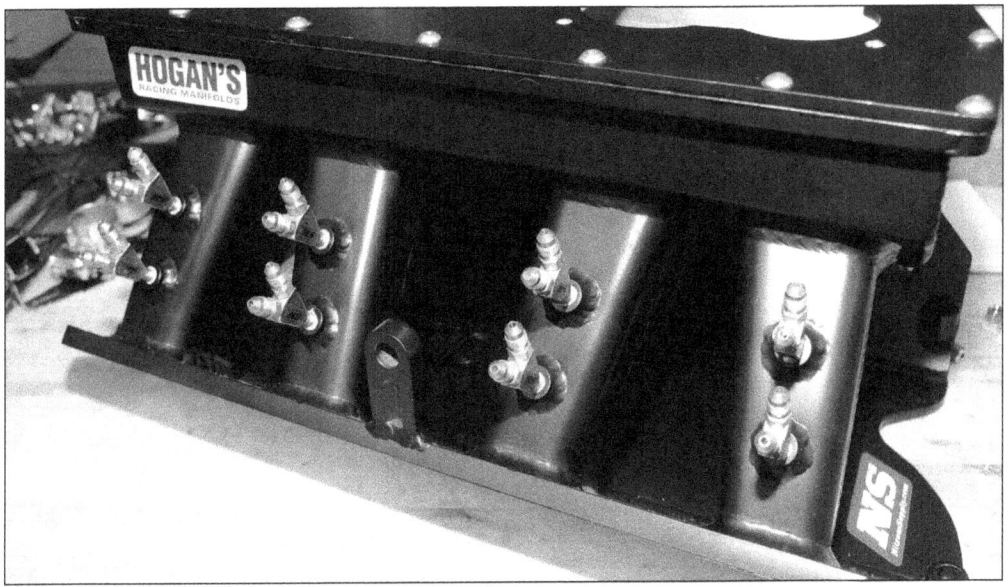

4 Here is the right side of this Two-Stage setup fully assembled.

CHAPTER 7

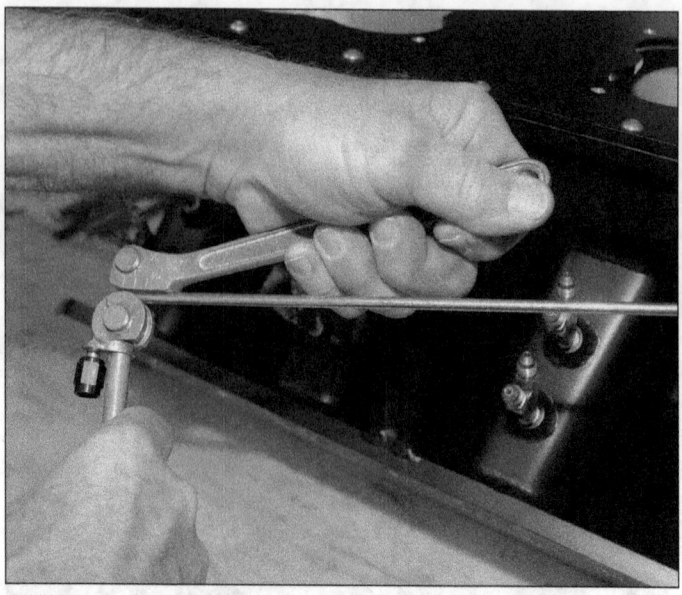 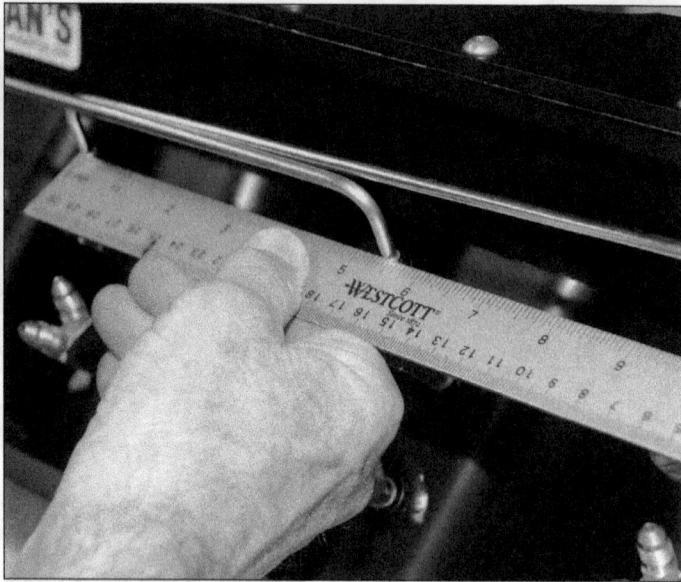

5 *Fabricating the 3/16-inch stainless-steel hard lines comes next. Check the first 90-degree bend for the top N$_2$O line.*

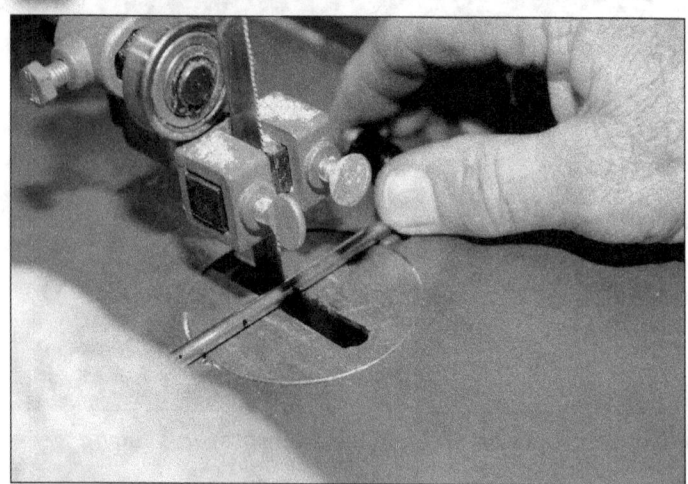 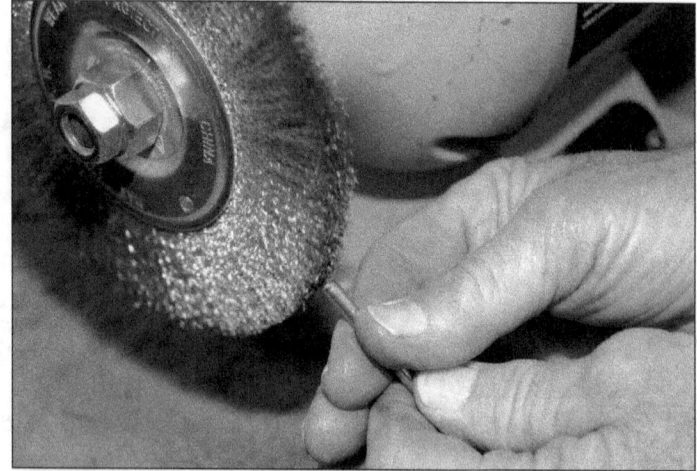

6 *Cut each individual line.* **7** *Deburr each line.*

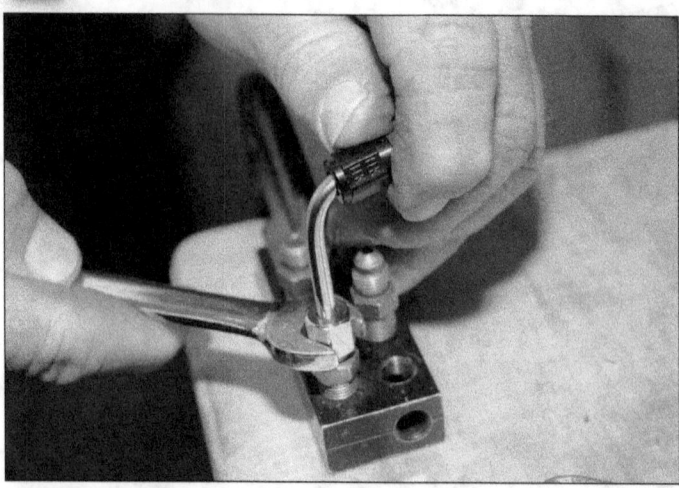 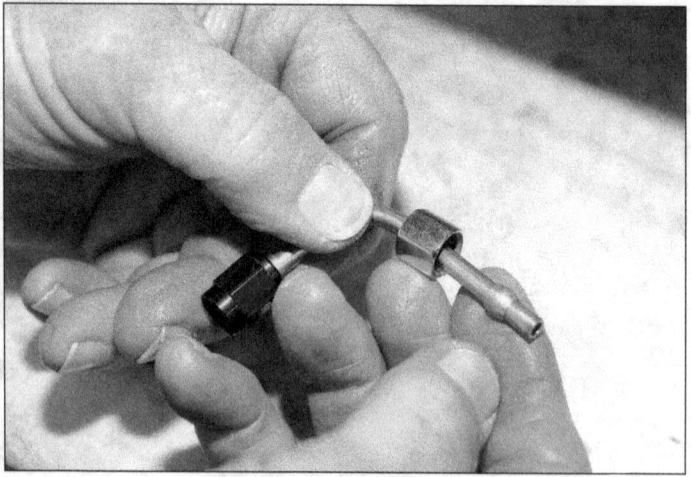

8 *Install the 3/16-inch fitting and flare the end of the line, on the end with compression fitting installed on the opposite end.*

HOW TO INSTALL AND TUNE NITROUS OXIDE SYSTEMS

MULTI-STAGE SYSTEMS

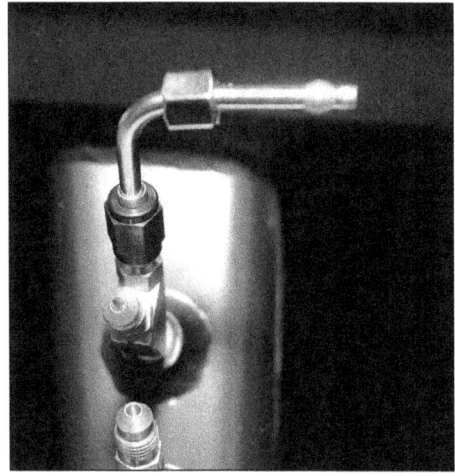
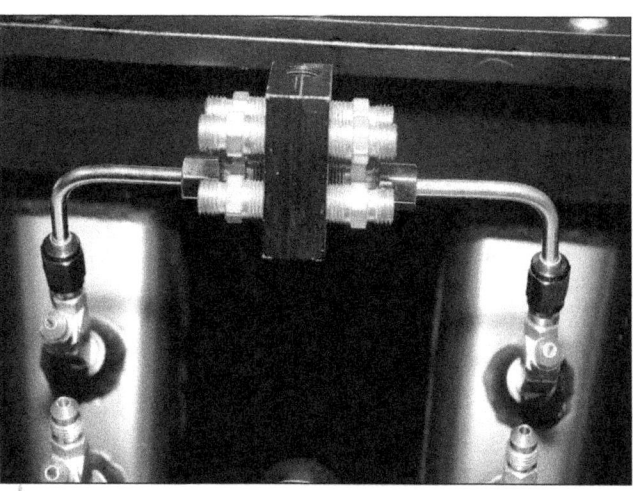

9 *Here's the first 2-3 intake runner set for the Fine Plume 1 Fogger nozzles.*

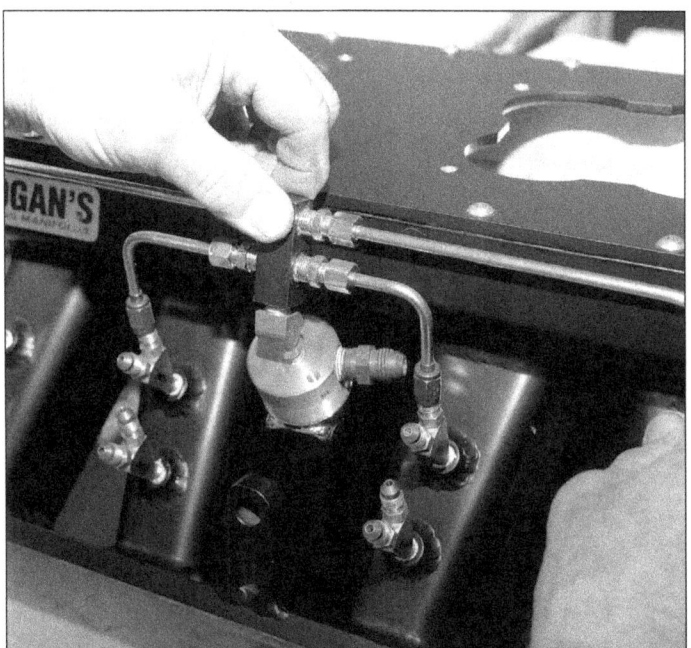
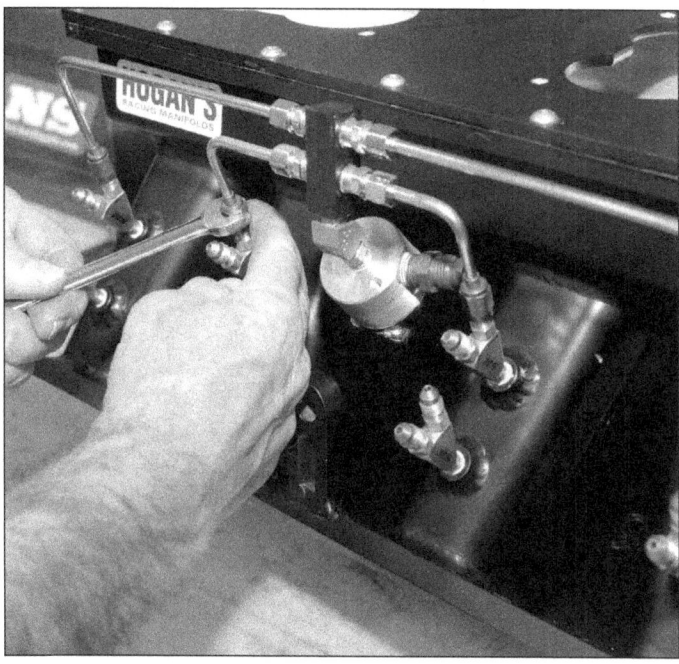

10 *Fabricate the outer set of Fine Plume 1 nozzle lines.*

HOW TO INSTALL AND TUNE NITROUS OXIDE SYSTEMS

CHAPTER 7

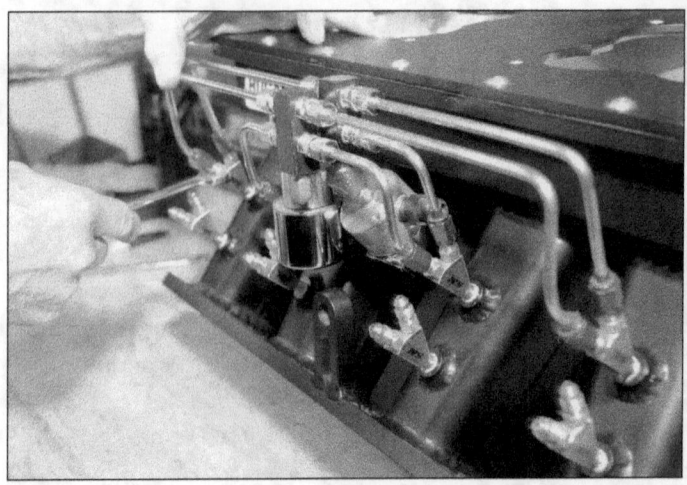

11 Fashion the top nozzle fuel lines and attach the fuel junction block via 7/16-inch coupling and compression fittings.

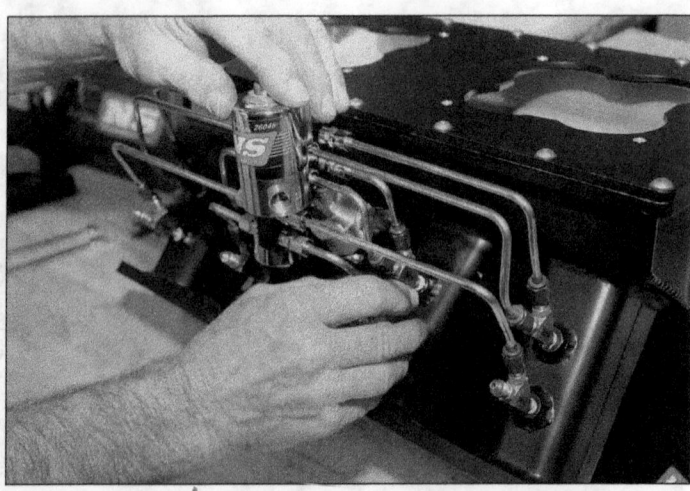

12 Note that the Fang N_2O lower lines have been fabricated, and Thurman is installing the fuel solenoid, which is actually marked "Gasoline."

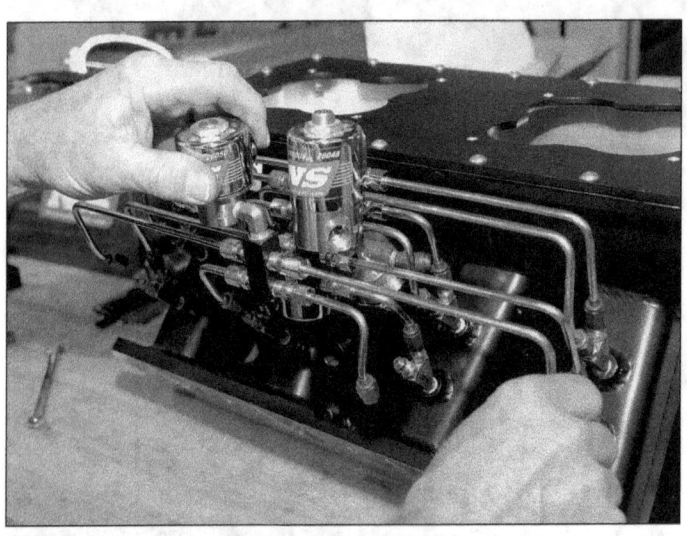

13 Install the N_2O solenoid next.

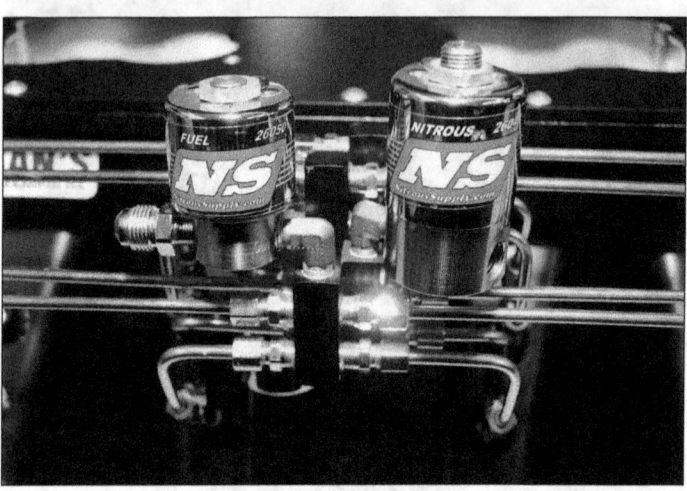

14 With everything plumbed, installed, and tightened, here's how one side looks.

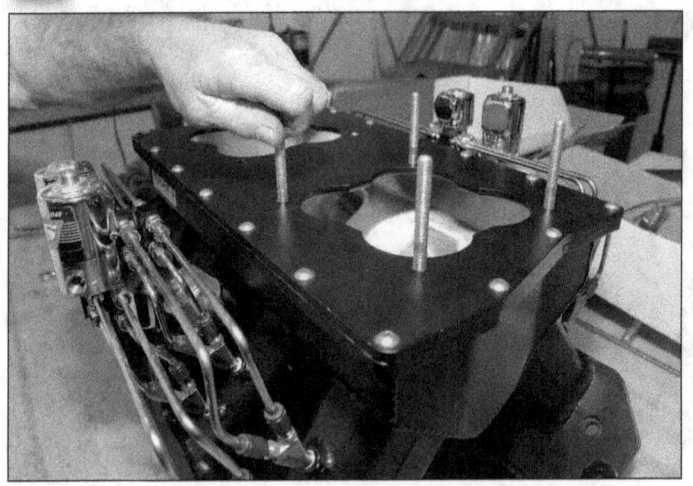

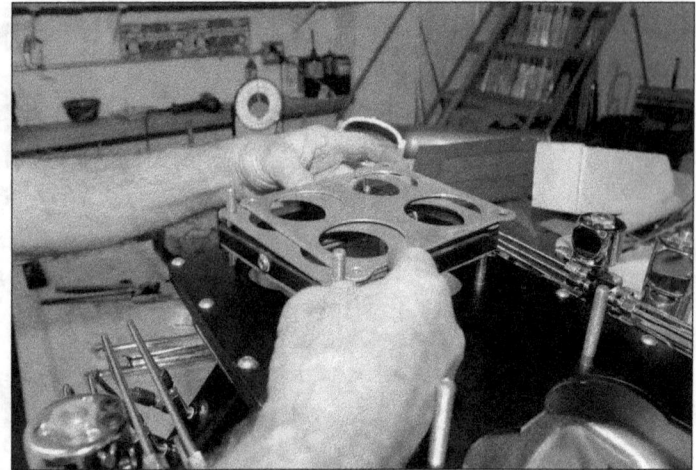

15 After repeating the hard-line fabrication process on the other side, screw in the Holley Dominator carburetor studs.

MULTI-STAGE SYSTEMS

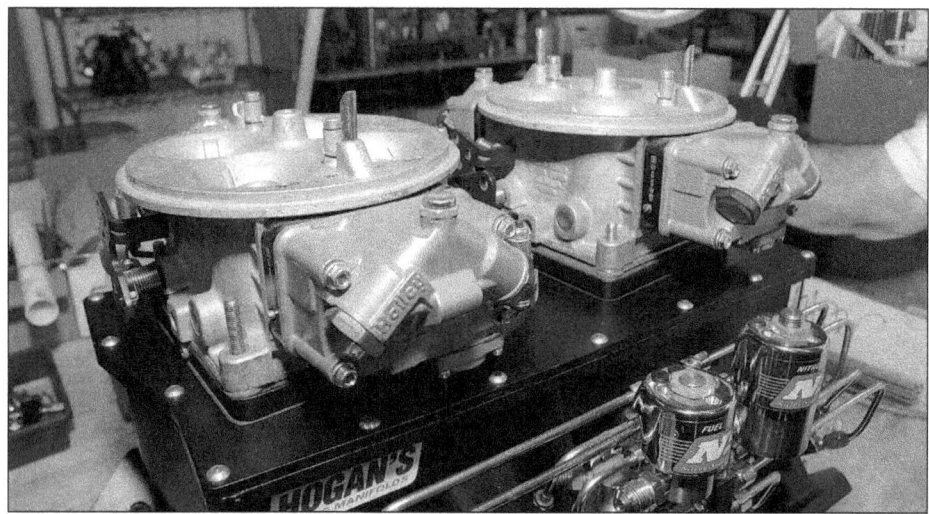

16 Install the Holley Dominator carburetors.

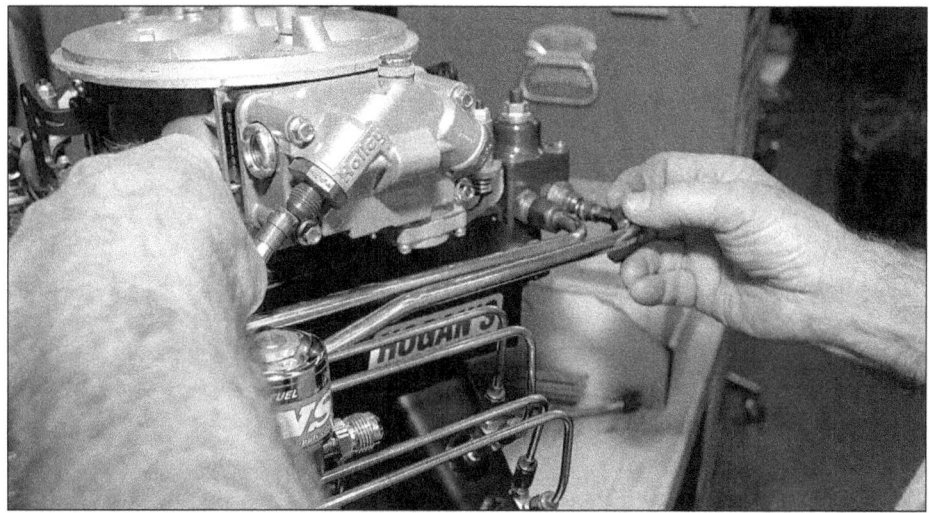

17 Fabricate the accompanying 3/16-inch fuel lines, running to the fuel regulators and Holley Dominator carburetors.

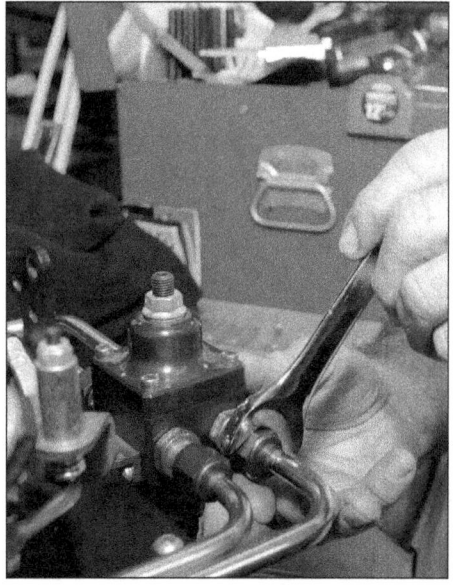

18 Tighten all lines snugly so there are no leaks.

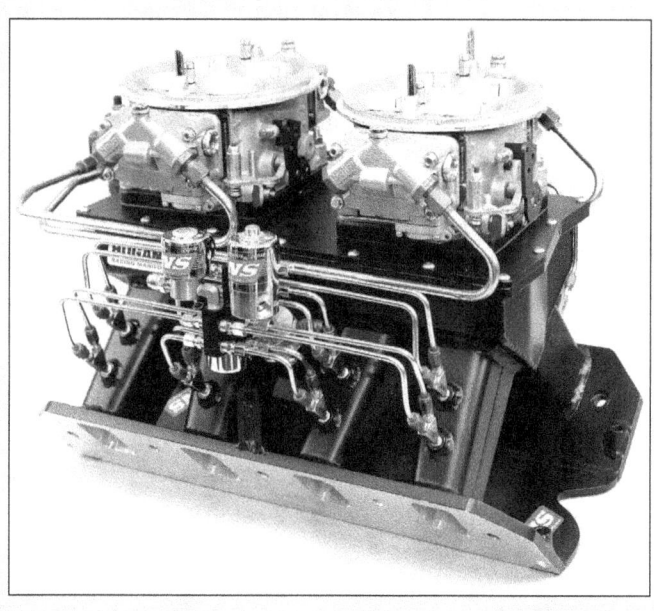

The finished product is ready for action.

CHAPTER 7

Eight-Second SS

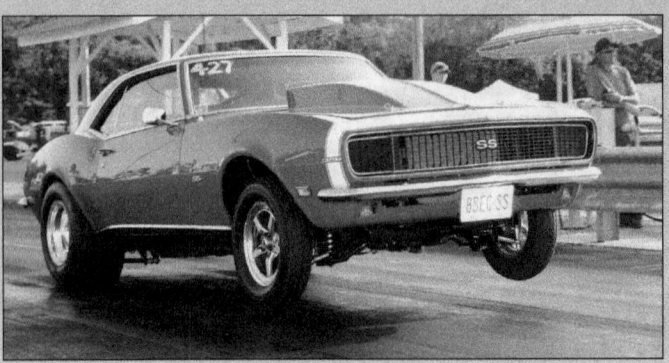

"Hard charging" is the only way to describe Greg Wong's 3,750-pound (with driver) 8-second, street-legal 1968 Camaro SS. Purchased in 1982 after he graduated from high school, Wong and his 1968 have progressively been lowering the street car ET record at Greg's home track, the IHRA-sanctioned Hilo Raceway Park. Would you believe this Camaro has run a best of 8.63 seconds at 158.32 mph at sea level?

Hawaiian Greg Wong first purchased his Matador-Red 1968 Camaro SS in 1982 after graduating from high school. After driving the Camaro around the Big Island for a couple of years, Wong regretfully sold it, but bought the car back again 15 years later. Ever since then, Wong and his 1968 have been inseparable and steadily knocking down Hilo Raceway Park's street car E.T. record to where it now stands, at 8.63 seconds at 154.34 mph. But that took a ton of hard work.

"The Camaro started off as a 10-second street car," says Wong. "Then I broke into the 9s with it. However, the quickest I could run was a 9.03 seconds at 153 mph, so I rebuilt the motor the following year and contacted Steve Johnson from Induction Solutions and sent my intake and fogger setup to him. Steve went through the entire system, and now the SS runs in the 8.60-second range. It is the quickest street-legal car on the Big Island!"

Powering Greg's Camaro is an owner-assembled, Magoo's Auto Parts–machined, 1989 vintage big-block 441-ci Chevy engine. Internally, the engine has been O-ringed, overbored .070 inch, and uses a set of Manley/Reher & Morrison H-beam connecting rods pressed onto a set of 14:1-compression Ackerly & Childs–equipped Ross nitrous pistons. Deep inside the beast you find a Reher & Morrison–grind roller cam featuring 302-degree intake, and 306 exhaust lobes with .740 inch of max valve lift. Also along for the ride are a set of Comp Cams roller lifters and pushrods. Cam timing is handled by a Crane double-roller multiple-index timing chain, while the crank trigger ignition and coil are MSD parts. Spark plugs are from NGK and Moroso Performance supplied the spark plug wires.

Bolted up top is a set of Magoo's shaved (114-cc combustion chamber) Reher & Morrison–prepared Brodix BB aluminum cylinder heads, equipped with 2.255-inch-diameter Manley stainless-steel intake and 1.880-inch-diameter exhaust valves. The upper portion of the valvetrain consists of Manley valvesprings and retainers, along with a set of Crane roller rockers and ARP rocker studs. The breatherless tall valve covers are obviously from Reher & Morrison.

Now here's where the estimated 1,200 hp worth of power gets made. A Holley Pro Dominator 2x4 intake and a set of 1,050-cfm Carburetor Shop/Holley Dominator carburetors serve as host to the Steve Johnson two-stage fogger N_2O system. "Steve blueprinted and flowed the entire system," says Wong. "He rebuilt the solenoids and set up the MSD Fuel Map."

Other items include GZ Motorsports Engine Pulleys, a CSI electric water pump, Moroso Performance solid motor mounts, and 1-1/8-inch Hooker Super Comp headers flowing into a set of 4-inch Flowmaster street mufflers. Backing all of this up is a Lakewood-contained, RAM Automotive single-disc clutch and RAM aluminum flywheel bolted to a Lenco SC1 4-speed transmission. Transmitting all that power back to a 4.29:1 geared Moser-prepared Ford 9-inch rear end is a Russell Iyo/R&R Machine custom-fabricated driveshaft.

Greg's brother, Royden Wong, who owns a pretty mean ATI Pro-Charged small-block 1968 Camaro of his own, prepared the chassis. For openers, Royden notched and mini-tubbed the rear frame rails, prior to installing the QA1 single-adjustable shock/CalTrac Split Mono Leaf–suspended Moser axle. Wheels and tires are Weld Aluma-Stars running either Mickey Thompson drag slicks or BFG street radial rubber.

MULTI-STAGE SYSTEMS

In the trunk are a pair of Nitrous Express 10-pound N_2O bottles, a narrowed 1968 Camaro gas tank, Induction Solutions' blueprinted fuel pumps, and an Optima gel-cell battery.

Inside, the Camaro uses a Wayne Rabang–installed eight-point rollcage, RJI Safety Equipment, and Auto Meter tachometer and gauges. With the exception of the humongous Harwood 4¾-inch cowl induction hood, and the slightly opened-up rear wheelwells, Greg's Camaro looks 100-percent stock because it is! Heck, it even still has the original working AM radio in it!

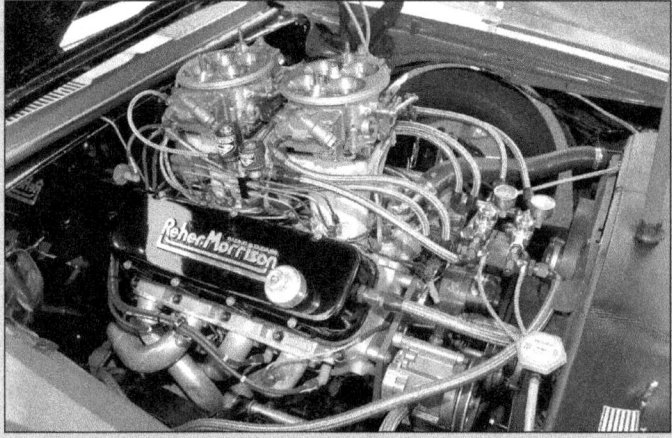
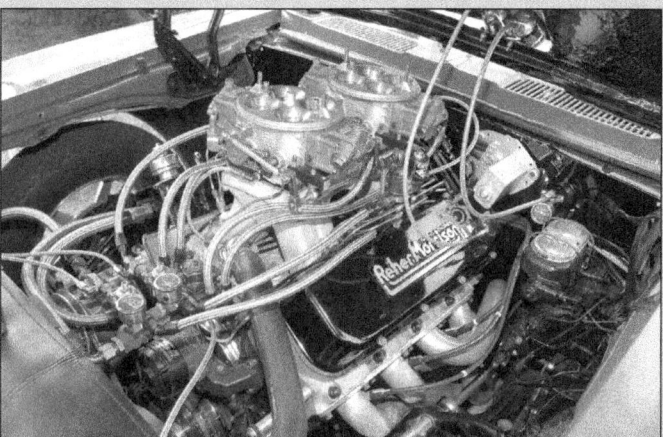

Wong's 1968 is powered by a Steve Johnson-Induction Solutions/Carburetor Shop 2x4 Holley twin Dominator/Holley Dominator intake, complete with Steve Johnson Induction Solutions blue-printed Dual Fogger nitrous setup bolted to a Wong-assembled 441-ci 1989 vintage 454 big-block Chevrolet engine. Internally, the big-block features Magoo's Auto Parts machining (balanced, decked, line-honed, and O-ringed). It has a GM forged-steel crank riding on Clevite engine bearings, a set of Manley H-beam connecting rods, eight 14:1-compression Ross nitrous pistons equipped with Ackerly-Childs piston rings, and a Reher & Morrison Racing Engines–grind nitrous cam. Bolted up top is a set of Magoo's Machined Brodix BB2 Plus big-valve cylinder heads featuring Competition Cams, Manley, and Crane Cams valvetrain components. Other items include a CSI electric water pump, GZ Motorsports engine pulleys, MSD Crank Trigger ignition, and Hooker Super Comp headers dumping into a Flowmaster muffler-equipped street exhaust system.

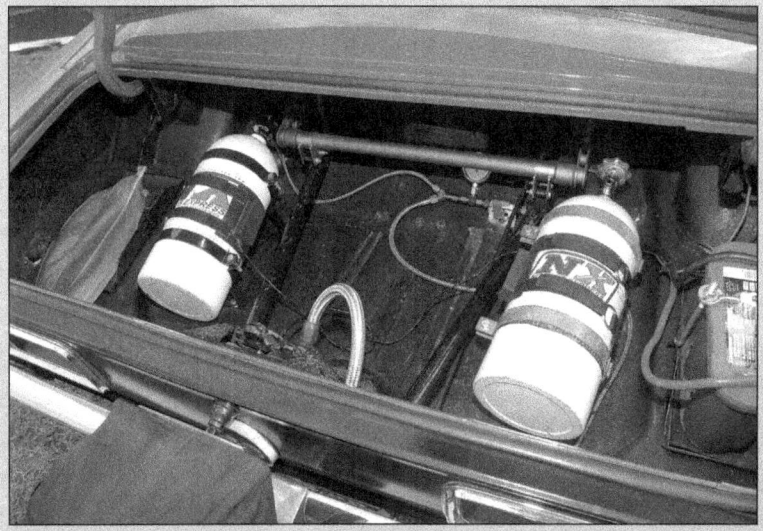

In the trunk is a narrowed 1968 Camaro gas tank sandwiched between Royden Wong–relocated rear frame rails. Wayne Rabang-installed the roll cage runners. A pair of dual Nitrous Express N_2O bottles, an Induction Solutions/Greg Wong fuel system, and an Optima battery are also on board.

CHAPTER 8

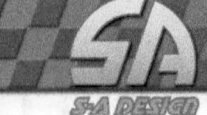

BAD-ASS 540-CI MERLIN III NITROUS BIG-BLOCK BUILDUP

Building an engine for use with nitrous oxide is not all that complicated, but it does require selecting the right parts. A World Products, Inc., Merlin III cast-iron big-block (PN 085010-4500) was selected as the foundation for this buildup. Manufactured to QS-9000 specifications, the four-bolt-main Merlin III (featuring 1045 splayed-steel billet main caps using ARP main cap bolts) uses a CNC-machined deck height of 9.80 inches and a bore of 4.50 inches. But with a wall thickness of .250 inch at a bore of 4.600 inches, it can be safely bored to an overall dimension of 4.625 inches. This block features the stock big-block Chevy cam location and uses off-the-shelf big-block Chevy cam bearings. It has expanded water jackets for superior cooling, a priority main oiling system, blind-tapped head-bolt holes, clearance for vertical bar lifters, uses solid oil pan rails with stock spacing and clearance for large stroke engines, and is 100-percent

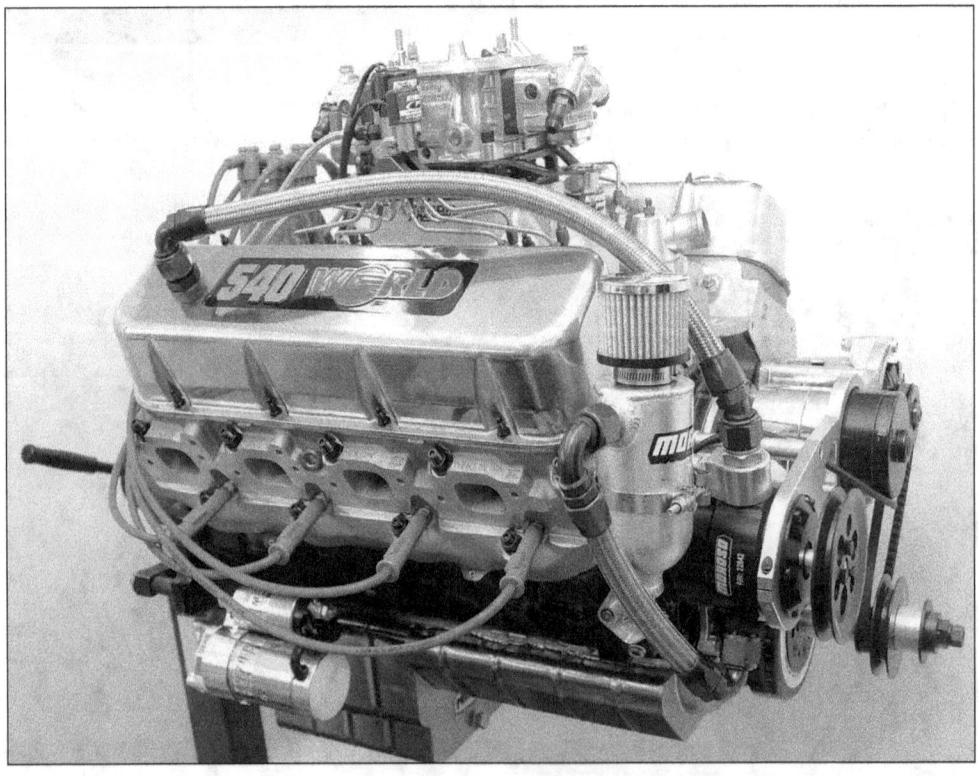

This four-bolt-main block features 1/2-inch main caps, a CNC-machined deck height of 9.800 inches, and a 4.500-inch bore. With a Lunati 4.250-inch Pro Series forged-steel crank, we're looking at a whopping 540ci!

compatible with original equipment manufacturer (OEM) GM parts.

When the time came to select a rotating assembly capable of handling more than 1,500 nitrous-assisted horsepower, engine builder Brad Lagman of QMP Racing Engines and project director James "Jimmy G" Galante let their fingers do the walking through Lunati Industries' catalog.

Fortifying the Engine

Because the objective is to produce in the neighborhood of 1,500 hp on nitrous, there are five main components that must be specified for N_2O use: the camshaft, crankshaft, connecting rods, pistons, and exhaust valves. Let's start with the camshaft.

Camshaft

For this application, the Lunati Cams (PN 50299ALUN) 55-mm big-journal roller cam was selected. The normal firing order on a big-block Chevrolet is 1-8-4-3-6-5-7-2. However, dyno testing shows that 1-8-7-3-6-5-4-2 evens out the firing order in the engine, and makes more horsepower. This is known as a 4-to-7 swap, and is a fairly common choice in competition engines. This particular cam features a lobe center of 111 degrees. The max valve lift is .823 inch on the intake, with 284 degrees of duration at .050 inch of lift, and .813 inch of max lift on the exhaust side, with 301 degrees of duration at .050-inch lift. These big-journal nitrous cams were built to withstand the torque stress from instant and often violent bursts of power, which could twist a normal cam.

However, in order to install one of these big-journal nitrous cams, it was first necessary for engine man Brad Lagman to line-bore the cam tunnel 2.478 inches in diameter using a BHJ fixture. Then Brad power-honed the enlarged cam tunnel .002 inch to achieve an overall internal diameter of 2.480 inches. Then a set of Timken TL5520 Caged Needle Roller Bearings were installed. These roller cam bearings are not only superior in design to normal insert-style bearings, they greatly assist in allowing the cam and valvetrain to achieve maximum RPM levels quicker with the nitrous.

Crankshaft

Crankshaft selection focused on a 4.250-inch-stroke Lunati Pro-Series forged-steel big-block Chevrolet unit (PN BP4211N), which was designed for high-performance street/strip applications. Lunati's Pro Series crankshafts are made in America and are manufactured out of high-quality 4340 aircraft-grade steel.

Connecting Rods

Connecting rods are another important component in the overall

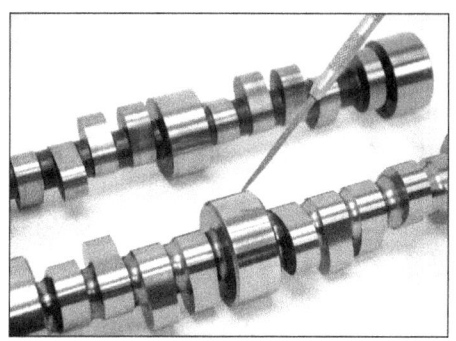

One of the key ingredients of our Bad-Ass N_2O Big-Block was a 55-mm Big Cam Journal Lunati N_2O roller cam (PN 50299ALUN) and kit, which included a set of Lunati flat-tappet roller-bar lifters (PN 72405LUN), Lunati Valvesprings (PN 74748LUN), Lunati Valve Retainers (PN 76739LUN), and 11/32-inch Lunati Valve Locks (PN 77114LUN). This cam features a lobe center of 111 degrees with .823/.284-inch maximum valve lift on the intake and .813/.301-inch on the exhaust at .050 lift. These big-journal cams were built to withstand the sheer torque stress from a sudden and violent burst of power that could twist a normal cam.

CHAPTER 8

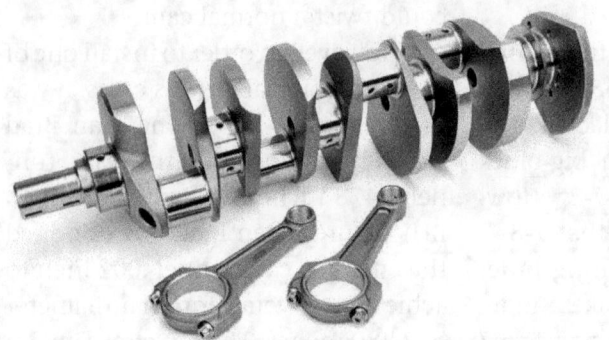

For our rotating assembly, we selected one of Lunati's Pro Series forged-steel, 4.250-ci big-block 4340 aircraft-grade steel-composition stroker cranks (PN BP4211N), along with a set of Lunati Pro Series 4340 alloy steel I-beam connecting rods (PN 6385FM) with ARP 7/16-inch cap-screw rod bolts.

strength and reliability of a nitrous oxide-assisted engine. "If you only intend on producing 1,000 hp or less, you can safely get away with a lower-grade connecting rod, but we chose to go with the best," said Galante.

Lunati's 6.385-inch I-Beam connecting rods (PN 6385FM) are the perfect complement to the Pro Series forged-steel crankshaft. These rods are forged from aircraft grade 4340 alloy steel and are heat treated, stress-relieved, shot-peened, and Magnafluxed to ensure the highest level of durability. Lunati's forged-steel big-block Chevrolet connecting rods are weight-matched to +/- 1.5 grams, and also come standard with 7/16-inch ARP cap-screw hardware.

Pistons

A set of Diamond Pistons was selected to compliment Lunati's Pro Series forged-steel crank and connecting rods. Forged from durable 2618 aluminum alloy, which can withstand higher cylinder head pressures and extreme temperatures created by doses of nitrous oxide, Diamond's Custom Dome N_2O pistons feature beefed up side skirts, wall thickness between .160 and .200 inch, a stiffening rib located under each wrist pin bore, and a thicker dome. These all add up to a piston that is 33 to 53 percent greater in sheer mass.

These pistons are also characterized by a series of gas ports, which penetrate the depths of the first ring groove behind the ring itself. This helps pressurize the top ring, force it outward, and create a tighter seal against the cylinder wall. The actual top ring groove itself is placed .300 inch down from the crown, which both physically and visually create the impression of a thicker piston dome, while protecting the top ring from the increased heat and cylinder head pressures that N_2O creates. This area also features .080 inch in thickness between the deepest point of the intake pocket and the widest point of the top ring grove, which helps avoid crushing the top ring land. Another of Diamond's nitrous tricks is eliminating the accumulator/pressure balance groove on the second ring land. Finally, this set of Diamond Custom Dome nitrous pistons was 100 percent coated with a green hard-anodized topcoat, and gray moly side coating that adds .001 inch on every surface it touches. Incidentally, this top coating is standard on pistons destined for use in nitromethane-fueled engines as well.

According to Galante, it is preferred to drop the compression ratio to 13:1. This way, when the nitrous oxide is being activated, the compression ratio shoots up to around 16:1 and higher. It is important to understand that any serious performance enthusiast wants to push the nitrous to the ragged edge. The use of exhaust gas temperature (EGT) sensors would certainly be a good idea

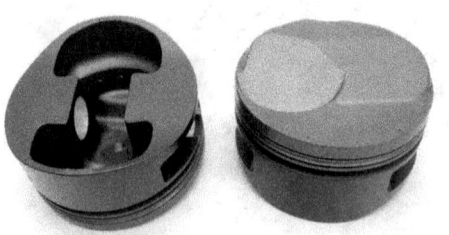 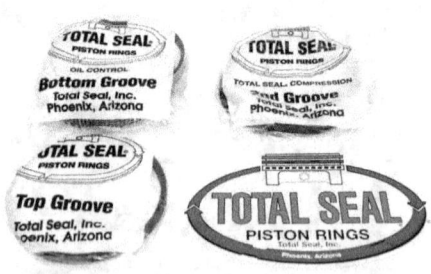

A set of Diamond Racing Custom Domed nitrous pistons (PN 0101B) was also selected for the build. Forged from durable 2618 aluminum alloy, these pistons are capable of withstanding high cylinder head temperatures and heavy doses of nitrous. They have beefed-up side skirts, a wall thickness between .160 and .200 inch, a stiffening rib located under each wrist pin bore, and a ticker dome, adding up to a piston that is 33 to 53 percent greater in sheer mass. The actual top ring groove is placed .300 inch down from the crown to protect the Total Seal top ring from increased heat. A series of gas ports also penetrate the depths of the first ring groove, which helps pressurize the top ring to keep it snug against the cylinder wall, and these pistons are thermal-coated with a green hard-anodized top coat and gray moly side coat to eliminate friction and to protect the piston.

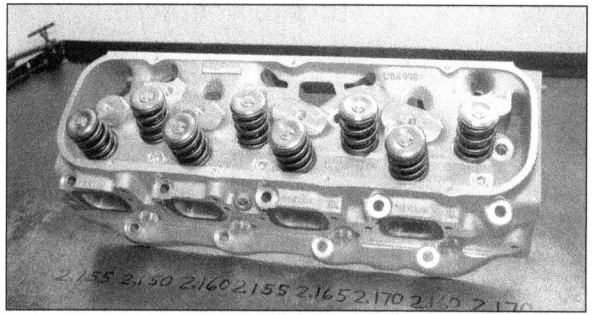

Also part of this combination is a set of Merlin III CNC-ported bare aluminum alloy cylinder heads (PN 20660). Like our Merlin III block, these heads were manufactured to QS-9000 quality standards using World Products Right Cast technology. Physical characteristics include screw-in rocker arm studs, manganese-bronze valveguides, standard spark plug location, CNC-ported 350-cc intake ports and 132-cc exhaust ports, high-efficiency-cut combustion chambers, and a thick deck for longer service life.

to make sure that you don't burn a piston from running the air/fuel/nitrous-oxide ratio too lean!

Cylinder Heads and Prep

A set of CNC-ported Merlin III aluminum alloy cylinder heads (PN 20660) was chosen to go along with this Merlin III Sportsman big-block. World Products offers the Merlin III BBC alloy cylinder head in a number of different ways, ranging from the machined bare head to complete cylinder head assemblies. However, since cylinder head porting specialist Mike Slover, proprietor of Slover's Porting Service, was going to perform a nitrous port and polish job on these beauties, we chose the CNC-machined Merlin III barehead model.

Features include screw-in rocker arm studs, manganese-bronze valve guides, all the correct bolt holes and accompanying OE engine-accessory brackets, 350-cc CNC-ported intake ports and 132-cc exhaust, standard spark plug location(s), and a thicker deck for longer service life.

"First of all," says Slover, "the overall size of the combustion chamber was enlarged to correspond with the 4.560-inch bore at 117 cc. The combustion chamber surfaces were polished, and all the sharp edges were removed. The bowls were blended, and the intake valveguide bosses were teardropped. The intake walls were opened up 20 percent using the intake gasket as a guide, and we also opened up the exhaust port an additional 20 percent. Basically, we opened up the exhaust as much as possible to enhance exhaust scavenging, which is crucial to a nitrous application. Since we're using a set of Jesel Shaft Rocker Arms (PN KPS-28787), the cast Merlin III rocker stud bosses were machined off to accept the two-piece interlocking Jesel rocker arm stands."

A set of Ferrea Extreme Duty Stainless-Steel valves, measuring 2.300-inch-diameter intake (PN F121P) and 1.880-inch-diameter exhaust (PN F1261P), was selected to fill out the valvetrain. A three-angle valve job was performed on the intake side, and a radiused valve job was performed on the exhaust side.

Because a nitrous motor builds up so much heat in the exhaust port, it's better to run a little more valve-to-guide clearance to keep the valves from sticking. A set of Lunati Triple Valvesprings (PN 74748LUN), Lunati Valvespring Retainers (PN 76739LUN), and Lunati Valve Locks (PN 7714LUN) were also part of this combination. A set of ARP Head Bolts secure the Slover-prepared Merlin III heads to the QMP-assembled Merlin III Sportsman block via a set of Cometic head gaskets. Finally, a set of World Products/Merlin III 540 polished-aluminum tall-deck valve covers (PN 07093-540W) keep everything covered.

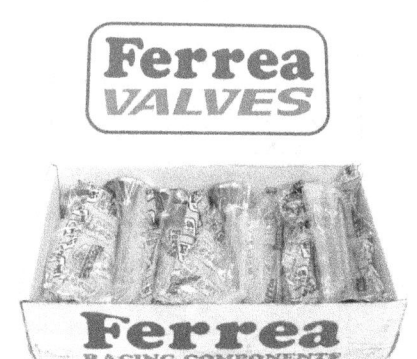

Other key valvetrain components included a set of Ferrea stainless-steel 1/32-inch-stem intake valves in a 2.30-inch diameter (PN F121P), and exhaust valve diameter of 1.88 inches (PN F1261P).

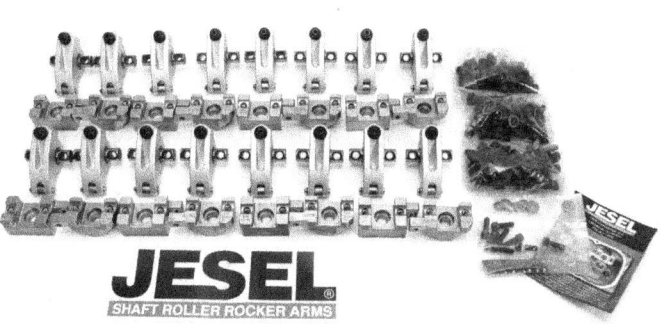

Also selected was a 1:7 Jesel Shaft Rocker Arm System (PN KPS-28787), which delivers trouble-free valvetrain service under extremely high RPM loads.

CHAPTER 8

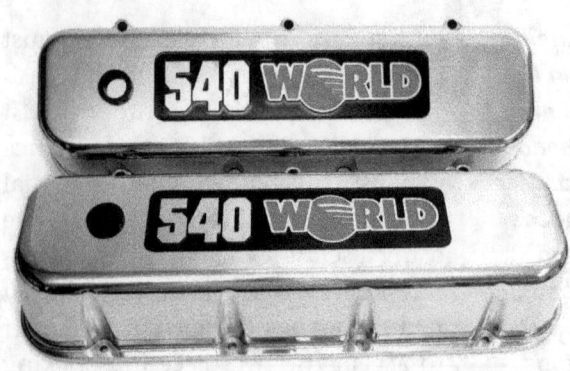

A set of World Products/ Merlin III 540 tall-deck polished-aluminum valve covers (PN 07093-540W) caps-off a fairly stout valvetrain.

Intake Manifold

Our first choice for an intake manifold was also on the World Products wish list. It was one of the Merlin III 4V single-plane cast-aluminum intake manifolds (PN 63040) topped with a 4150 Holley Ultra Dominator 4-barrel carburetor (PN 688634).

Project: Wilson Manifolds & Nitrous Pro-Flow Merlin III Two-Stage Plate and Fogger Intake Buildup

James "Jimmy G" Galante wanted to produce from 1,300 to 1,500 hp on nitrous oxide using a fogger and wet-plate system. He shipped the Merlin III intake to Wilson Manifolds/Nitrous Pro-Flow, and CEO Keith Wilson and nitrous and fuel injection specialist Rob "Junior" Klein took it from there.

"A multiple-stage N_2O system serves two purposes," says Wilson. "With drag racers, the first part of the run is typically the most important part of the equation. The idea is to get a heavy vehicle, such as the 1967 Nova Top Sportsman car this engine was intended for, launched and accelerating as quickly as possible without losing traction or wheel-standing the car. Most single-stage plate systems can deliver up to about 350 hp, and most single-stage fogger systems can deliver up to 500 hp. Depending on the motor combination, some racers want to induce more nitrous oxide than their single-stage systems can flow, therefore they use a multiple-stage system.

"Multiple-stage systems also help to create a traction control for the car. Instead of launching on a 500-shot with a single-stage kit and spinning the tires, the car left on 250-shot with the first stage, and then timed out the second stage to, let's say, .800 second, when he fired the second stage of 250-shot. This allows the tire to begin rolling at launch using a smaller degree of horsepower. By the time the second stage is activated, the car is already moving and the hit of nitrous is so intense that it introduces more power while not overpowering the tire."

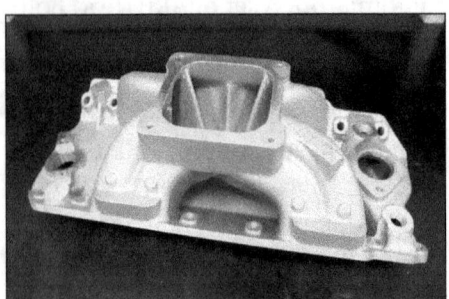

The stock World Products/Merlin III single-plane intake with 4,500-style Holley Dominator-flange (PN 63040), featuring a 9.800-inch-tall deck. Stock out of the box, these manifolds are most efficient when operating in the 2,500- to 7,500-rpm range, and have excellent low-end throttle response. Note that these intakes are equipped with pre-cast fuel injection bosses.

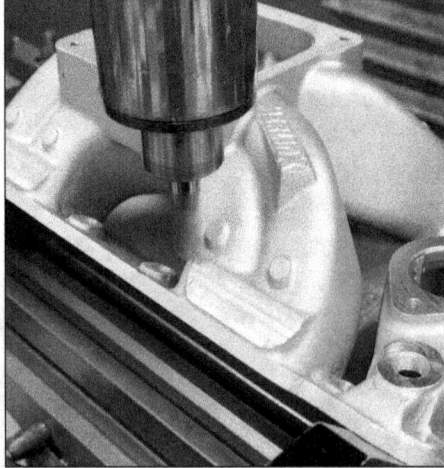

1 *Because the nozzle location actually changes, Wilson Manifolds & Nitrous Pro-Flow technician Rob "Junior" Klein machines off the stock casting pads on the mill.*

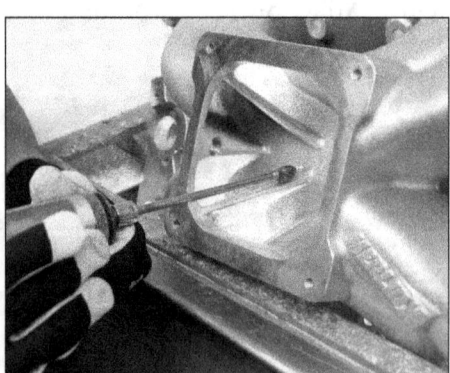

2 *Next Klein gave the intake plenum an intermediate-style porting job. In the process, Klein modified the roof angles and reshaped the dividers for enhanced fuel distribution over the stock intake. Klein says this is always advantageous when using a plate system.*

BAD-ASS 540-CI MERLIN III NITROUS BIG-BLOCK BUILDUP

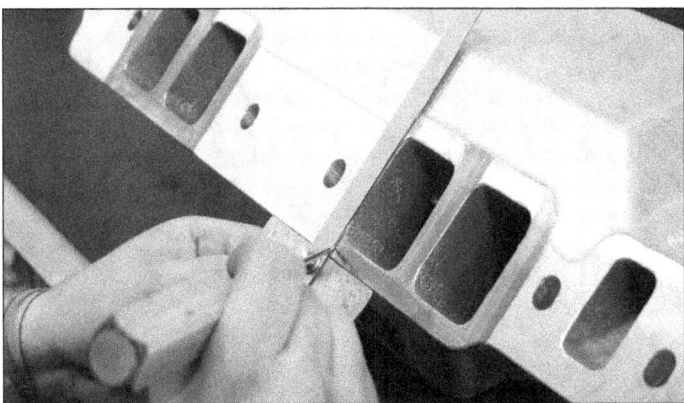

3 Klein scribes the outside of the port openings, which allows the installer the ability to locate the center of the port for proper nozzle placement.

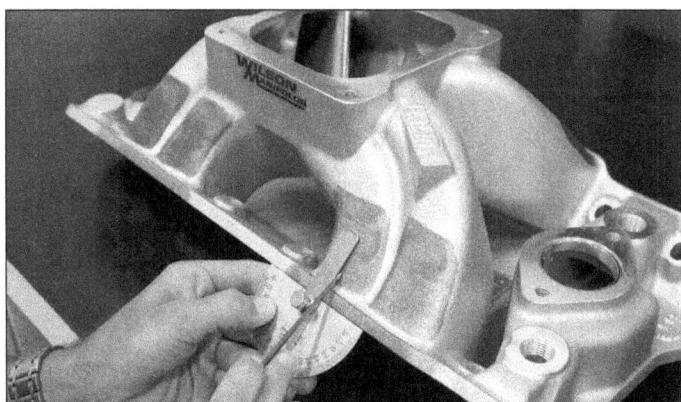

4 The installer transfers his marks to the outside and center of the port scribe lines to the topside of the intake, which sets the nozzle height above the intake flange.

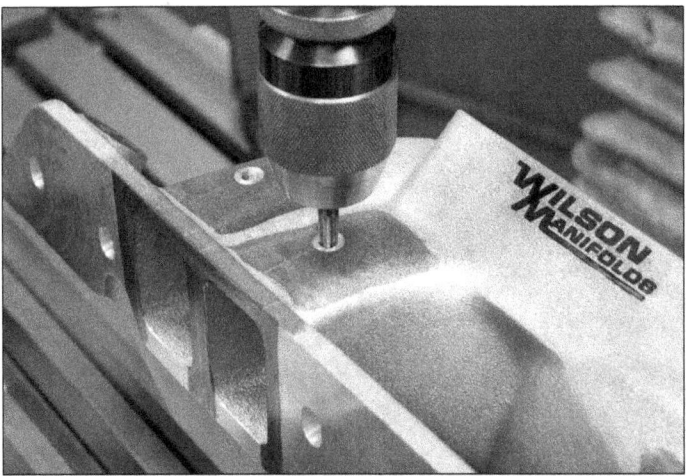

5 Klein drills the new locations for the nozzles and begins the tapping sequence.

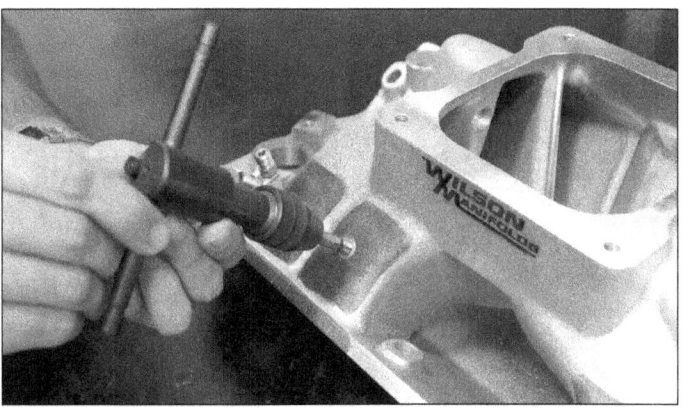

6 Klein hand-taps the new holes to their final depth. This is done by hand to ensure each nozzle is placed at the correct depth, but depths may vary due to casting thicknesses.

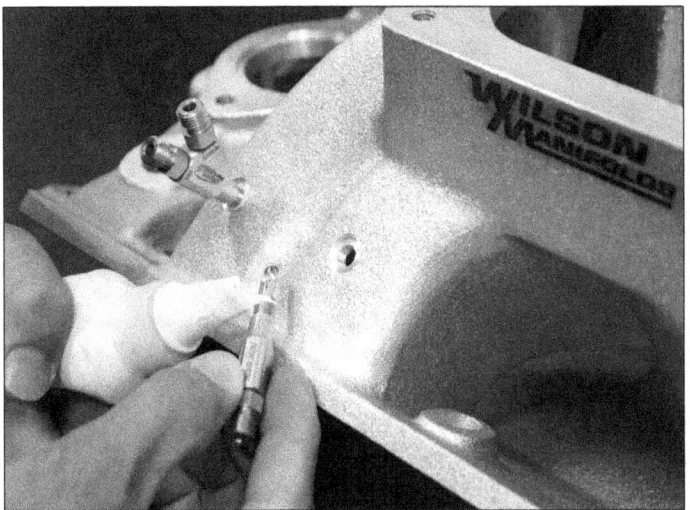

7 Placement of the Wilson Manifolds & Nitrous Pro-Flow V-force nozzles begins. Klein applies a small dab of Teflon paste on each of the threads.

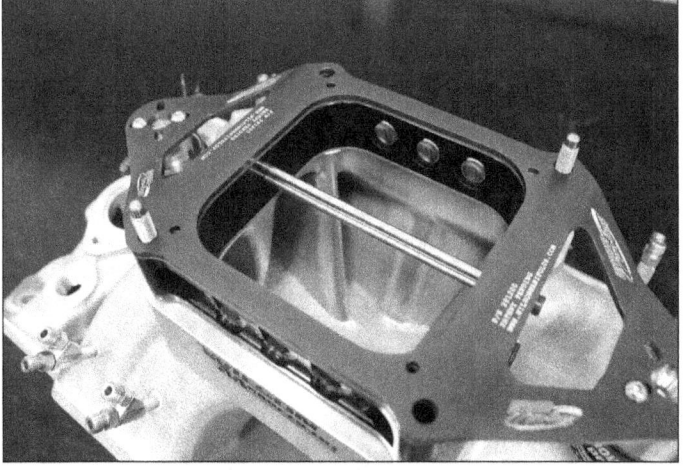

8 During the placement of the carburetor spacer and solenoid bracket, the bracket is placed front-to-back rather than side-to-side, to accommodate the fogger setup that will be installed.

HOW TO INSTALL AND TUNE NITROUS OXIDE SYSTEMS   71

CHAPTER 8

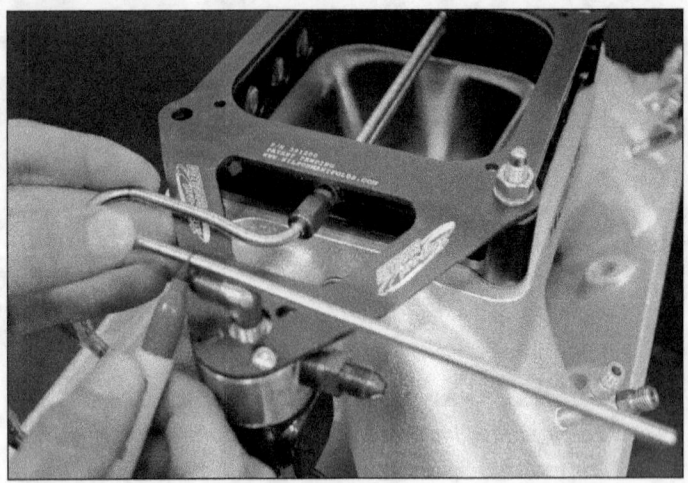

9 Klein fabricates the hard lines for the plate system that connect the spray bar and the solenoid.

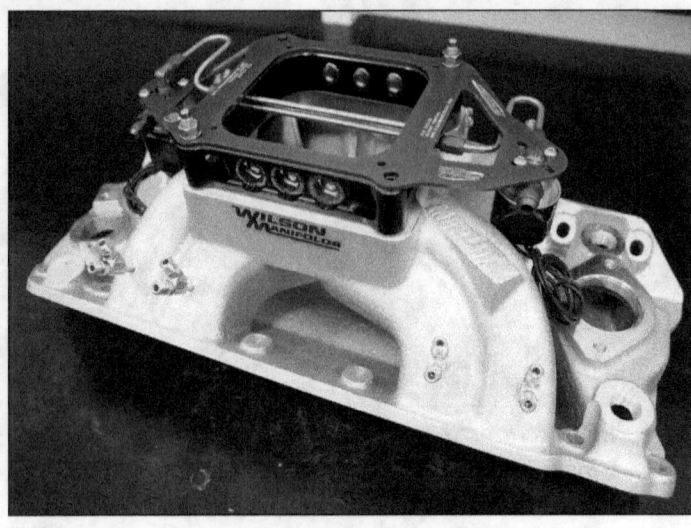

10 The layout of the solenoids and N_2O lines.

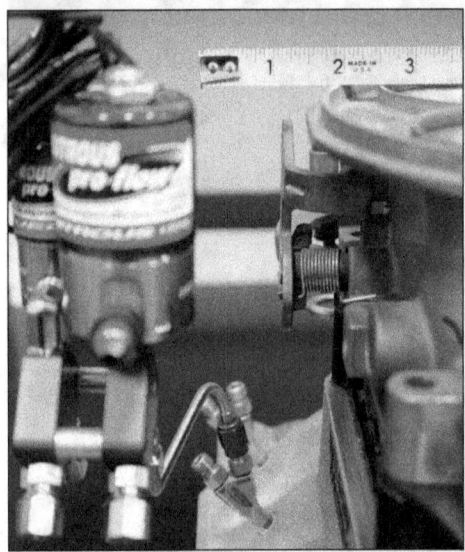

11 Depending on the type of throttle linkage, an appropriate distance is required from the carburetor so that the Wilson Nitrous Pro-Flow fogger does not interfere with the throttle linkage.

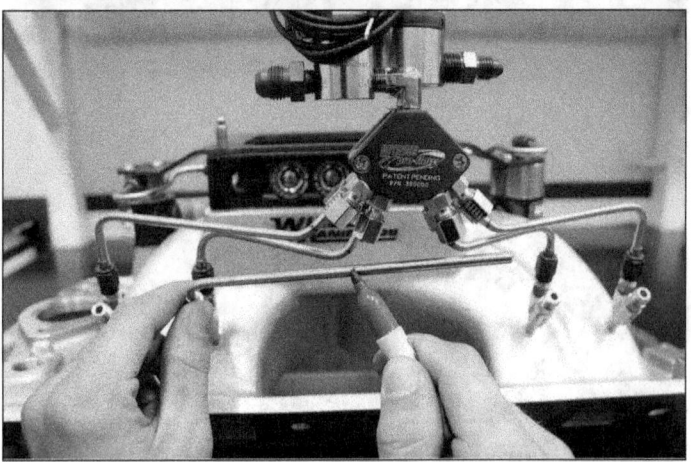

12 The installer plumbs the fogger, marking each tube so that the proper fitment or bend is achieved.

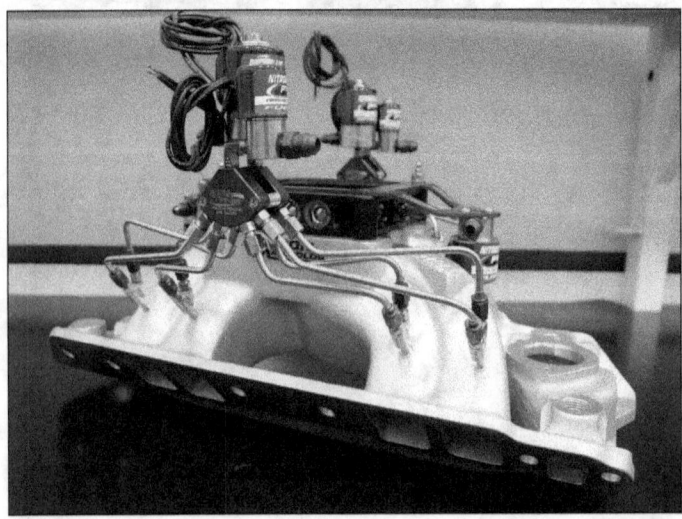

13 A shot of the Merlin III/Wilson Manifolds & Nitrous Pro-Flow 4V intake with plumbing process complete.

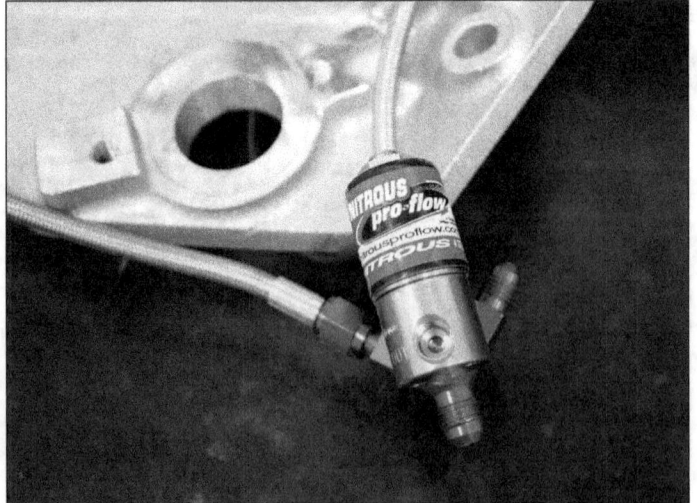

14 The nitrous purge and distribution block, which supplies the three accompanying solenoids.

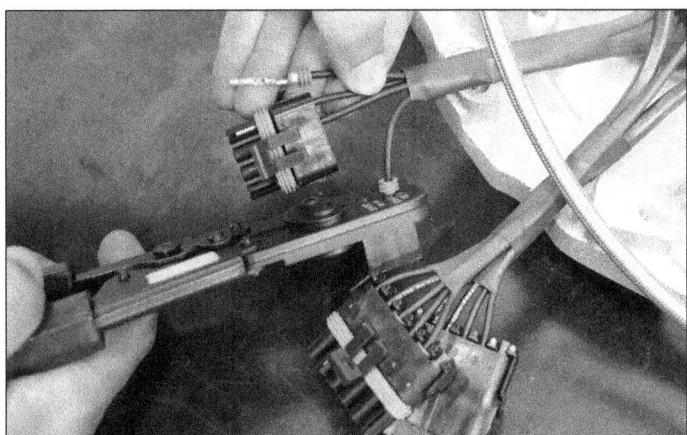

15 Klein shows how the wires are terminated at the weather pack connector. All wires are heat shrunk for cleanliness and overall appearance.

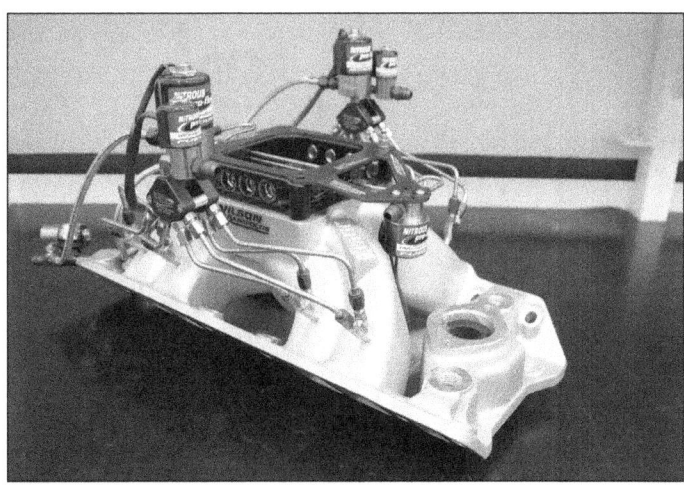

16 The completed Wilson Nitrous & Pro-Flow two-stage fogger-plate 4V manifold.

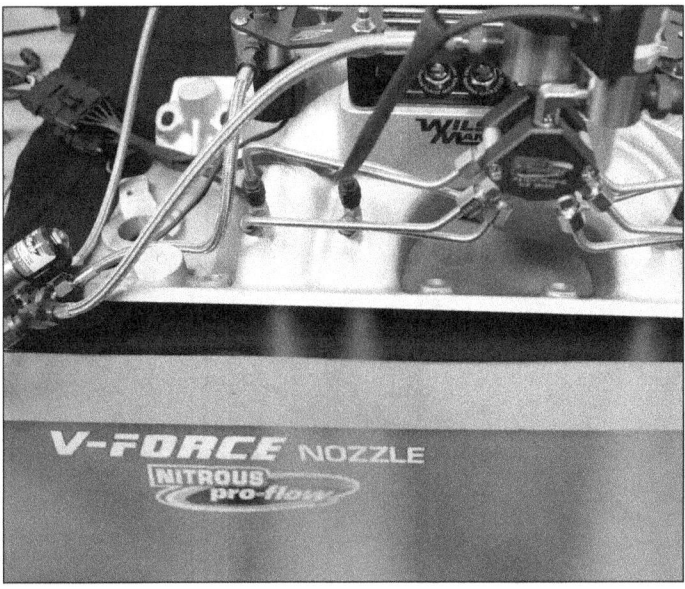

17 With everything buttoned together, Klein test-fires the fogger system.

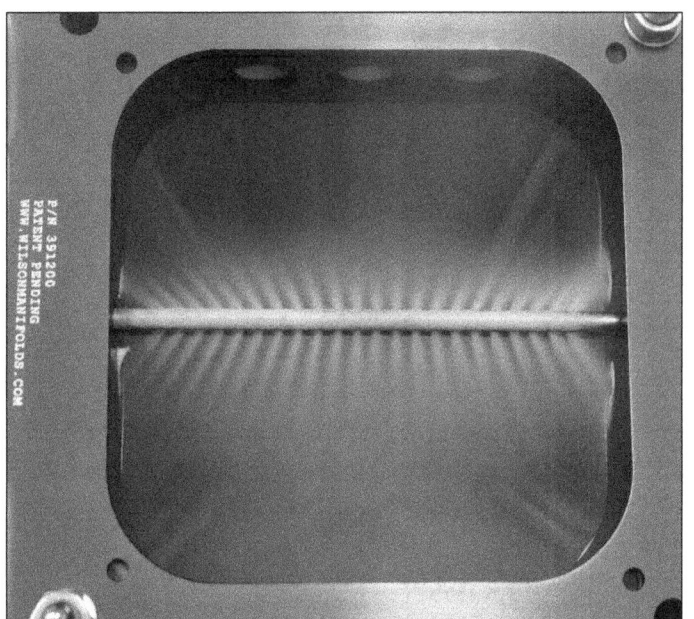

18 Testing of the plate system.

The Supporting Cast

Engine timing on this Nitrous 540 big-block was handled by a Jesel Olds-style Belt Drive (PN KBD-32000), along with an ATI Super Damper (PN 91731). Engine cooling was handled by one of Don Meziere's 55-gpm Polished High Flow Water Pumps (PN WP300U). Another important component was the inclusion of a Moroso Performance breather tank and vacuum pump kit (PNs 85465 and 63838, respectively), which was designed to interface with the Meziere Competition water pump.

On the bottom end, a Milodon high-volume oil pump (PN 18760), matching oil pump pickup (PN 18201), Milodon 8-quart Drag Race oil pan with side kick-out (PN 31187), and ARP oil pump driveshaft (PN 135-7901) were all teamed together to provide adequate and reliable lubrication. Ignition duties are handled by an MSD Pro Billet big-block Chevrolet distributor with internal billet trigger (PN 85501), a set of MSD Super Conductor spark plug wires (PN 31809), and an MSD Digital-7 (with boost retard) ignition box (PN 7531). QMP Racing Engines master technician Robert Bieschke performed the actual engine assembly.

CHAPTER 8

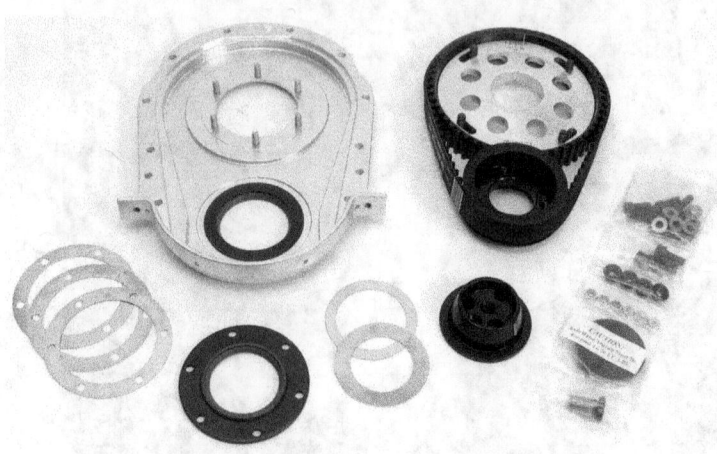

Valve timing is handled by a BB & DRCE Olds-spec Jesel Belt Drive (PN KBD-32000).

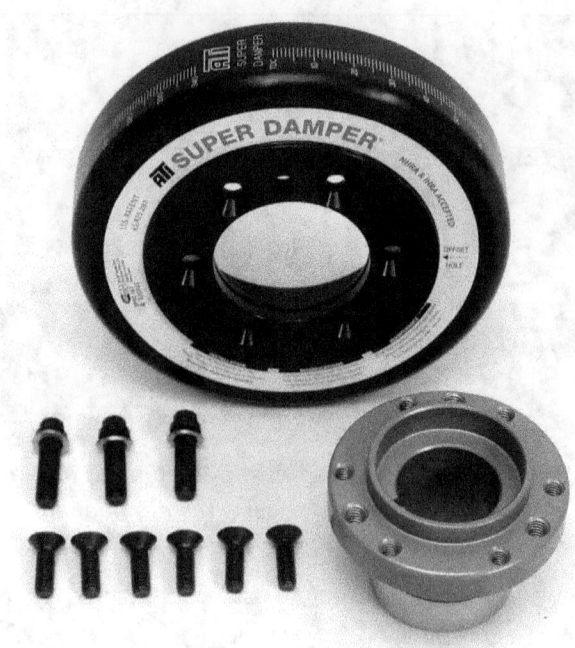

An integral part of this Merlin III's balancing act is an ATI Super Damper (PN 91731).

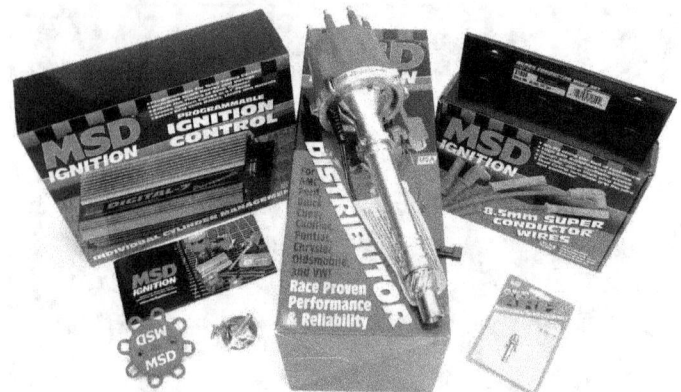

Ignition is handled by an MSD Pro Billet distributor (PN 85501), firing a set of MSD 90-degree spark plug wires (PN 31809), and Digital-7 Plus ignition box (PN 7531).

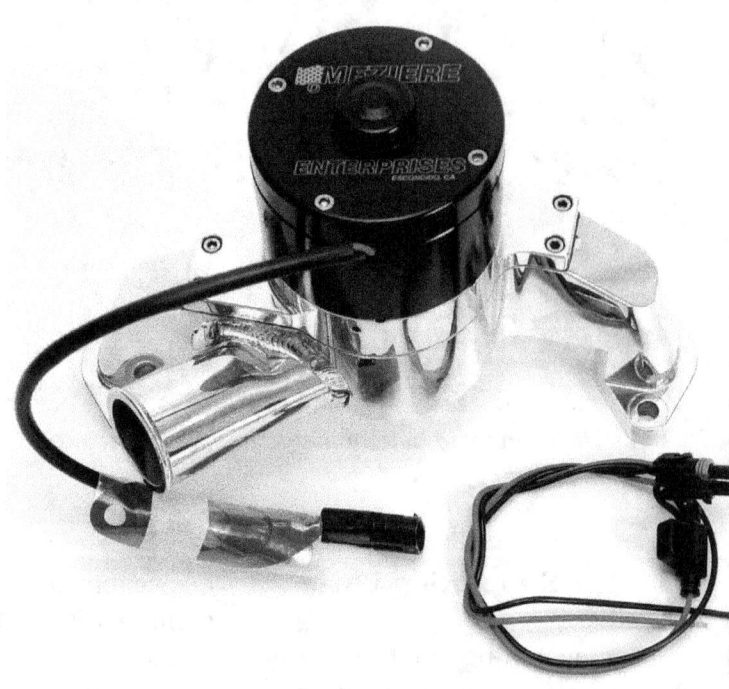

Engine cooling is handled by a polished Meziere High Flow Water Electric Pump (PN WP300U).

Our Bad Ass N_2O Big-Block's bottom end is protected by a Milodon High Volume Oil Pump (PN 18760), Milodon Oil Pump Pickup (PN 18201), and 8-quart Milodon Drag Race oil pan with side kick-out (PN 31187). Other key components include an ARP Oil Pump Stud Kit (PN 230-7004), and ARP BBC Oil Pump Driveshaft Kit (PN 135-7901).

Project: Final Assembly

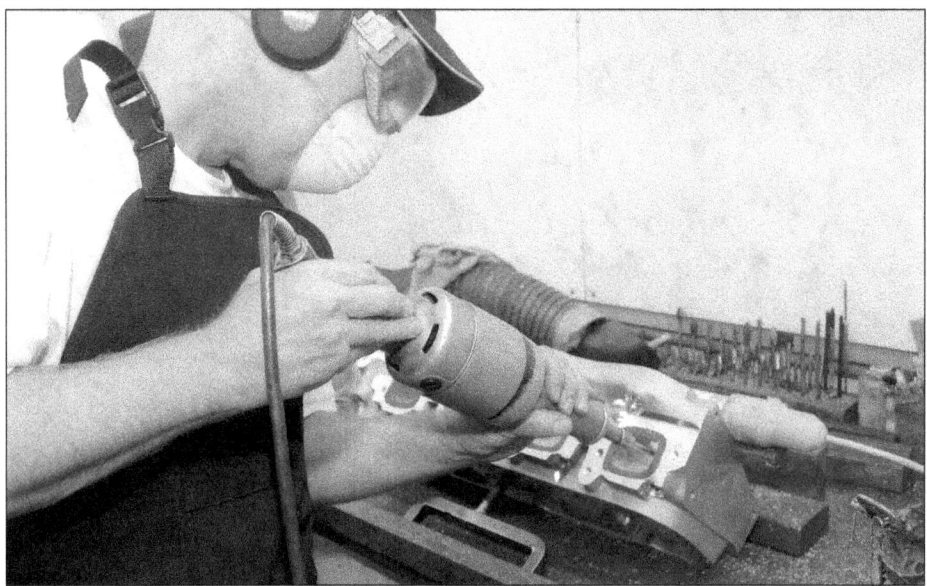

For nitrous-prepping the Merlin III big-block cylinder heads, Mike Slover, of Slover's Porting Service, was the man with the plan.

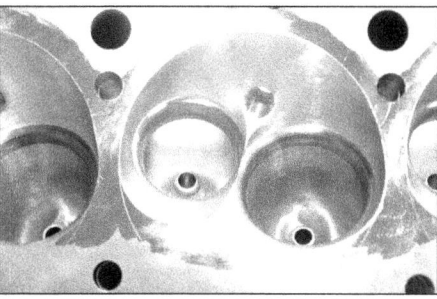

1 First, Slover used a 100-grit wheel to final-polish the combustion chamber, eliminating any sharp edges in the process. He treated the intake side to a three-angle valve job, and then radiused the exhaust. He also blended in the combustion-chamber fuel bowls, and tear-dropped the valveguide bosses on intake and exhaust.

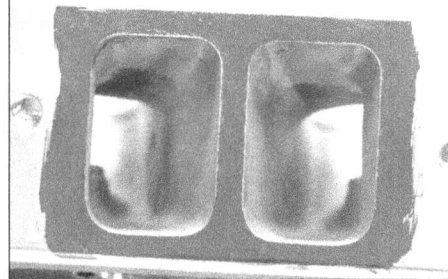

2 Using the Fel-Pro head gasket as a guide, Slover straightened the walls and opened up the intake side approximately 20 percent using a 60-grit final-finish polishing wheel.

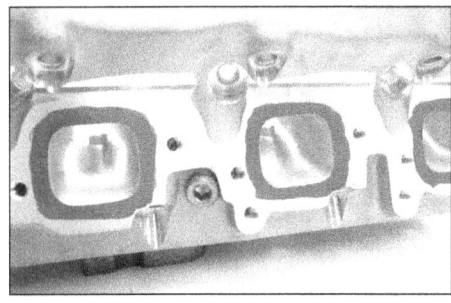

3 Slover likewise opened up the exhaust (approximately 12 percent) to enhance exhaust scavenging using a 100-grit final-finishing wheel.

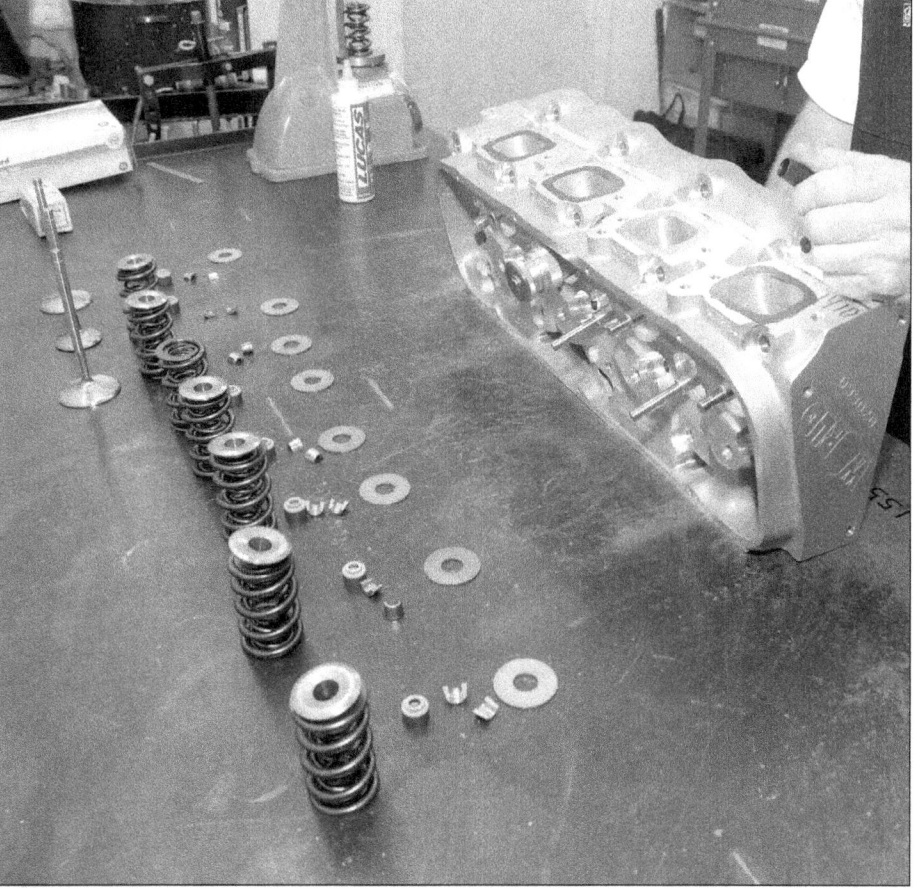

4 After lapping-in the Ferrea stainless-steel valves, Slover began initial valvetrain setup.

CHAPTER 8

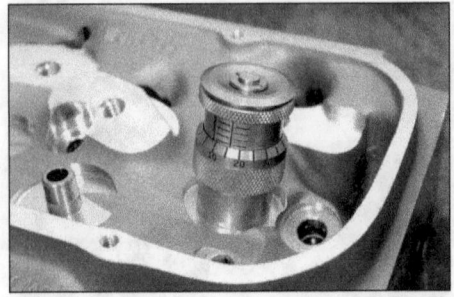

5 And with Lunati valvesprings in place, Slover arrived at an overall installed height of within .0015 inch.

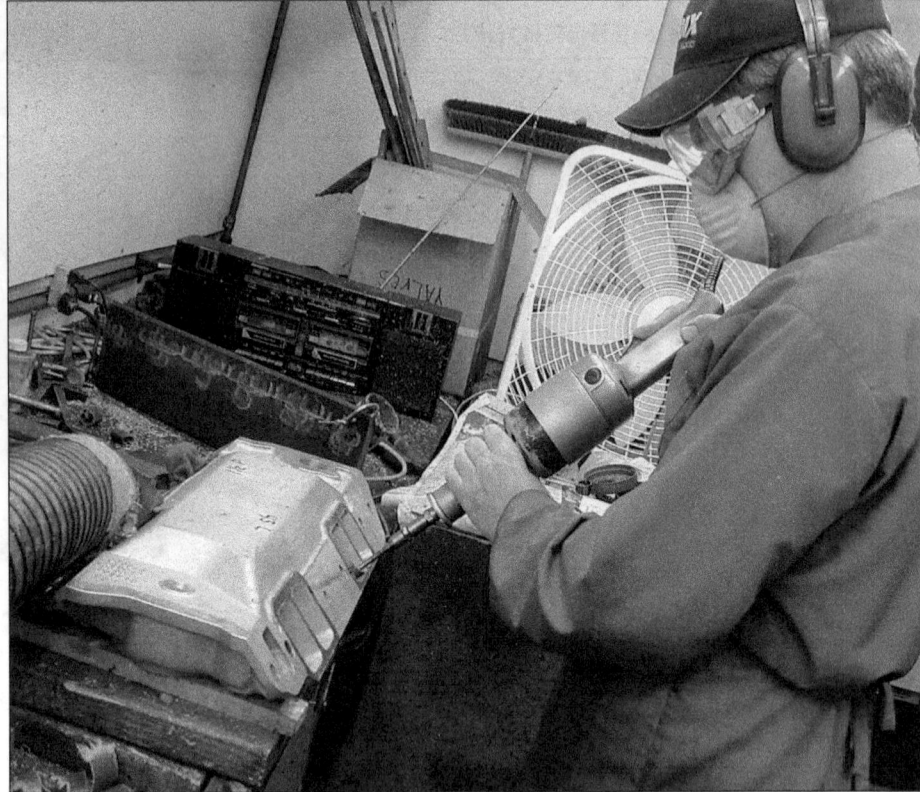

6 Back from Wilson Nitrous Pro-Flow, Slover disassembles the highly modified Merlin III intake, and does a final port and polish on the intake ports to match them up to the Merlin III cylinder heads.

Block Machining & Pre-Assembly Preperation

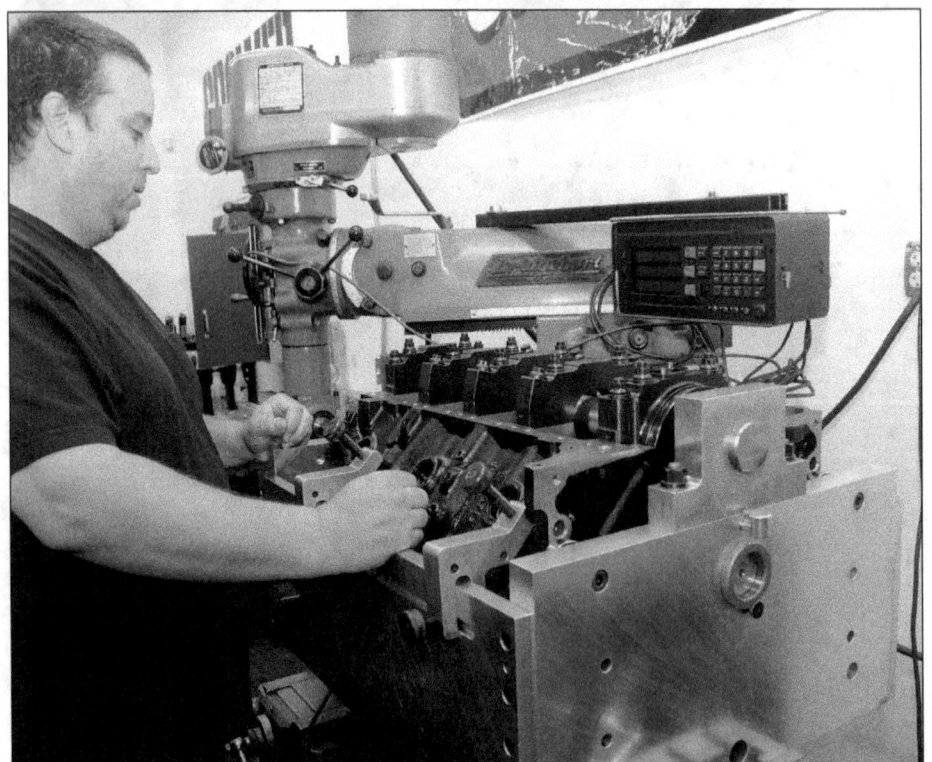

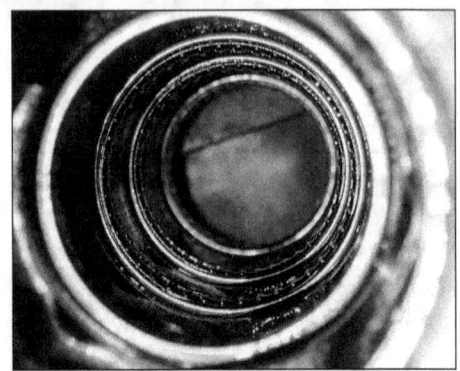

1 In order to install one of these big journal nitrous cams, it was first necessary for engineman Brad Lagman to line bore the cam tunnel 2.478 inches in diameter using a BHJ fixture. Then Lagman power-honed the enlarged cam tunnel .002 inch to achieve an overall inside diameter of 2.480 inches. Then a set of Timken TL5520 Caged Needle Roller Bearings was installed, which is not only superior in design to normal cam bearings, but they also greatly assist in allowing the cam and valvetrain to achieve maximum RPM levels quicker on the nitrous.

76   HOW TO INSTALL AND TUNE NITROUS OXIDE SYSTEMS

BAD-ASS 540-CI MERLIN III NITROUS BIG-BLOCK BUILDUP

Big-Block Engine Assembly

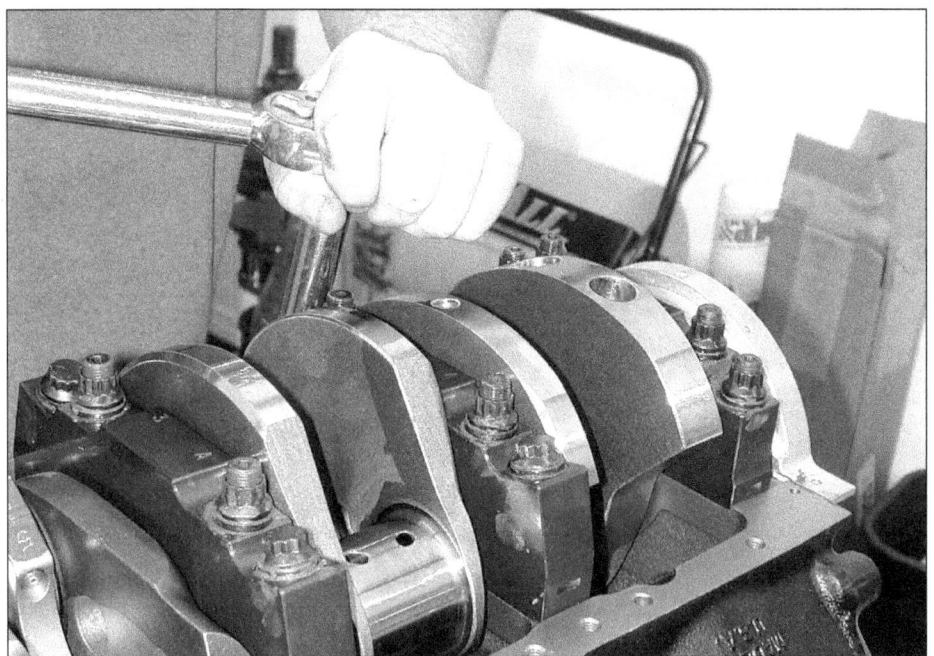

1 QMP Racing Engine's Robert Bieschke was on deck for the actual long-block engine assembly. After planting the Lunati Pro Series forged-steel crank, he torques the Merlin III's four-bolt main caps to 100 ft-lbs.

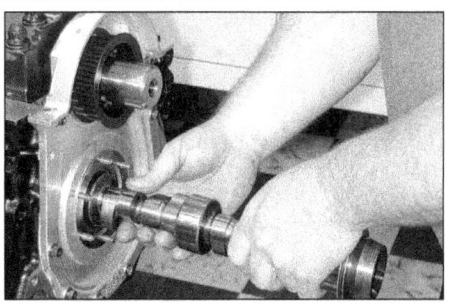

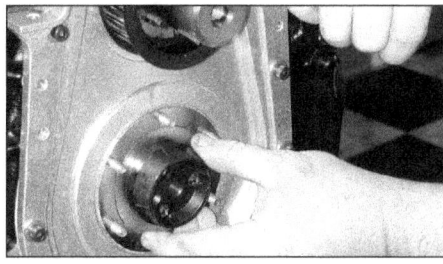

2 At this juncture, Bieschke installs the Lunati 7-4 Swap mechanical roller cam using plenty of assembly lube. The cam thrust bearing gets installed next.

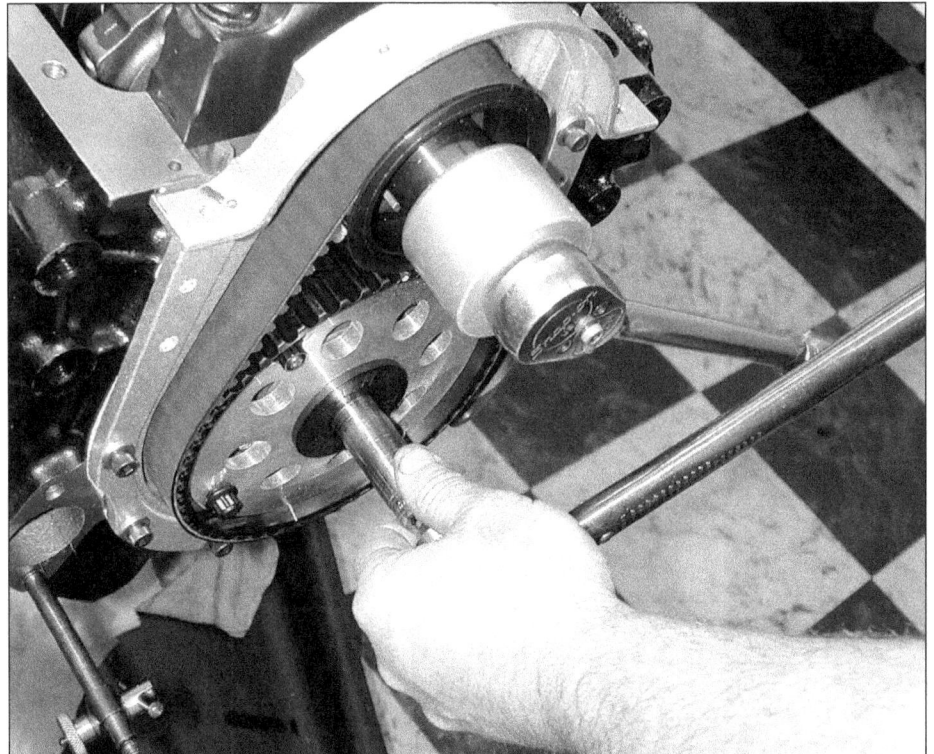

3 The cam installation is followed with the installation of the Jesel BB & DRCE Olds-style Belt Drive gear onto the Lunati Pro Series crank snout, followed by installing the cog belt and timing gear.

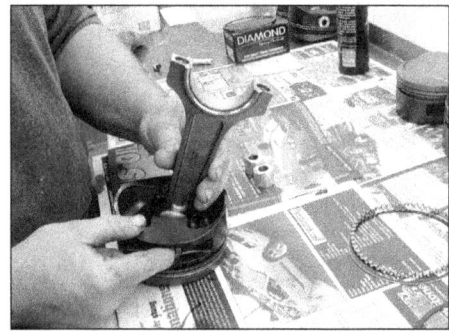

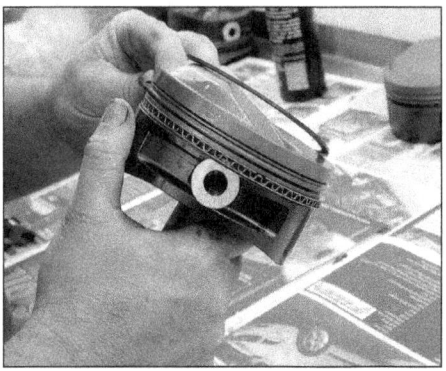

4 Hanging the Lunati I-beam connecting rods and Total Seal-equipped Diamond Racing nitrous pistons comes next.

HOW TO INSTALL AND TUNE NITROUS OXIDE SYSTEMS

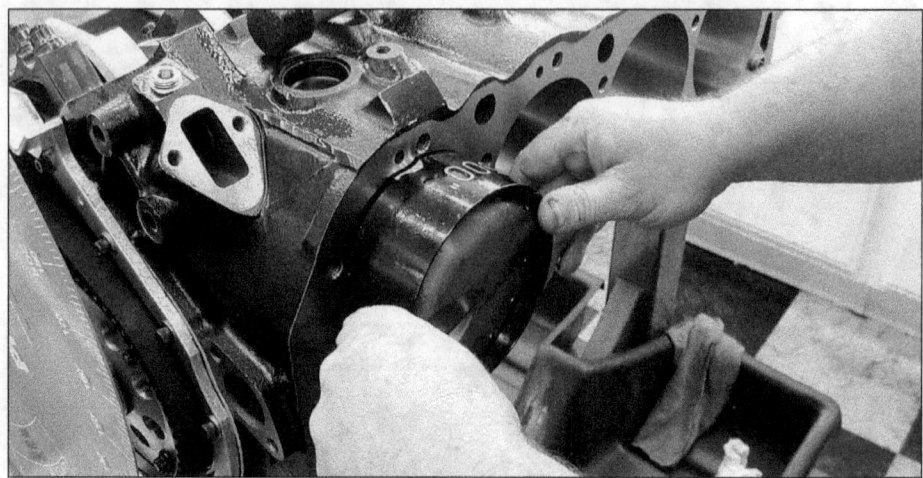

5 *In go the rod and piston assemblies one at a time.*

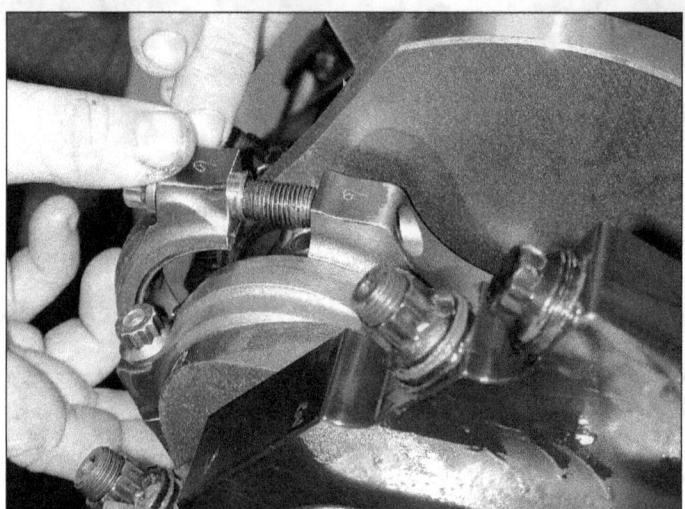
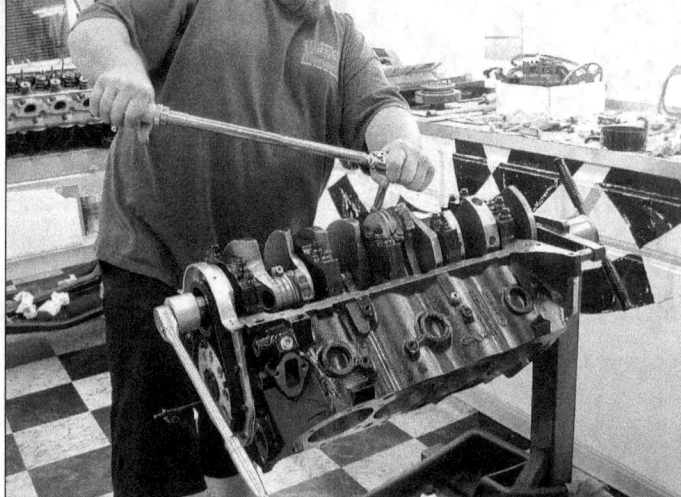

6 *The Federal Mogul-equipped Merlin III main caps are installed and final-torqued to 64 ft-lbs while the rod caps are final-tightened to 95 ft-lbs of torque.*

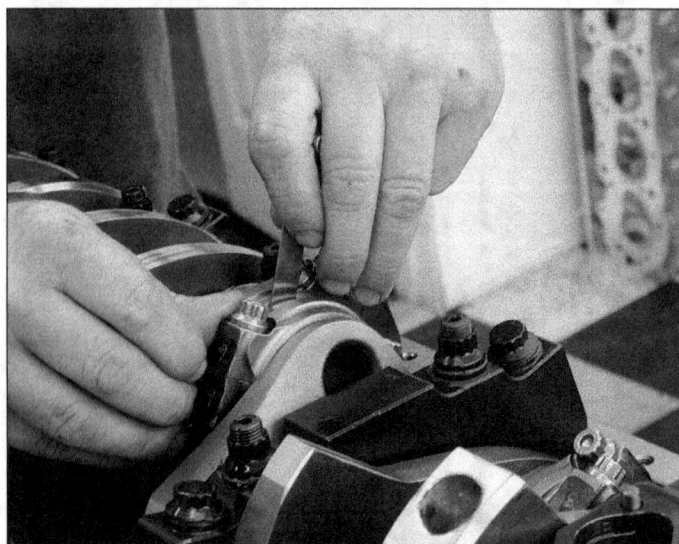
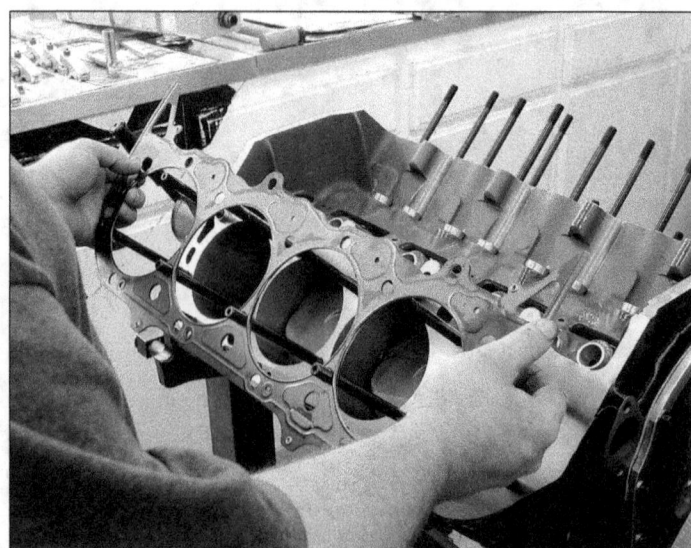

7 *Side-to-side connecting rod clearance is checked and an average of 0.023 to 0.025 inch is achieved.*

8 *After installing the ARP Head Studs Bieschke installs the Cometic high-performance head gaskets.*

BAD-ASS 540-CI MERLIN III NITROUS BIG-BLOCK BUILDUP

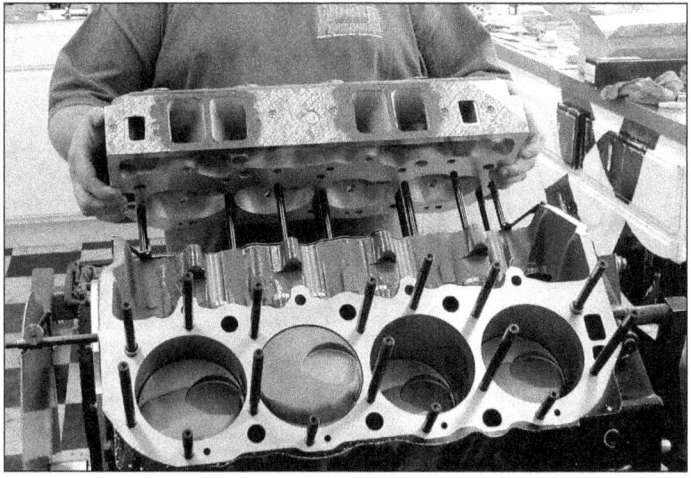
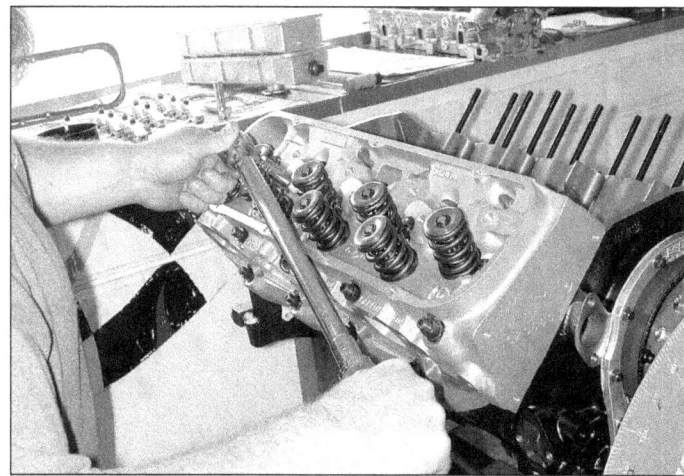

9 On goes the left-side Merlin III alloy cylinder head, followed by some anti-seize applied to the 1/2-inch ARP head studs. Then the head is final-torqued to 75 ft-lbs.

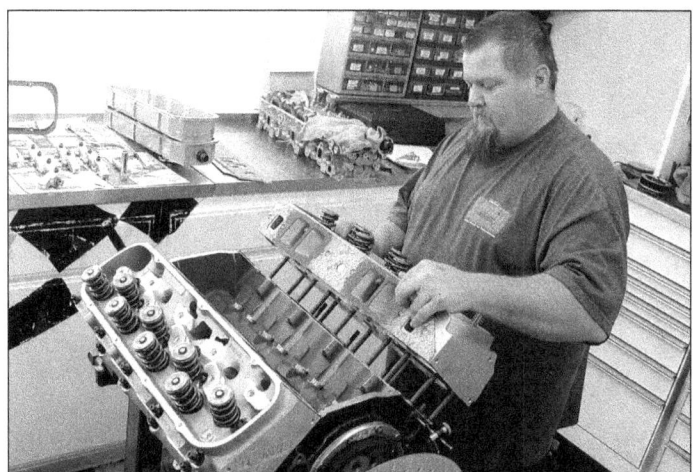
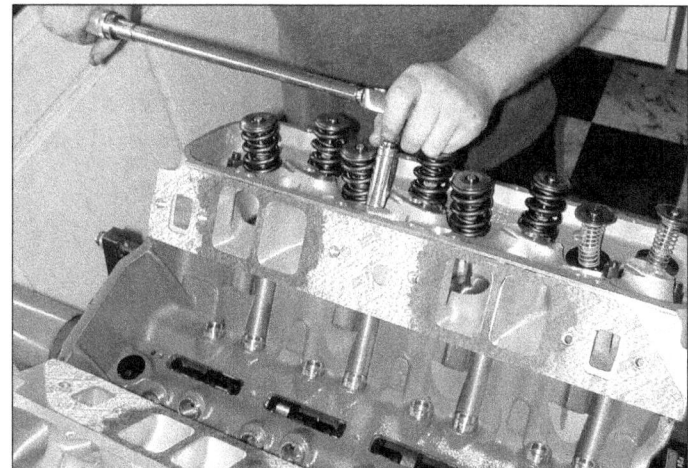

10 The right-side cylinder head is likewise installed and final-torqued to 75 ft-lbs.

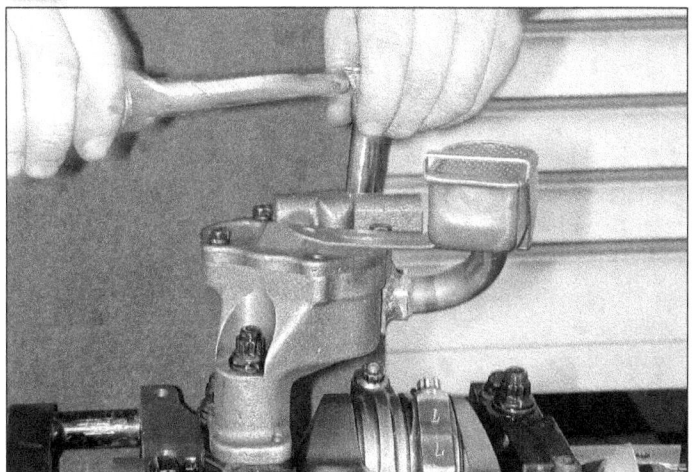

11 With the engine flipped back over, Bieschke installs the ARP Oil Pump Drive BBC 12-point stud kit, followed with the installation of the ARP Oil Pump driveshaft and Milodon High Volume Oil Pump Pickup.

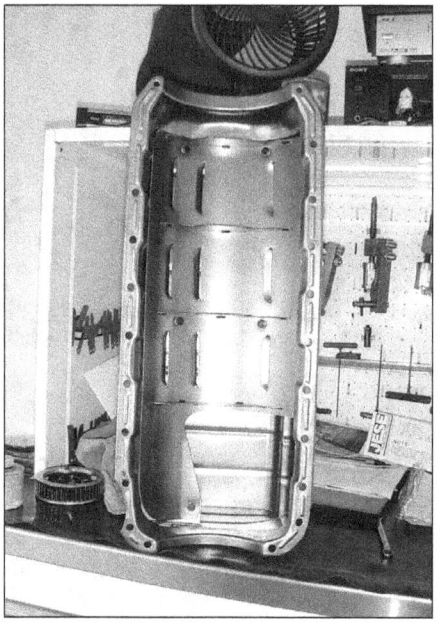

12 Due to the fact that this is an aftermarket four-bolt-main block, the oil baffle inside the pan required minor clearancing.

HOW TO INSTALL AND TUNE NITROUS OXIDE SYSTEMS

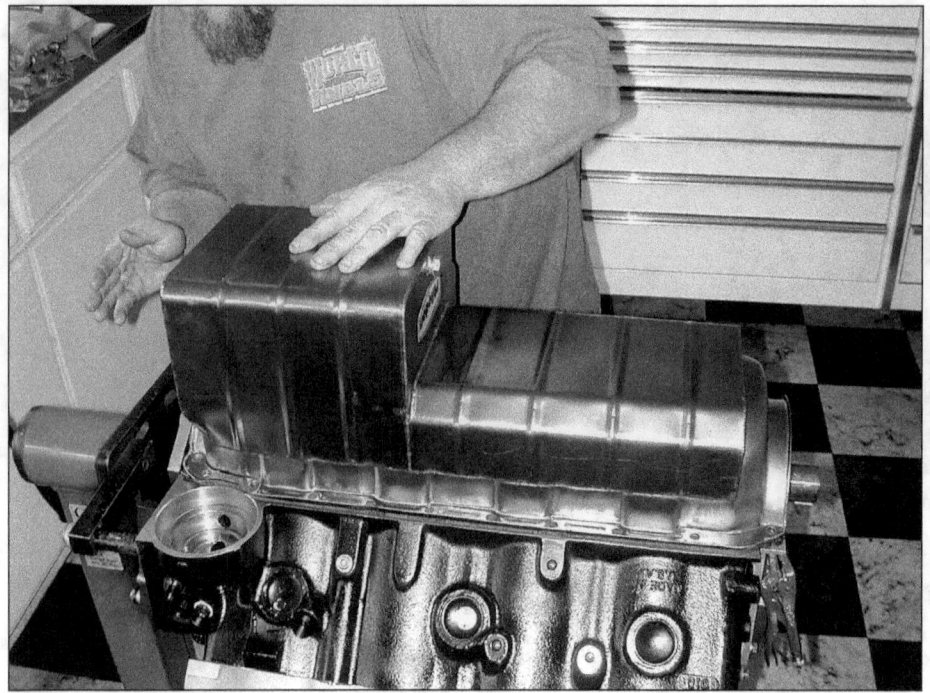

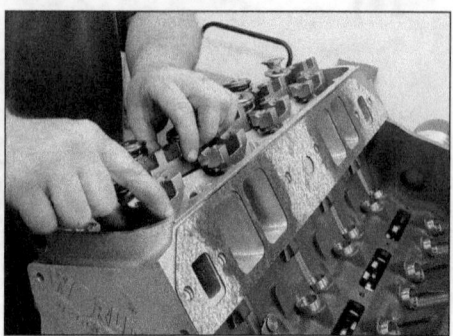

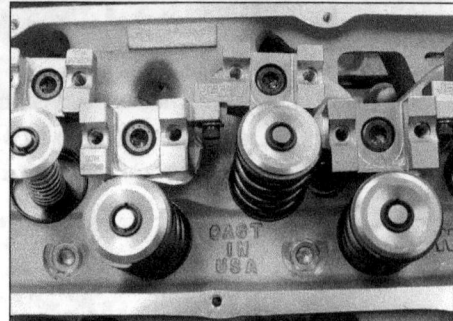

13 After installing the oil pan gaskets, Bieschke installs the Milodon oil pan using ARP's Oil Pan Stud kit.

14 Installing the Jesel rocker arm stands comes next.

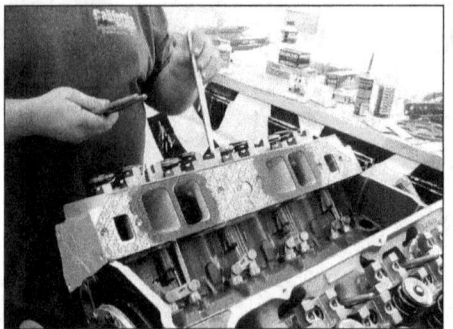

15 Next the Trend Performance pushrods, which measure 8.350 inches in length on the intake and 9.200 inches on the exhaust, are installed.

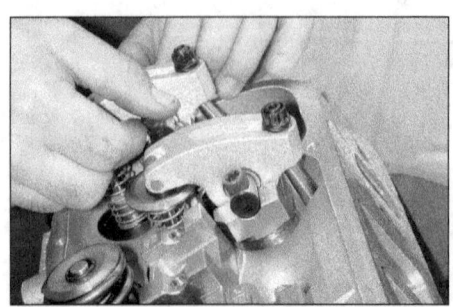

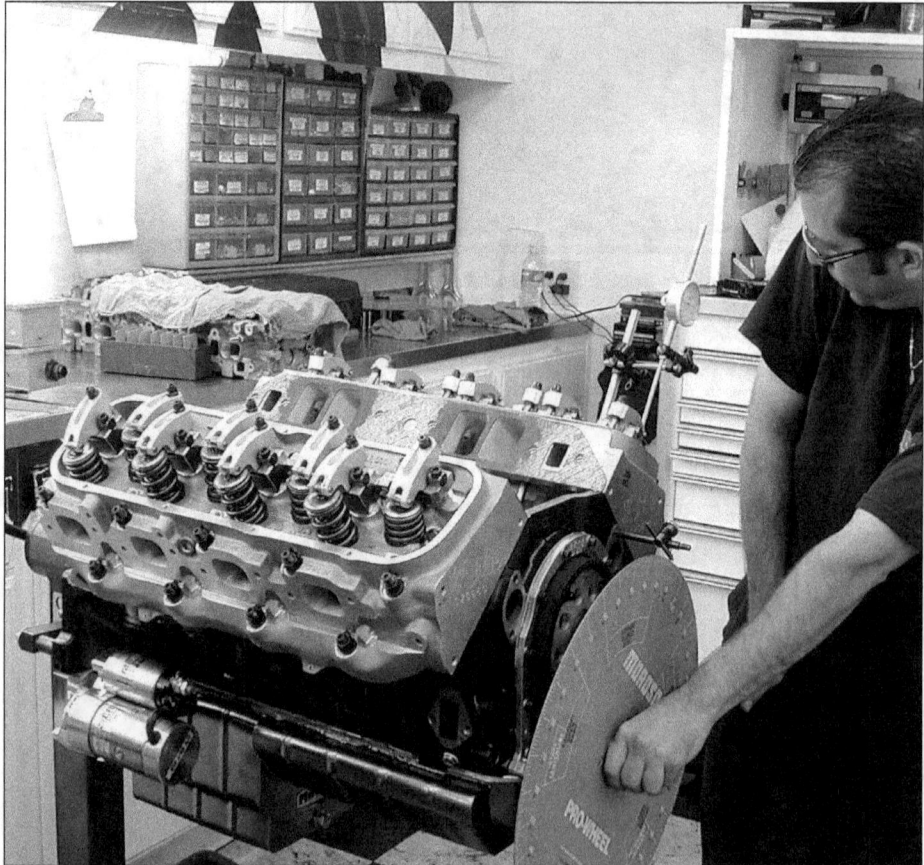

16 Installation of the Jesel 1.7-ratio-shaft rocker arms is next.

17 QMP's Mike Consolo degrees-in the Lunati cam at 10 degrees.

BAD-ASS 540-CI MERLIN III NITROUS BIG-BLOCK BUILDUP

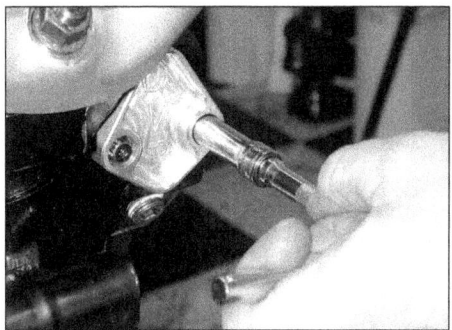

18 One of QMP's billet-aluminum fuel block-off plates being installed.

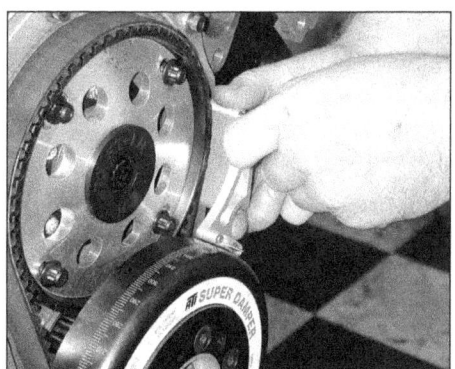

19 The ATI crank snout hub, ATI Super Dampener, and QMP billet-aluminum pointer are installed.

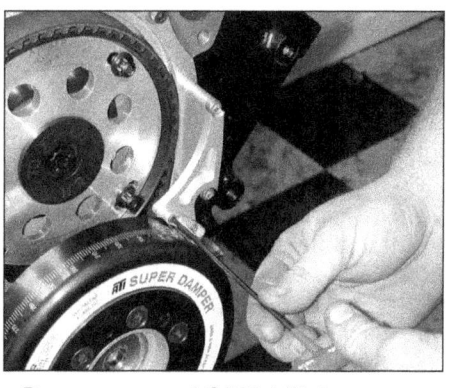

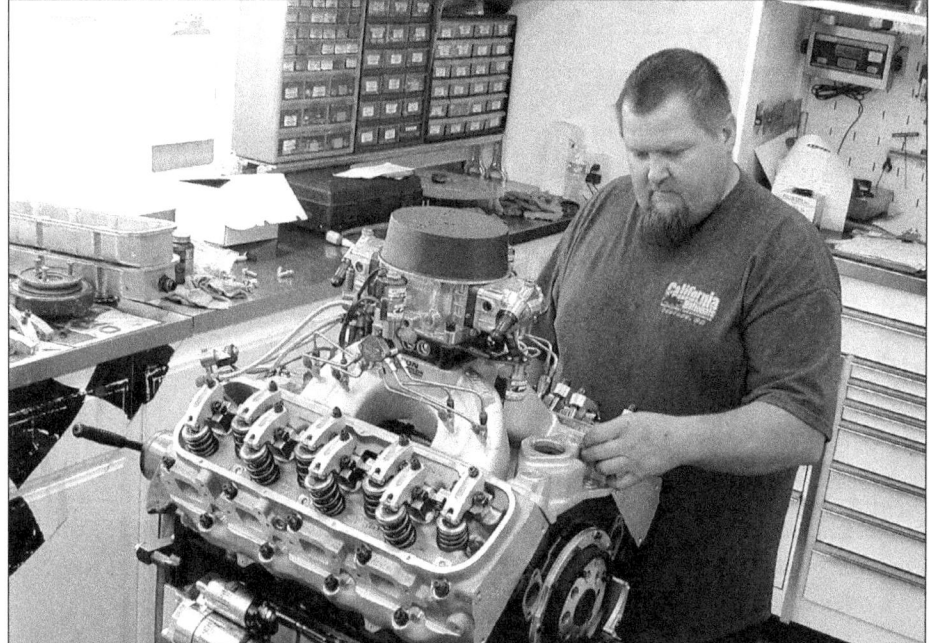

20 Bieschke installs the Mr. Gasket intake manifold gaskets followed by the Wilson Manifolds & Nitrous Pro-Flow/Merlin III two-stage nitrous intake, using a set of 3/8-inch ARP stainless-steel 12-point hex-head bolts.

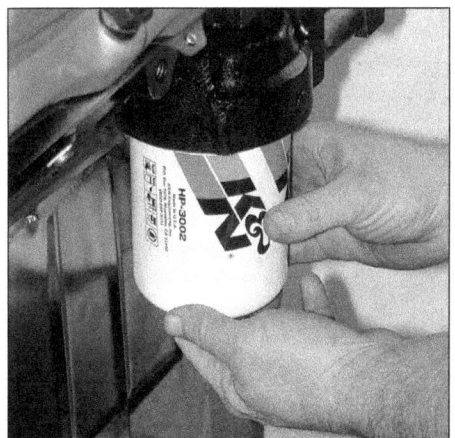

21 Then one of K&N's high-performance oil filters and 20W-50 Lucas Engine Break-In oil gets poured in.

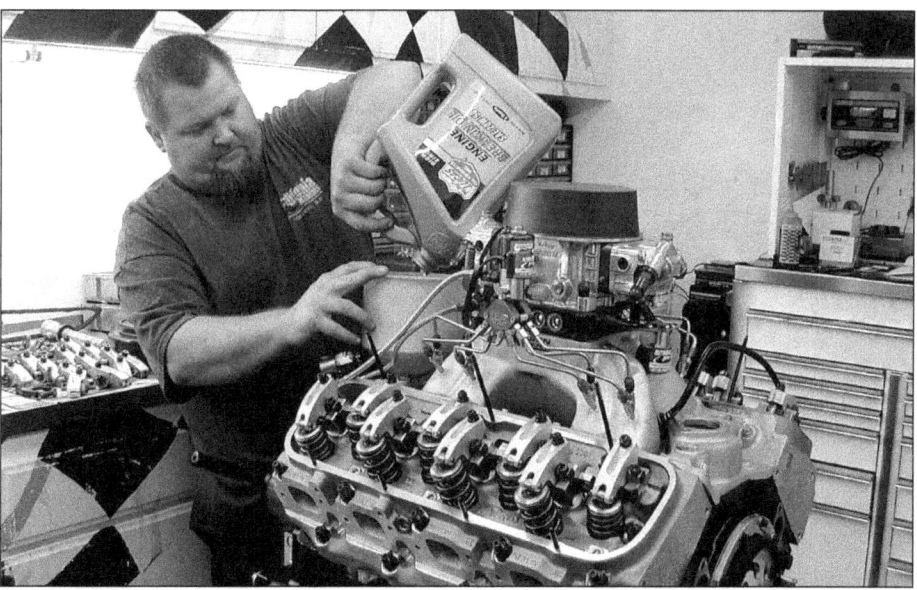

HOW TO INSTALL AND TUNE NITROUS OXIDE SYSTEMS

CHAPTER 8

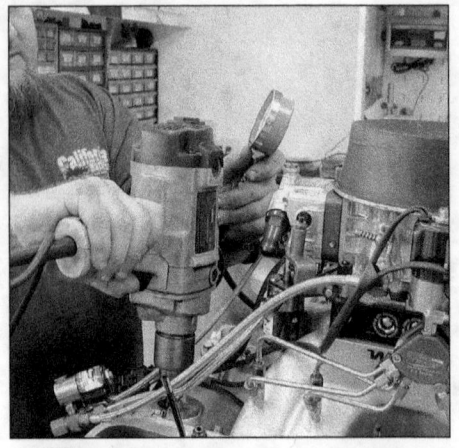

22 Oil Pressure is checked and approved at 80 psi.

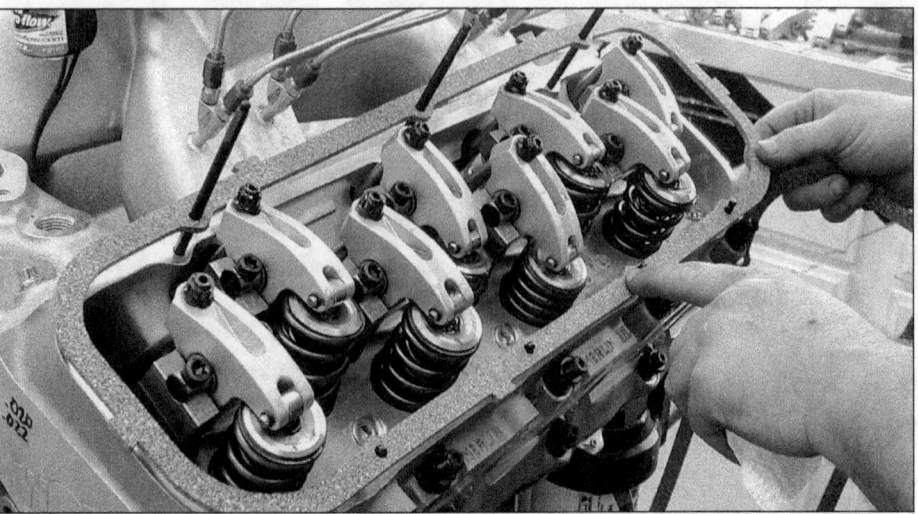

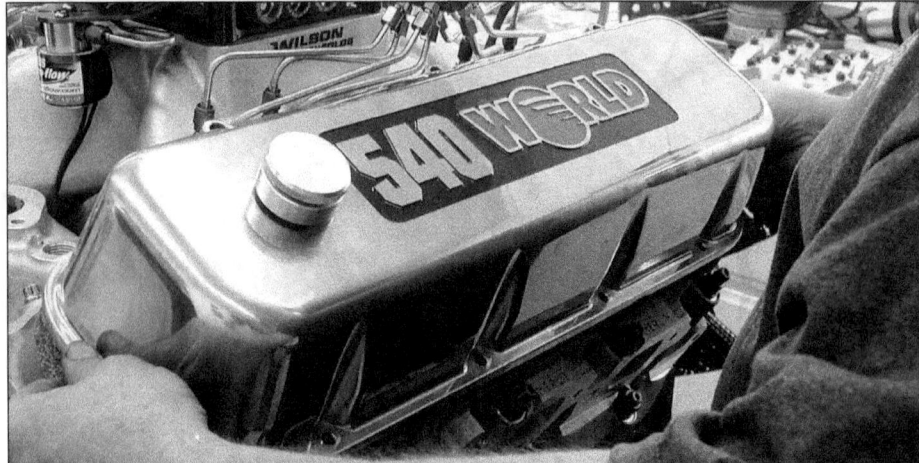

23 On go a set of Mr. Gasket cork valve-cover gaskets and World Products Merlin III polished-aluminum tall-deck valve covers, using an ARP valve cover stud kit.

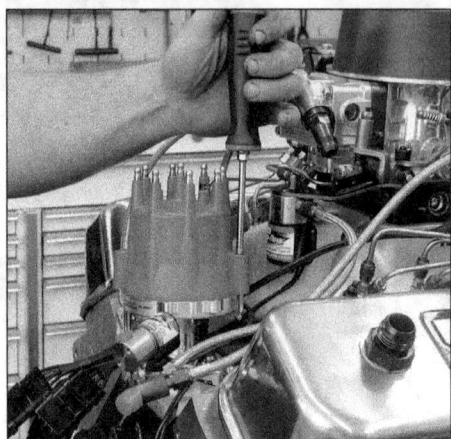

24 Installation of the MSD Pro Billet distributor is secured in place via a set of ARP 12-point distributor bolts.

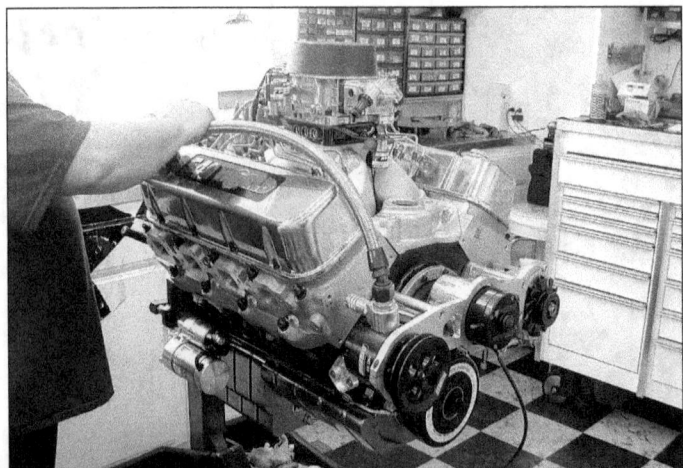

25 Bieschke hooks up the 1-inch-diameter DMP braided stainless-steel line that runs from the valve cover breather to the Moroso vacuum pump.

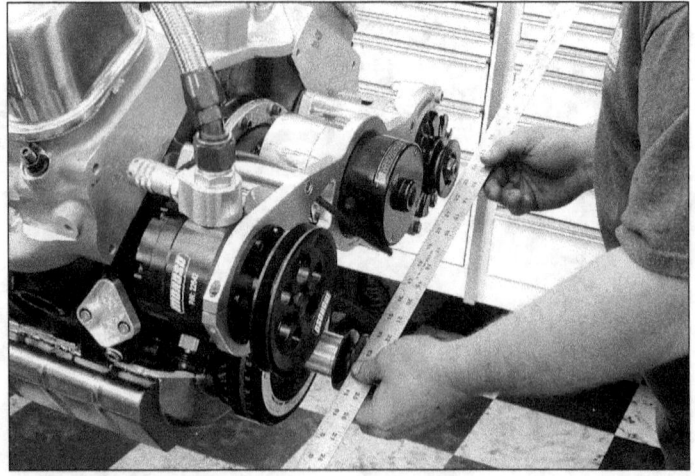

26 The Meziere High Flow Electric Water Pump and Moroso Vacuum Pump and billet-aluminum alternator/vacuum pump brackets are installed and aligned.

BAD-ASS 540-CI MERLIN III NITROUS BIG-BLOCK BUILDUP

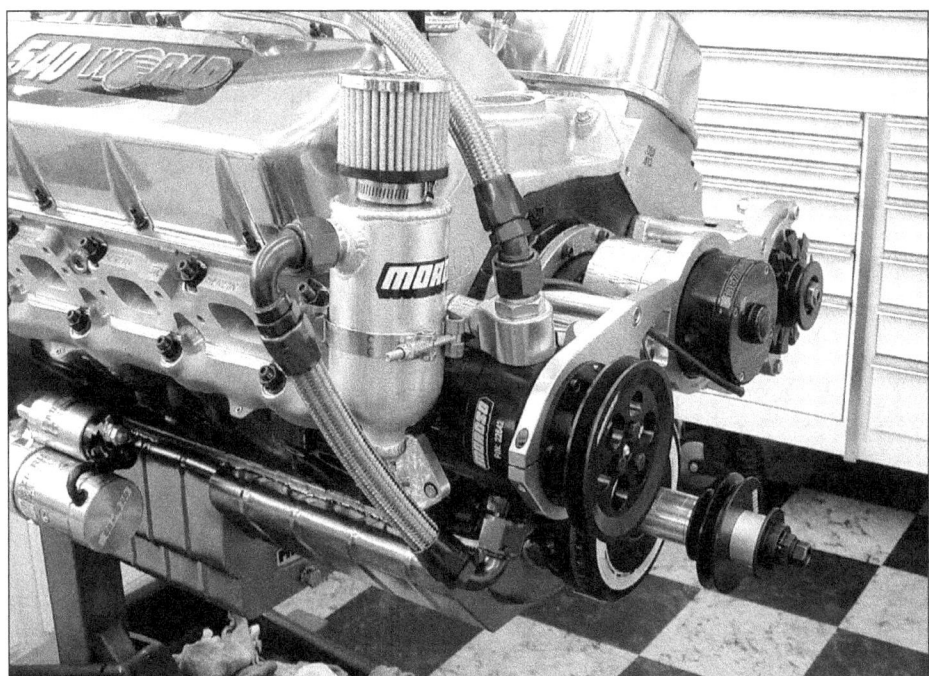

27 *Finally, the Moroso Vacuum Pump breather tank and short line to the actual pump is installed.*

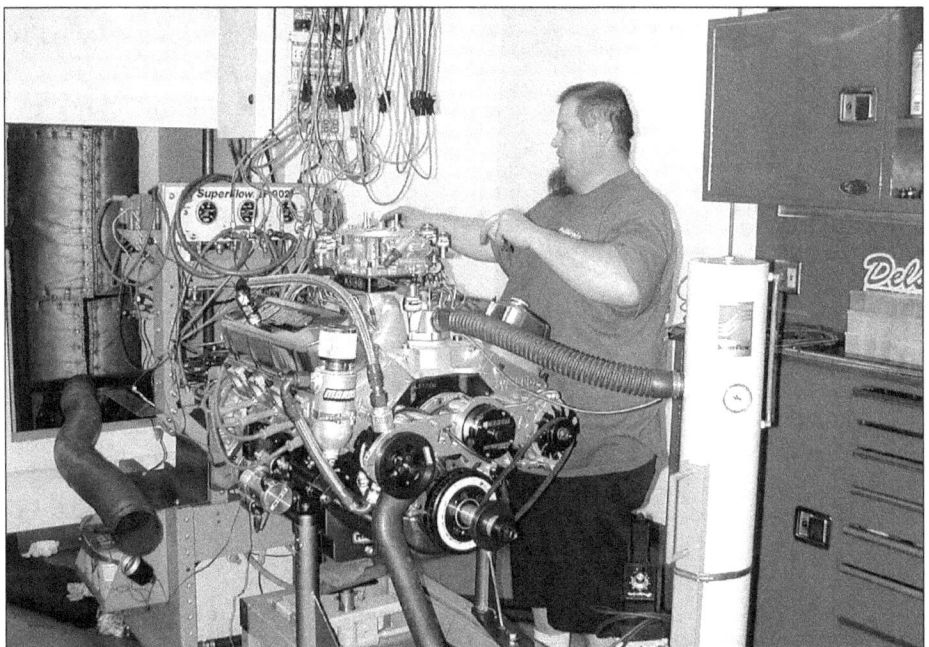

28 *Bieschke installs the Merlin III on the QMP's Superflow SP 9002 dyno. Although not able to test the engine on two-stage nitrous because the sudden surge in torque and horsepower far surpasses the dyno's limitations and could spell disaster, testing was done solely on the engine producing 891 hp at 7,200 rpm and 678.8 ft-lbs at 6,300 rpm. Not a bad start. The tune-up is entirely different after installed in the engine bay of a car like Galante's 1967 Nova Top Sportsman racer. Horsepower should be around 1,300 to 1,500, depending on timing, jetting, fuel pressure, and fuel distribution.*

One Year Later

"It's been more than a year since I started this 540-ci Merlin III big-block project," says James "Jimmy G" Galante, "and it has been a real eye opener! Up until now, my only experience with nitrous oxide was when I installed a 150-shot non-adjustable Fogger kit on one of my friend's race cars and he loved it. Nonetheless, I was still a neophyte when it came to the subject, and with all the time and expense I have wrapped up in this project, my two greatest concerns were: Will this thing produce the power and torque I think it will and do so without blowing the darned thing up?"

The initial dyno test on the engine was very promising. After being broken in by QMP Racing Engines technician Robert Bieschke, our Merlin 540 cranked out 891 hp at 7,200 rpm, and 678 ft-lbs at 6,300 rpm on Lagman's Superflow engine dyno.

It was explained that there was no need to dyno the engine on nitrous because the tuning is entirely different than what it will be after the engine is installed in a race car. When the nitrous is activated on a multiple-stage system, the torque and horsepower curve can shoot up so fast that it's difficult for the dyno to control the horsepower.

The system is a basic two-stage plate and direct port nitrous system setup by Wilson Manifolds/Nitrous Pro-Flow. Both stages are a wet-style system using fuel and N_2O at the same time, and Wilson Manifolds & Nitrous Pro-Flow provided me with a port jetting map as a guideline to suggest what jets to use in conjunction with its patented V-Force nozzles, as well as to provide a guide to how much nitrous

CHAPTER 8

and fuel flow to equal a given horsepower equation.

Valve lift and cylinder head design are also critical to this equation. I mean, if the cylinder head's ports are not big enough to handle the volume of air necessary to make this thing breathe, you're not going to realistically produce the horsepower numbers you're looking for, which explains why Slover's Porting Service performed so much work on our Merlin III cylinder heads.

That's also where solenoid and nozzle placement and proper jet sizing really come into play. The professional nitrous oxide racer takes this to the highest level, pushing the laws of physics, and risking blown-up, burnt-up, and exploded engines to get the right tune-up. Since money doesn't grow on trees, I'll be more than happy to follow Wilson's map until I get a better handle on the subject. Also remember that nitrous oxide timing can be just as critical as fuel pressure. The timing on a race engine without N_2O is usually set to full advance of the total amount of timing desired during a full cycle of operation. When running a multiple system such as this one, it becomes necessary to adjust or incrementally retard the timing each time you activate it. And just how do you do that?

We chose the MSD Programmable Digital-7 ignition control box, with boost retard (PN 7531). This unit is set up to handle all timing and RPM limiting in one box, and is one of the most advanced units on the market. In fact, you can even alter the timing from one cylinder to another cylinder.

Exhaust gas temperature (EGT) sensors are used when you really want to get serious about tuning N_2O for maximum power. These individual sensors (one per cylinder) measure each cylinder's exhaust gas heat, and tell you if your engine is operating at maximum combustion efficiency or burning itself up. Cylinders that run hotter than others can be retarded through the ignition timing controller to manage the overall temperament of the engine. Changing nitrous jetting on certain cylinders to control excessive heat buildup is how you prevent runaway detonation, and that's the beauty of having EGT information.

When pushing these systems to efficiently flow as much nitrous as the engine/car can handle, pay close attention to the details. Wiring and fuel distribution must be perfect. Do not use butt connectors and push locks when setting up your wiring loom. Use a high-quality connection like a weather pack connector or equivalent—it is much safer.

Furthermore, fuel systems cannot be mismatched or poorly planned. When using a multiple-stage N_2O system, be sure to use a separate fuel regulator for each stage. In other words, you need a total of three regulators: one for the carburetor, one for the first stage (or plate), and one for the second-stage fogger nozzles. It's also best not to mix and match parts from different manufacturers. Use all same-brand, same-type parts to ensure they are designed to work seamlessly together as a complete system.

Wilson Nitrous Pro-Flow 8-Cylinder Direct-Port-Jetting Map

First Stage

HP	Nitrous Jet	Fuel Jet	Timing Retard (degrees)	Flow Jet Nozzle	Fuel Pressure (psi)
100	18	18	4	36	6–7
125	20	20	5	40	6–7
150	22	22	6	44	6–7
175	24	24	7	48	6–7
250	28	28	10	56	6–7
300	32	32	12	64	6–7
350	36	36	14	72	6–7
400	40	40	16	80	6–7
500	42	42	20	84	6–7

Second Stage

HP	Nitrous Jet	Fuel Jet	Timing Retard (degrees)	Flow Jet Nozzle	Fuel Pressure (psi)
100	18	18	3.00	36	6–7
125	20	20	3.75	40	6–7
150	22	22	4.50	44	6–7
175	24	24	5.25	48	6–7
250	28	28	7.50	56	6–7
300	32	36	9.00	64	6–7
350	36	36	10.50	72	6–7
400	40	40	12.00	80	6–7
500	42	42	15.00	84	6–7

CHAPTER 9

EFI, WET AND DRY

The three basic concepts of an Electronic Fuel Injection (EFI) nitrous oxide system—wet plate, wet manifold—and dry manifold, are nearly identical to their carbureted cousins.

Wet-Plate Systems

First you have the wet plate, which is similar to a carbureted nitrous plate with its fuel and N_2O jet ports. These plates get sandwiched between the EFI throttle body and the intake plenum. This is the most commonly used N_2O street application. Most brand-name N_2O kit manufacturers currently offer nitrous wet-plate EFI applications, usually covering the 75- to 125-hp index.

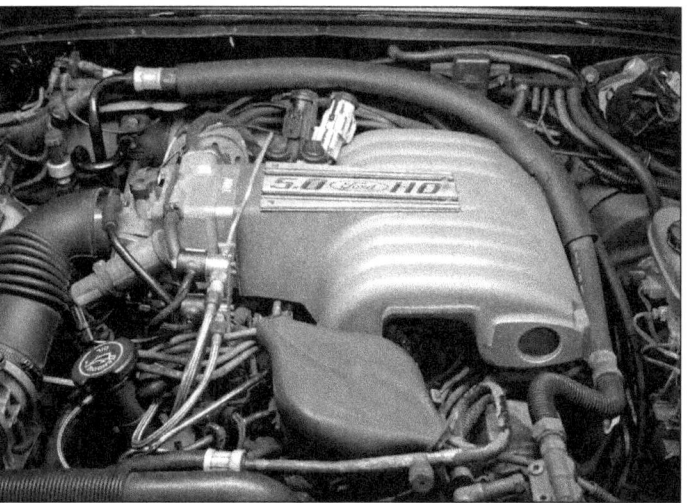

Ford's 5.0L EFI H.O. (High Output) pushrod V-8 engine is very popular when it comes to adding a nitrous kit. Various N20 kit designs have been developed from 1986 to 1995, the most popular of which are the wet plate applications. Shown is TNW's 5.0L Wet Kit which sandwiches the nitrous plate between the 5.0L intake plenum and throttle body. Other companies such as Holley-NOS, Holley-systeMAX, Edelbrock Nitrous, 10,000 RPM Speed Equipment, and Nitrous Express market kits that feature a wet plate that bolts between the base of the EFI intake manifold and EFI intake plenum. Either design is quite efficient producing on average an additional 100 to 300 hp.

Nitrous Express

Nitrous Express offers both a 5.0L EFI (PN 20102-10) as well as two mod-motor EFI nitrous plate kits for the two-valve SOHC Ford V-8 (PN 20946-10) and three-valve SOHC Ford V-8 kit (PN 20947-10). Both offer horsepower increases of 50 to 150.

Next are NX's 50- to 300-hp and 50- to 600-hp bolt-on spray bar kits for the 5.0L set. However, with these two applications, when you start tickling the 150 to 200 range of horsepower, you must make some serious internal component modifications if you want your 5.0L to live!

NX also markets an MAF combination throttle-body/MAF-nitrous housing in 60- to 150-hp trim for both the GM LS and LT-1 engines (PNs 20110-10 and 20931-10, respectively).

Finally, NX's new 2010 5th-Gen V-8 Camaro Plate System is available (PN 20931-10) and capable of producing 35 to 150 hp—a 200 upgrade jet kit is also available. An installation article on one of these systems is located later in this chapter.

NOS offers 150- to 300-hp wet-plate kits for the 5.0L; there are three including Edelbrock

CHAPTER 9

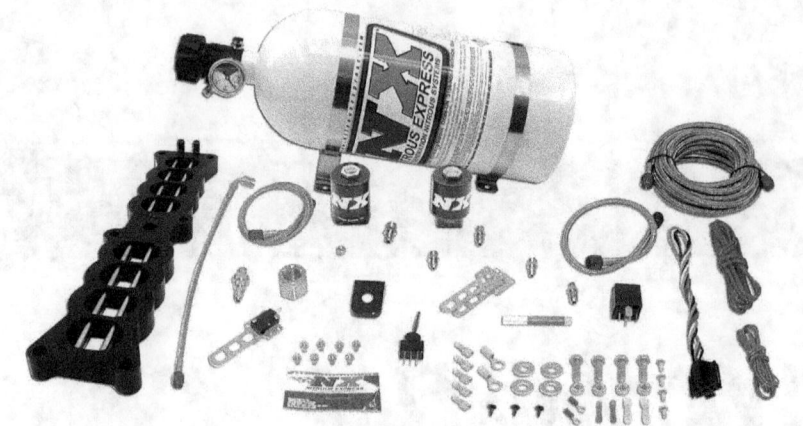

Nitrous Express seems to have the 1985–1995 5.0L EFI arena covered with its patented Phase 3 Gemini Twin 5.0 Plate, with settings from 50 to 300 hp on each stage. Intake applications include a stock 5.0L (PN 20100), Ford Racing GT40 (PN 20101), Edelbrock Performer & RPM (PN 20202), Edelbrock Victor (PN 20103), TYFS Street 5.0L (PN 20104), TFS Rplate (PN 20105), and 5.0L Holley SysteMAX (PN 20106).

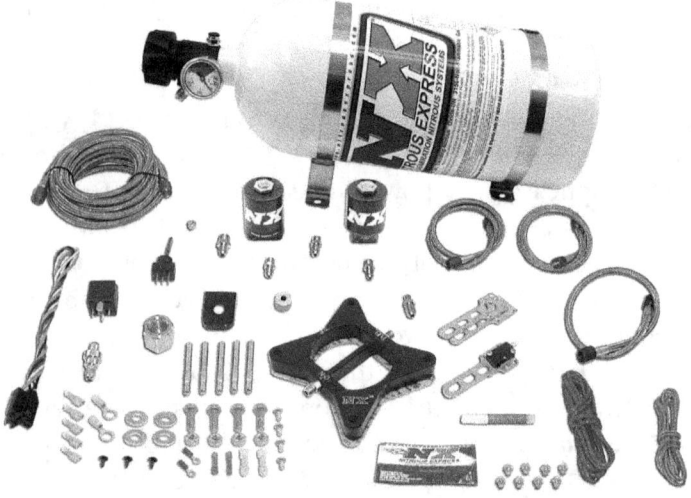

NX also offers plate kits for the Ford 2V SOHC (PN 20946-10) and 3V SOHC modular motors (PN 20947-10), both capable of producing 50 to 150 hp.

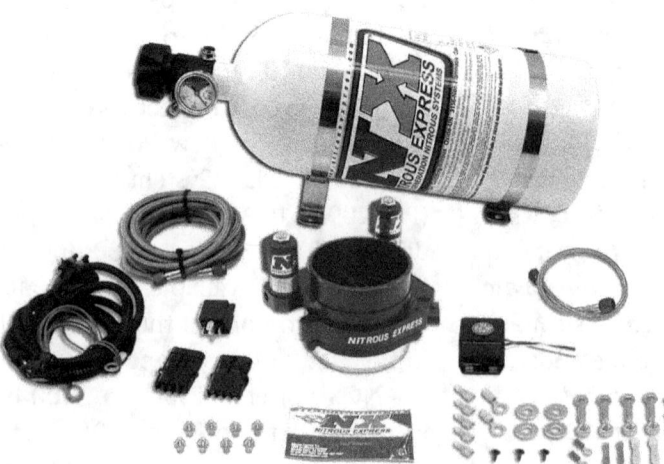

NX combination throttle body/MAF nitrous housing is available in 60- to 150-hp trim for the GM LS and LT-1 engines (PNs 20110-10 and 20931-10, respectively).

Performer and RPM, and the Holley SysteMAX intakes (PNs 02117NOS and 02119NOS, respectively). NOS also offers applications for the DOHC and SOHC Ford three-valve and four-valve engines (PNs 02121NOS and 02120NOS, respectively), a Chevrolet LS1 Camaro/Firebird/Corvette C5-V-8 application (PN 05168NOS), a 2005-and-later C6 Corvette application (PN 05169NOS), and GM Tuned Port applications (PN 05151NOS, 1985–1992 5.0/5.7L, and 1985–1991 5.7l Corvette). Did I exclude your particular wet-plate application?

10,000 RPM Speed Equipment

The 10,000 RPM Speed Equipment Company still keeps its hand in the game with 5.0L pushrod V-8 Mustang EFI plate systems available for both the stock High Output intake plenum (PN 1094-5.0) and the upscale GT40/Cobra's (PN 1095-GT40) intakes.

Edelbrock

Edelbrock Nitrous markets its 80-hp 1986–1995 5.0L kit (PN 70400). It also offers the 100- to 150-hp Pro-Flo/Pro-Flow 2 4V EFI Performer RPM kit (PN 70070) for the four-valve Cobra modular engine, and a 50- to 100-hp 2005–2009 4.6L 2V Ford SOHC kit (PN 70410). Mopar enthusiasts can take advantage of Edelbrock's 5.7L and 6.1L Gen-III Hemi Wet Kits (PNs 70217 and PN 70410, respectively).

Nitrous Outlet

One of the new players on the market worth mentioning is Late Model Restoration Supply's 1996–2004 2V Mustang GT Plate Kit, manufactured by Nitrous Outlet. It boasts horsepower increases of 50 to 100.

EFI, WET AND DRY

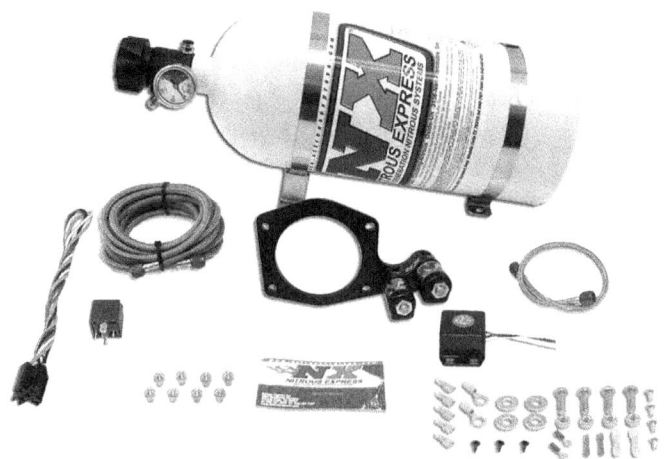

NX's new 2010 5th-Gen V-8 Camaro Plate System is available (PN 20931-10) and capable of producing 35 to 150 hp; a 200-hp upgrade jet kit is also available.

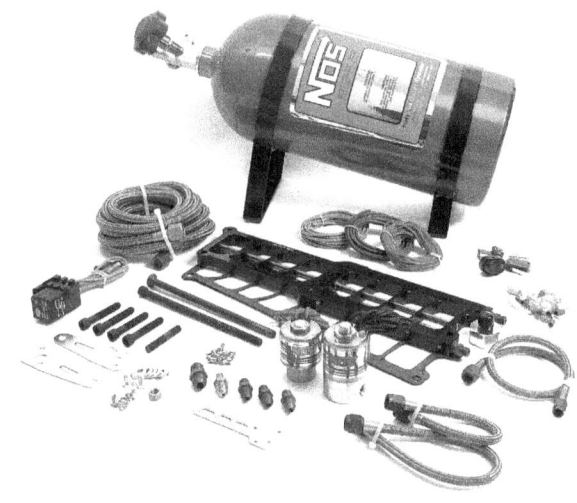

NOS offers three 150- to 300-hp wet plate kits for 5.0L Edelbrock Performer and Edelbrock Performer RPM (PN 02117NOS) and Holley SysteMAX intakes (PN 02119NOS, shown). NOS also offers applications for the DOHC and SOHC Ford 3V and 4V engines (PNs 02121NOS and 02120NOS, respectively).

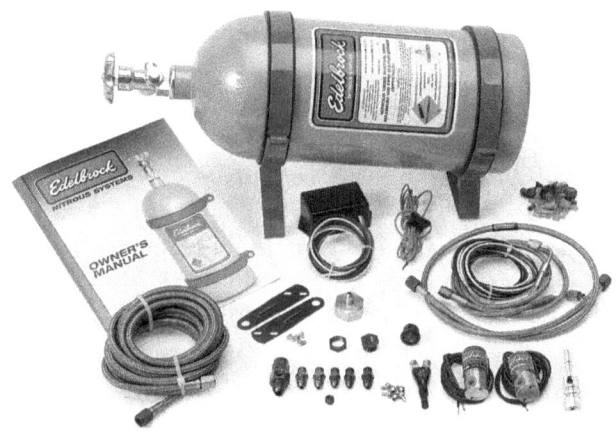

For Mopar fans, there are the Edelbrock Nitrous 5.7L and 6.1L Gen III Hemi Wet Kits for cars (PN 70216), and for 5.7L Hemi trucks (PN 70217), power rated at 40, 60, and 80 hp. Also on the roster is Edelbrock Nitrous 2003–2007 5.3L Hemi truck wet kit (PN 70410) power rated at 40, 60, and 70 hp.

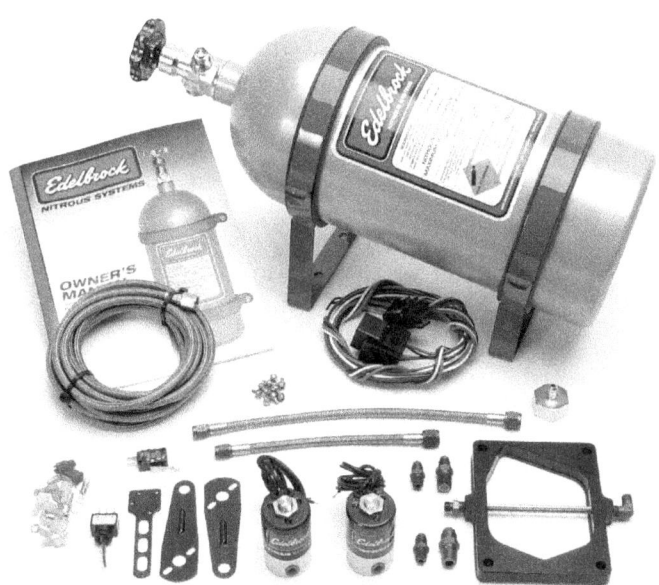

The Edelbrock Nitrous 80-hp 1986–1995 5.0L kit (PN 70400). The company also offers 100- to 150-hp Pro-Flo/Pro-Flow II 4V EFI Performer RPM kit (PN 70070, shown) for the 4V Cobra modular engine, and a 50- to 100-hp kit for 2005–2009 4.6L 2V Ford SOHC (PN 70410).

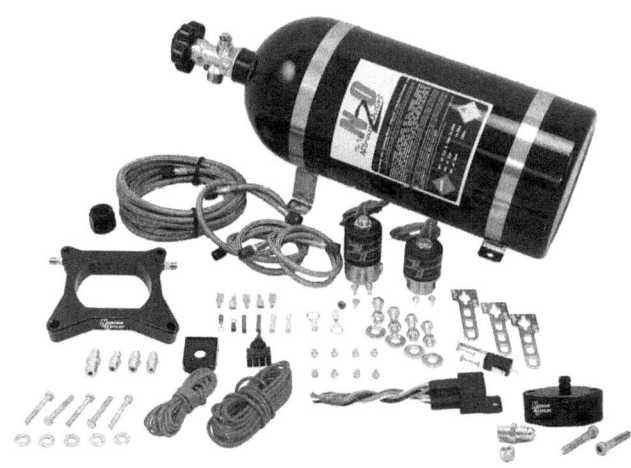

One of the new players on the market is Late Model Restoration Supply's 1996–2004 2V Mustang GT Plate Kit, manufactured by Nitrous Outlet, which boasts horsepower increases of 50 to 100 hp. No part number is available as of this writing.

CHAPTER 9

Wet-Manifold Systems

The second most commonly used EFI N_2O kit is the spray nozzle kit available in either wet or dry applications. Dry applications consist of a sprayer nozzle only, which injects N_2O into the intake tract while the fuel injectors (in some applications, larger volume fuel injectors) may be called on to enhance fuel delivery. This was the original design pioneered in the late 1980s by NOS, and it is still offered in Stage-1 (PN 15115NOS) and Stage-II applications (PN 05115-IINOS).

Alternately, the wet design features a spray nozzle that delivers both fuel and N_2O simultaneously to the engine when inserted into the air intake tube. Today, this is most commonly used on modern engines like the Ford 4.6L two-, three-, and four-valve engines; GM's LS1-LS7 engines; and Mopar's 5.8 to 6.1L Gen-III Hemi-engine series.

ZEX Nitrous Products

ZEX Nitrous Products seems to offer the most sophisticated wet-sprayer kits, with its 2005-to-current Mustang 3V wet system 75 to 175 hp (PN 82034), ZEX 1999–2004 Mustang GT 2V wet system (PN 82217), and 75- to 125-hp Mustang Bullitt wet kit (PN 82023), the 75- to 125-hp 1999–2004 F-Series Ford Truck system (PN 82240), and even the 55- to 100-hp kits for the 2005–2010 Mustang V-6 (PN 82242). These are all big sellers, especially when combined with the ZEX electronic throttle-position sensor (TPS) and the ZEX advanced-design Nitrous Management Unit, which replaces the fuel and nitrous solenoids used by competing brands.

ZEX also markets sprayer kits for Chevrolet's LS- and LM-series engines. These include kits like the LSX Nitrous System for GM LS1-LS7 engines (PN 82235-75-175), the Gen-III LS1-LS6 High Output Nitrous System with an advertised power increase of 100 to 250 hp (PN 82087), and the Silverado Nitrous System (75- to 125-hp) for 1999-and-later 4.8L, 5.3L, and 6.0L GM Vortec V-8-powered Chevrolet trucks and SUVs (PN 82231).

ZEX offers three Mopar sprayer nitrous-kit applications, which all feature a special 58-psi high-pressure fuel system with revised jetting. Leading off is the ZEX 75- to 125-hp Hemi Truck Nitrous System (PN 82176), designed for the 2003-and-later Chrysler Hemi-engine trucks. Then there's the company's Charger/Magnum/Chrysler 300-C Nitrous Kit (PN 82177), which delivers 75 to 125 hp to 5.7L/6.1L Hemi engines. And this kit also fits 6.1L SRT8 engines, producing an advertised 500-plus hp! Now SRT8 Hemi-Jeep Grand Cherokee enthusiasts can take advantage of ZEX's 75- to 125-hp kit (PN 82241).

Nitrous Oxide Systems

Nitrous Oxide Systems offers a generic single-sprayer Power Fogger system for V-8 engines in 75-, 100-, and 125-hp settings in either standard, eight-cylinder EFI (PN 05131NOS), or Drive-By-Wire EFI applications (PN 05135NOS). Then there's the NOS 75- to 100-hp kit for 1994-to-current 3.4L/3.8L V-6 (PN 05175NOS), the LT1 Camaro/Firebird EFI kit (PN 05176NOS), the LT1 Camaro/Firebird with 58-mm NOS Throttle Body EFI kit (PN 05176TNOS), the 2.8L/3.4L V-6 TPI (PN 05120NOS), and the all-years Duramax Diesel EFI nitrous kit (PN 02519NOS).

The NOS 75- to 150-hp Ford EFI systems begin with a Power Stroke Diesel kit for all years (PN 02159NOS), the Stage 1 5.0L Mustang kit (PN 05115NOS), and Stage 2 5.0L Mustang kit, which contains a high-volume fuel pump. Also note that NOS offers a pair of Stage 1 to Stage 2 5.0L Conversion Kits, (PNs 0015NOS and 0016NOS, respectively) with the second being an accessory kit including a nitrous pressure gauge, fuel pressure gauge, nitrous bottle heater, progressive nitrous controller, and NOS purge valve. NOS also offers a 1996–1998 2V/4V SOHC/DOHC Kit (PN 05171NOS), and a 1999–2002 2V SOHC engine kit (PN 05116NOS).

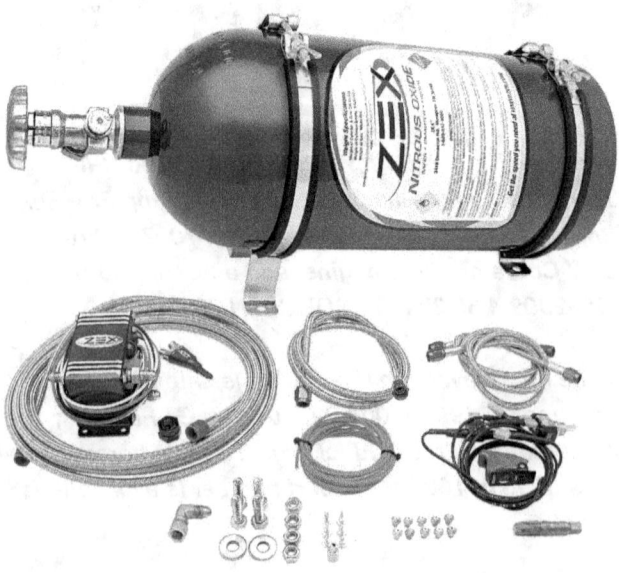

ZEX LSX wet-spray nitrous system is adjustable from 75 to 175 hp and fits LS1 LS2, LS6, and LS7 engines (PN 82307) and features a ZEX Wet Nitrous Management Unit. Note: This kit may also interface with certain GM LM-Series truck engines. Check with the manufacturer.

EFI, WET AND DRY

Nitrous Express

The Nitrous Express Fly-By-Wire Stage 1 EFI sprayer kits are quickly becoming the company's best sellers. To date, V-8 applications include a Universal Fly By Wire Kit (PN 20919), and a Chrysler SRT8 and Hemi System (PN 20918-10), shown being installed in Chapter 9, and a 2010 Camaro Single Nozzle System Fly-By-Wire Kit (PN 20930). All NX Fly-By-Wire Systems include NX's patented Shark Nozzle, your choice of a 5-, 10-, 15-, or 20-pound composite bottle, stainless-steel bottle brackets, an NX-exclusive Autolearn TPS Switch, a pair of Lightning Solenoids, and N_2O line.

The NX Stage 1 EFI Nitrous Systems are for all other applications ranging from a 35- to 150-hp Universal EFI kit (PN 20915), 35- to 150-hp GM All EFI kit (PN 20920), the NX Dodge All EFI 35- to 150-hp kit (PN 20921), and the All Ford 35- to 150-hp EFI kit (PN 20922). NX also offers 35- to 250-hp Race EFI kits for Ford and GM (PNs 20113 and 20118, respectively). NX TBI kits include All GM 35- to 150-hp (PN 20118), and Dodge TBI (PN 20213).

Dual-nozzle systems are also available from Nitrous Express for Ford, GM, and Dodge/Dodge Viper applications. The company also offers similar applications for dual-stage EFI setups, which are not to be confused with dual-nozzle setups because the dual-stage features quad solenoids for the two separate stages of N_2O being applied.

Wilson Nitrous Pro-Flow

Wilson Nitrous Pro-Flow markets a 2005–2006 sprayer application for the 4.6L three-valve mod-motor Mustang V-8 (PN 308710), which produces up to 200 hp. Also note that this kit can be adapted to fit the 2008–2010 4.6L three-valve engines with a slight modification to the solenoid brackets.

When installing any sprayer nozzle N_2O kit, placement of the sprayer nozzle into the air intake tube is absolutely critical. The nozzle must be located dead center to the throttle body, especially in twin-bore throttle body applications like the 2001 Mustang Bullitt, so that the sprayer directs the flow of both fuel and nitrous in an even plume pattern; this avoids a lean condition.

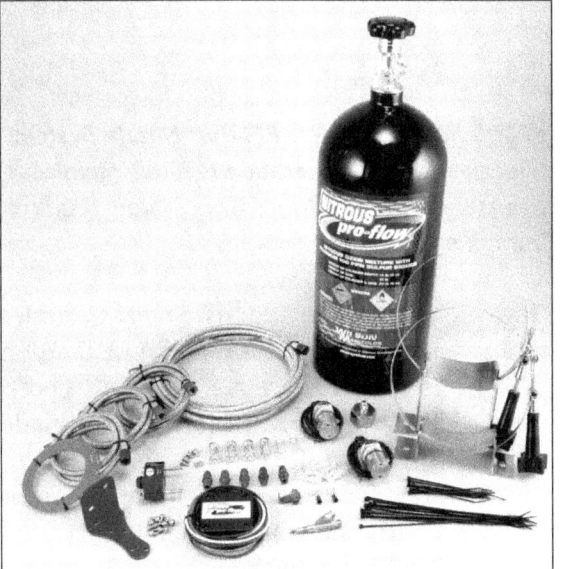

Wilson Manifolds & Nitrous Pro-Flow manufactures a 75- to 200-hp N_2O kit for the 4.6L, 2005–2006 SOHC 3V Mustang V-8s (PN 308710). With slightly modified solenoid brackets, this kit also fits the 4.6L, 2008–2010 3V Mustang modular motors.

Dry-Manifold Systems

The third-place usage category is the dry-manifold nitrous oxide system. It's called that because the fuel nozzles are placed directly into the intake ports of the intake manifold with absolutely no fuel/nitrous mixture going through the intake plenum. The dry manifold approach has become very popular on today's high-tech engines and, due to its design, is less visually detectable. The top nitrous kit manufacturers offer "straight wet," meaning single-nozzle design, or "wet/dry," meaning both nitrous and fuel EFI kits.

Edelbrock

Edelbrock Nitrous offers a 40- to 80-hp Universal wet/dry kit (PN 71820), or 50- to 70-hp Universal Wet Kit with return-style fuel line (PN 71000). Specific applications also include a Ford Performer EFI Dry kit and a GM Performer EFI wet/dry kit. Edelbrock also offers Super Victor Direct Port universal nitrous systems in three E-Series Power Nozzles: Super Victor four-cylinder (PNs 71835/6), Super Victor V-8 (PNs 71831/71850/71852), and E-Power Nozzle applications. Finally, there's the Edelbrock Super Victor V-8 Direct Port nitrous kit with E3 nozzle (PN 71848).

Nitrous Oxide Systems

Nitrous Oxide Systems offers two 100- to 300-hp MPFI applications for the 4.6L SOHC Ford Mustang: Deluxe (PN 08100NOS) and Standard (PN 08101NOS). Nitrous Oxide Systems also offers an F-Body LS1 Dry NOSzle Direct Port EFI Kit (PN 08301NOS).

CHAPTER 9

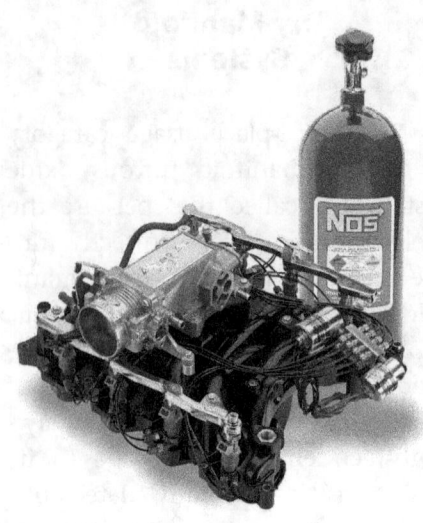

Nitrous Oxide Systems offers two 100- to 300-hp Multi Port Fuel Injection MPFI applications for the 1996–2004 4.6L Ford Mod-Motor Mustang: Standard (PN 08101NOS) and Deluxe (PN 8100NOS). The difference is that the latter includes a fuel safety switch, electronic WOT switch, and a window switch for added safely. While these kits are capable of delivering an adjustable 100 to 300 hp, anything over 150 hp is not recommended without modifying the engine internally as well as upgrading the stock fuel system.

ZEX Nitrous Products

EFI Dry Kit applications from ZEX Nitrous Products (a division of Competition Cams) run from A to V—Acura to Volkswagen. For hardcore American V-8 aficionados, there are dry applications for the 1993–1996 Chevrolet Corvette (PN 82018/82018P). Then there are ZEX's 1986–1994 5.0L Mustang kits (PN 82015/82015S), and a 1993–1997 Pontiac Firebird/Trans Am dry application (PN 82014/82014P). All of these kits offer 75 to 125 hp. Also on the table is ZEX's Small-Block Chevrolet Direct Port Nitrous System, offering 75 to 300 hp (PN 82062), and a Big-Block Chevrolet Direct Port Nitrous System (PN 82063).

Nitrous Express

Nitrous Express (NX) made a name for itself with its exclusive patented nozzle, solenoid, jet, and bottle valve designs. The NX nozzles are recognized for their outstanding atomization capabilities with both fuel and nitrous. The solenoids made by NX are also of an exclusive design, and boast only one 90-degree turn in their design. NX claims that reduced turbulence in the flow path through

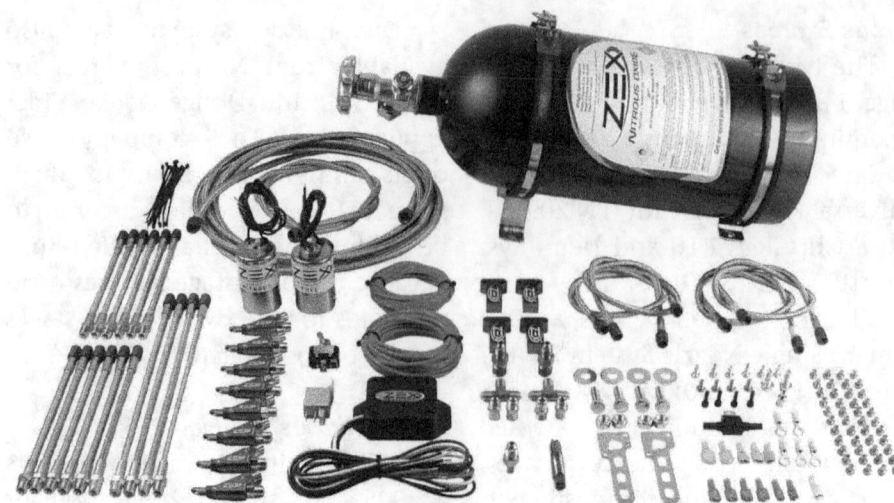

ZEX Nitrous Products offers a Chevrolet Small-Block Direct Port Nitrous System (PN 82062) and is fully adjustable from 75 to 300 hp. ZEX also offers a Chevrolet Big-Block Direct-Port application (PN 82063), also fully adjustable from 75 to 300 hp.

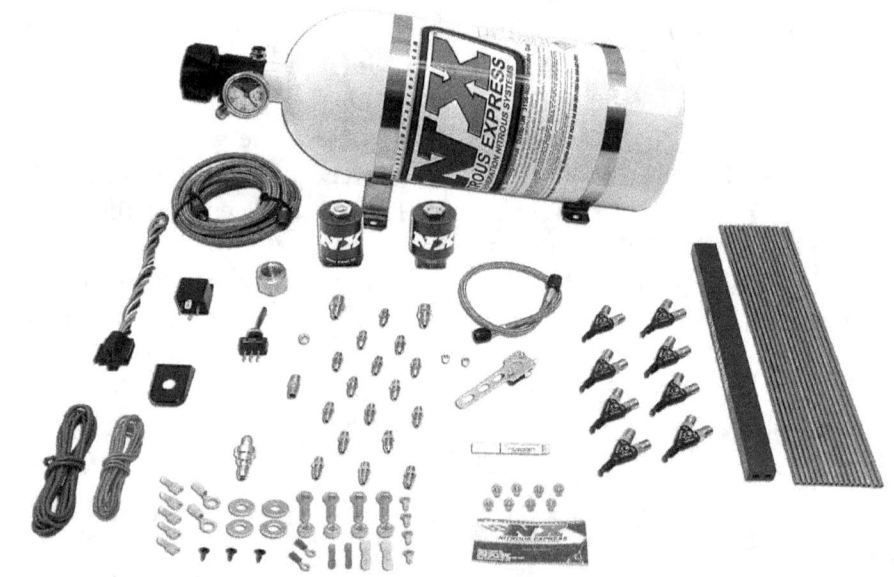

Nitrous Express' adjustable 50- to 300-hp LT1/LT4 Pro EFI Port Nozzle System (PN 80010) features NX Piranha Nozzles, a next-generation fuel rail, stainless-steel hard lines, and all the necessary electrical hardware. This system requires the drilling and tapping of the LT1 intake.

Mustang Illustrated, Fall 1987: Small-Block Nitrous Shootout EFI Versus Holley

What better way to test a product like Nitrous Oxide Systems' new 75- to 100-hp Fogger EFI for the EEC-IV-governed 5.0L Mass Air Flow Mustang pushrod V-8 engine than to pit it against your own top-of-the-line carbureted system or, in this case, systems? That's exactly what happened in Fall 1987 when Nitrous Oxide Systems resident dyno-tech Louie Hammel tested a 1985-model 5.0L 302 4V small-block Ford V-8 engine (the last of the line of carbureted Ford small-blocks) against a 1987 5.0L Ford EFI small-block.

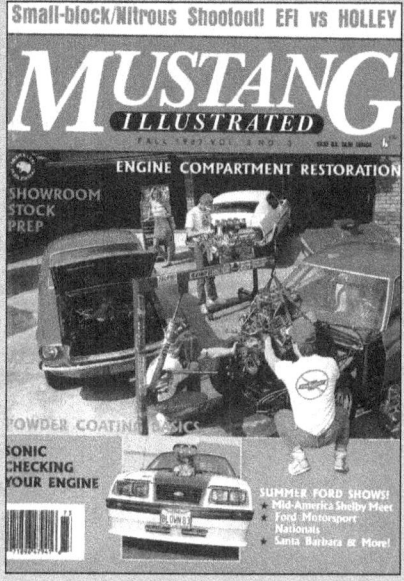

The data gained from this shootout might very well have signified a changing of the guard, so it was determined that both Nitrous Oxide Systems' Top Shot and Power Shot 5.0L street nitrous systems be given, well, a fair shot!

Prior to installing either of the kits, a baseline was achieved using NOS' Superflow dyno. In stock form, the factory rating on Ford's 1985 vintage 5.0L was an advertised 205 hp. However, numbers can sometimes be deceiving.

Superflow Dyno Baseline

RPM	Torque	Horsepower
2,000	266	101
2,500	275	131
3,000	280	160
3,500	291	194
4,000	283	216
4,500	264	226
5,000	233	222

Carbureted With 75- to 150-hp Top Shot Module

RPM	Torque	Horsepower
2,500	396	188
3,000	378	216
3,500	365	243
4,000	347	264
4,500	273	234

Carbureted With 100- to 150-hp Power Shot System

RPM	Torque	Horsepower
2,500	423	201
3,000	412	235
3,500	400	266
4,000	376	286
4,500	347	297

Stock 5.0L 302 EFI Factory-Rated at 225-hp

RPM	Torque	Horsepower
2,000	276	105
2,500	288	137
3,000	298	170
3,500	293	195
4,000	275	210
4,500	246	211

5.0L EFI With 75 to 100 NOS Wet Fogger Nozzle

RPM	Torque	Horsepower
3,000	433	253
4,000	376	285
4,500	338	290

Mustang Illustrated magazine editors concluded that installing these systems onto the respective carbureted and fuel injected Ford small-blocks produced noticeable horsepower gains of approximately 33 percent. And because that peak horsepower between the Power Shot–equipped carbureted 5.0L Ford V-8 engine and the Fogger-equipped 5.0L EFI V-8 engine was within 7, the one-year-old MAF-governed 5.0L Ford EFI small-block system had plenty of growth potential. Obviously, this has been illustrated time and time again over the past 25-plus years.

CHAPTER 9

Common EFI Fuel System

By Adam Campbell, former technical advisor at The Nitrous Works

When setting up an EFI fuel system, complete with a supplemental inline fuel pump, fuel inlet, and fuel return lines, there are a number of common misconceptions and/or mistakes that people often make. Along with advice and comments, the following are some of the typical reasons for bad assembly results.

Not Following the Manufacturer's Recommendations

This includes substituting components and plumbing. Quite often a customer questions the line size specification called for in the plumbing chart. Improvising is also a problem; technicians are constantly being asked, "The diagram says it has to be mounted here, but why can't I mount it there?"

Restrictive Plumbing

Due to lack of space under certain cars, an installer may get line-happy and use too many 45- and 90-degree fittings. Heck, on some cars, I've even seen 180-degree bends.

Match your line size with pump volume. Running a big pump with standard-size or under-size fuel lines—in an effort to save money, or because it may be all you have—could spell real trouble. Line size should match the specification called for in the directions provided with the pump. Remember, you want your fuel and return lines to be as free flowing as possible.

Too Small a Vent or None at All

Most owners expect the stock vent on their fuel tank and/or vent feature on their gas cap to provide proper ventilation for a high-pressure EFI system; but it doesn't work and here's why. Let's say you have a 5-gallon gas can and you start to pour the fuel out of it. What happens if you place your finger over the vent? Fuel flow slows to a trickle or stops entirely. This is the same principle with either a gas tank or a fuel cell. You can have the best pump in the world but, if you cannot get the air into the tank or cell to displace the fuel, it overworks the pump and reduces the volume of fuel that the pump is supplying to the fuel regulator.

Faulty Return Line Plumbing

In an effort to save time and money, I've seen situations where owners run their return line back into the bottom of the sump of the tank, right next to the bulkhead area they are using for the fuel feed. Think about this for a moment! Most electric fuel pumps are pusher pumps and they are not designed to pull, meaning they need to be gravity fed. Mounting the pump lower than the outlet on either a gas tank or fuel cell achieves this. But when you take your return line (which is under pressure) and plumb it right next to where your gravity-feed line is, you start pushing the fuel away from the pickup. This creates all kinds of fuel delivery problems, with pump cavitation being the greatest of them.

Other issues include the actual length of a fuel return line. A full-length return line must be properly sized to return fuel in the most efficient manner, meaning that it must be pressure regulated. Too small a return line can restrict flow and volume, which exerts excess pressure at the fuel bypass. Also when a full-length return line is used, it must be plumbed into the top of the fuel cell or gas tank but cannot return fuel below the existing level of stored fuel in the tank. Otherwise, the low pressure of fuel in the return line could cause problems in regulating the fuel pressure. With fuel pumps that utilize a return line directly on the fuel pump, the return line is still run to the top of the tank or fuel cell but it must also extend down into the fuel supply far enough to avoid aerating the existing fuel supply.

Race Pumps on Street Cars

Fuel pumps that are rated for Competition Use Only should not be used in street applications for continuous duty. Several aftermarket manufacturers offer very-high-volume fuel pumps that are not intended for normal street driving due to the excess heat these situations can generate. In addition to the heat emanating from the pavement, high-volume and deadhead-style fuel systems also create a lot of heat internally. They can heat up both the fuel and the pump, creating delivery issues and eventual pump failure. Consequently, high-volume dual-purpose pumps can also suffer from the same issues when improperly plumbed or when improperly installed.

Mistakes and Misconceptions

But there is a wide variety of Continuous Duty Cycle street fuel pumps on the market. They are designed to operate inline, complementing the existing fuel delivery system, in-tank, working in concert with the existing OE fuel pump. In some rarer cases they operate as a completely dedicated independent system with the latter being generally for custom-assembled, nitrous-assisted fuel systems, and/or all-out competition use.

Mismatched Parts

This is a common problem when upgrading any fuel system—mixing existing components with new ones. Generally speaking, fuel system components and line sizes need to be matched for a specific application and horsepower range. Let's say your old engine produced 500 hp and your fuel pump and regulator were rated at 650 cfm. But after, let's say, the introduction of nitrous oxide, a turbocharger, or a supercharger your engine is capable of producing 800 hp. Simply changing out the fuel pump for a bigger one does not adequately supply the new combination because the fuel regulator and fuel line sizes need to be changed as well.

Some situations have arisen where there is an existing bypass regulator and a fuel pump with an internal bypass (or one that has its own bypass) located directly off where the pump is installed. In the latter situation, you are now faced with two return lines, prompting the installer to plug one. Neither of these components was intended to be used in this manner, and now you have a problem. When in doubt, call the manufacturer.

Upgrading the Fuel Pump but Not the Lines

A fuel pump with increased volume capability also requires a larger volume of fuel supplied to its inlet side. Electric fuel pumps should always be fed with a line that is one size larger than the one that runs forward in order to avoid pump cavitations. Fuel volume and fuel pressure are not directly related, and fuel pressure can often be confused with having adequate fuel volume. Yes, it is possible to show adequate fuel pressure yet still have inadequate fuel volume.

Another common misconception, when installing a fuel pump that requires a larger feed line than the tank or fuel cell is equipped with, is that two smaller lines can be run in tandem. The aim is to feed the pump and provide more volume because flow is increased when the lines' volumes are combined. This is simply not the case. In fact, it is possible that one line can (for any number of reasons) run dry, thereby cavitating the pump, and causing a loss in volume.

Debris in Newly Fabricated Fuel Lines

When fabricating new fuel inlet and return lines, always flush them out prior to actually hooking them up to the remaining components in your fuel system. All it takes is the slightest piece of debris to affect the internal workings of an electric fuel pump, fuel pressure regulator, or fuel injector. Once new lines are installed into the system, always check for leaks, and immediately repair any if found. Teflon tape is not recommended, as even the smallest wayward particle can find its way into a fuel pump or fuel regulator. If you must use a sealer, use a Teflon paste, and only in very small amounts.

Fuel Lines Too Close to the Exhaust

Running fuel lines too close to headers or the exhaust system is downright dangerous. When fuel becomes overheated, it vaporizes or percolates the fuel, causing a vapor lock that stalls the engine—and that's the best-case scenario. With high-pressure EFI systems, if a fuel line fed by a high-pressure fuel pump fails, a fire is almost a guarantee. Fuel lines should be kept as far away from a heat source as possible and, when in doubt, use a thermal heat wrap.

No Fuel Filter or a Very Restrictive One

Always use a fuel filter with any high-performance fuel system. Gas tanks contain fuel sediments that can break free from the surface of the tank and work their way into the fuel line. If not for a fuel filter, this foreign debris ends up clogging your high-dollar fuel pump, fuel pressure regulator, or, even worse, clogs a fuel injector. The same thing can be said for running a fuel cell. The foam rubber inside a cell can deteriorate over time, and the fuel filter becomes

CHAPTER 9

Common Mistakes and Misconceptions CONTINUED

a failsafe. Remember, it's always cheaper to replace a fuel filter than it is a pump, fuel pressure regulator, or an entire engine.

Restrictive fuel filters can also cause delivery problems and premature pump failure. If the inlet side of the fuel pump does not get enough volume of fuel it can cavitate. For example, a fuel pump is rated at 280 gph, while the fuel filter is only rated at 130 gph. Based on those numbers, what do you think occurs? The fuel filter restricts fuel delivery.

Another misconception concerns the micron rating of a fuel filter. It is a common misconception that the higher the number, the superior the filtering properties. This is not the case; the micron rating describes the size of the particle that can pass through the filter. An 8-micron fuel filter has much better filtering capabilities than one rated at 80 microns, for example.

No Relay or Inadequate Wiring

Installing a higher-volume fuel pump energized by existing OE electrical wiring may be courting disaster. It's not that it can't be done, but it is not recommended. Always follow the manufacturer's recommendations when it comes to providing the proper amount of voltage or it can affect overall fuel pump performance and damage the unit over time. Many older-model cars were wired with fuel pump relays in the dash as opposed to in the rear by the pump. Using existing wiring can create a voltage drop to the pump and create issues like low pump pressures, blown fuses, and melted wires.

The best way to use a relay is to run a wire from the battery to the relay, then from the relay to the pump and use the switch in the car (instead of the pump) to turn the relay on. When this circuit is complete, it allows the battery sufficient voltage to have the shortest run to the pump for maximum volume and pump efficiency. A 12-gauge wire is generally recommended for the power feed on a pump and a 16-gauge wire is recommended for the switch wiring to the relay.

Warning: Not using a relay at all eliminates the failsafe in the system, possibly melting the wiring or even causing an electrical fire!

Switching from EFI to Carburetion

Converting an EFI car to carburetion may look easy, but there is a lot more to it than you may think. EFI systems traditionally use smaller-diameter higher-pressure fuel lines, which do not work well with carbureted fuel pumps. Conversely, lower-pressure larger-diameter fuel lines, traditionally used on carbureted applications, don't work well either. Then, of course, you have the whole engine-management picture to consider as well. A word to the wise: don't do it!

---

its solenoids is worth power. The exclusive bottle valve design is also well regarded for its excellent flow characteristics. By getting more measurable power gains from similarly-sized components, efficiency is NX's claim to fame.

Nitrous Express offers a 50- to 300-hp LT1/LT4 Pro EFI System port nozzle application under PN 80010.

Nitrous Supply

Although Nitrous Supply does not offer a specific LT1/LT4 or LS1-LSW7 dry-intake-system kit per se, the company will build one for you.

Also note that some of the more sophisticated N_2O setups, particularly the dry systems, may call for a fuel injector upgrade to provide adequate fuel delivery/fuel pressure to the system, especially in the higher horsepower ranges. Quite typically, stock EFI systems operate at 35 to 40 psi. But some of these kits may require as much at 80 psi, so check with the manufacturer if you need to perform a fuel injector upgrade.

Electronic Fuel Injectors

Whenever you increase airflow capacity in an internal combustion engine as with nitrous oxide, it is necessary to induce more fuel into the induction system to maintain the proper air/fuel ratio (AFR). How do you do that? You upgrade to larger-volume fuel injectors!

OE fuel injection systems are either Mass Air Flow or Speed Density designs. With a mass-air-flow system, the mass air sensor (MAS) measures the mass of air being inducted into the engine via an electronically-heated platinum sensor wire inside the mass airflow meter. The wire sends a signal to the electronic control module (ECM), which is simultaneously measuring throttle position sensor (TPS) and O_2 sensor readouts. The ECM processes all of this data (these systems are termed self-compensating) and ultimately fires the electronic fuel injector. A Mass Air Flow system can adapt to atmospheric conditions, and subsequently make the necessary adjustments or changes in the engine rather quickly, which makes them ideally suited for day-to-day driving conditions.

A Speed Density system uses the speed of the engine, the density of the air, and the manifold vacuum airflow, or volumetric efficiency (VE), to process information via a preprogrammed fuel map. This process is officially known as mapping and functions on an overall average. As a result, the computer's calculations are based on the map of VEs. Most aftermarket EFI systems offer a range of performance options other than OE, such as changing the exhaust, installing a supercharger or turbocharger, and, yes, adding nitrous oxide. Speed Density appears to be the most popular of the two from a high-performance perspective because it re-maps, incorporating those changes into the system.

But remember that the size (fuel injectors are rated in pounds per hour at a specific fuel pressure) and type (ohm-resistance rating) of fuel injector upgrade chosen must be compatible with the car's Electronic Control Module (ECM), or you can fry the drivers in the ECM! There are two kinds of electronic fuel-injector control circuits (drivers): Saturated (high impedance, designed to function on a certain voltage, like those used on OE) and Peak and Hold (low-impedance/low-current).

Saturated

There are myriad electronic fuel injectors on the market, manufactured by the likes of Bosch, Denso, Ford Motorcraft, Lucas, MSD, RC Engineering, Rochester, etc., and choosing the proper fuel injector can be a tricky proposition.

For example, in street applications—situations where you drive your car on a daily basis—the 12-volt, high-resistance Saturated-type injector is used because it maintains a low current flow in the injectors and drivers to keep them cool and promote longer life. Though response time is slower and less suited for high-performance applications, they are still suitable for nitrous. In fact, the Saturated type may be just the right thing for, let's say, a street-driven 5.0L Mustang equipped with an 80-100-125-hp dry N_2O kit.

Of course upgrading to a larger fuel injector usually requires a larger-volume fuel pump. The static flow rate changes if the fuel pressure is increased, and either re-flashing or installing an aftermarket high-performance computer chip is also required. Check with the N_2O kit manufacturer for recommendations.

Peak and Hold

Fuel injection systems that are intended for racing use peak-and-hold fuel injectors, which operate on 12 volts but feature low resistance through a high current driver circuit. The peak current is used to kick or lift the injector off its seat quickly; then the lower current holds it open until the ECM closes it. There are two basic drivers used in peak-and-hold injectors: the 4-amp peak/1-amp hold and the 2-amp peak/0.5-amp hold. Both have a quicker response and a longer duty-cycle time—up 7.5 milliseconds, or a 75-percent-longer duty cycle—which is perfect for nitrous.

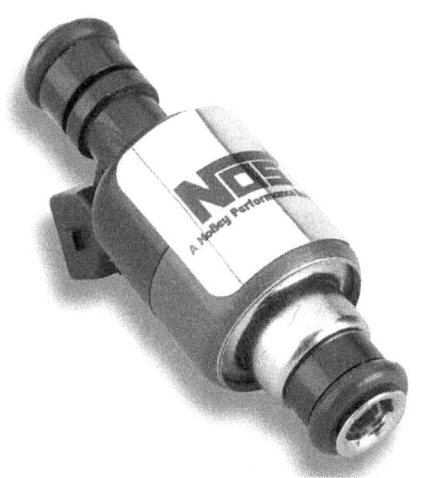

Here is a shot of a Nitrous Oxide Systems High Volume electronic fuel injector, which is available in all popular applications.

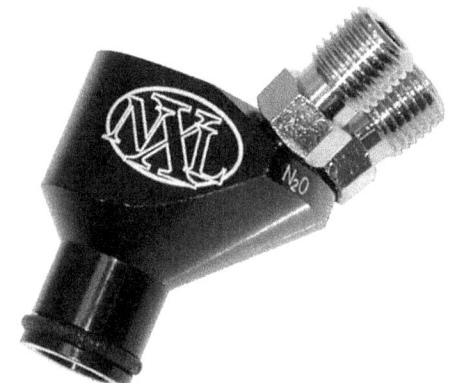

Although not considered an actual electronic fuel injector itself, Nitrous Express "GM/Ford NXL Nozzle (PN 75001) allows "nitrous-ites" the option of injecting pre-jetted quantities of both N_2O and fuel directly into the fuel injector port of the engine. This wet-nozzle setup can be used as a standalone, or in conjunction with an air intake sprayer nozzle or throttle body plate system. Pretty cool, eh?

CHAPTER 9

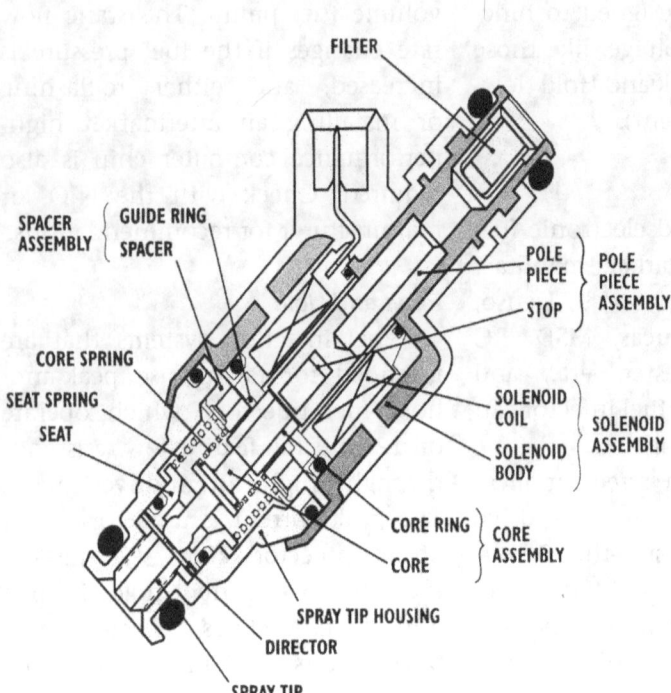

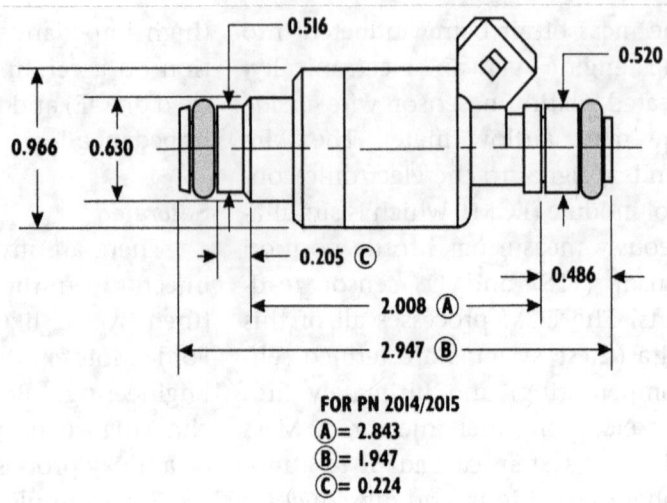

This illustration shows the overall dimensions of an "average" domestic and Honda-specific electronic fuel injector. It's hard to believe that such a small component (you can conceal one in the palm of your hand) does such a phenomenal job delivering expertly timed and precise doses of fuel from 30 to 109 lb/hr pressure flow ratings!

This cutaway drawing, which applies to an MSD "Domestic Application" electronic competition fuel injector (available in 4/1A/2 ohm Peak and Hold Driver, in 75 lb/hr and 96 lb/hr applications) and to a Saturated 12V/12 ohm Circuit Driver electronic fuel injectors (available in 50 lb/hr saturated and 38 lb/hr applications), clearly shows its precise internal construction. These MSD injectors feature stainless-steel ball-and-seat metering, which creates maximum internal sealing. MSD's Multec metering design produces superior fuel charge flow for consistent fuel delivery at any RPM. A six-hole injector metering orifice produces a totally atomized and compact 10- to 15-degree spray pattern. Fuel flow rates are set and calibrated during manufacturing, and recessed delivery holes resist fuel clogging and injector formation so cleaning is required. Most domestic electronic fuel injectors pretty much share this design. Fuel injection longevity, quality, and performance are generally distinguished by quality of materials and workmanship in construction.

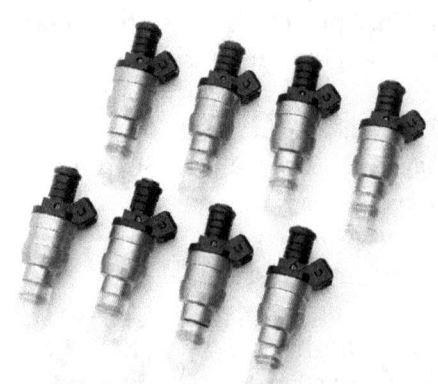

Ford Racing offers a total of nine high-impedance "EV-Series" electronic fuel injector upgrades for its 302-351W Pushrod V-8 and 4.6L SOHC 2-, 3-valve, and 4.6L to 5.4L DOHC four-valve V-8 engines. Flow ratings range from 24 to 80 lb/hr at 11-12-18 ohms on USCAR applications, and 11-18 ohms on Jetronic/Minitimer all-injector flow rates are quoted at a delta pressure of 39.15 psi. When converting to a delta pressure of 43.5 psi, multiply the flow rate by 1.054.

This cutaway view of an NOS electronic fuel injector branded as the "NOSzle" clearly shows the inner workings of the injector. Applications include the 1996-2004 Ford 2V mod motor when used with NOS 100-300 Adjustable HP systems as well as a GM LS1 F-Body NOSzle Direct Port EFI application power rated at 125 to 300 hp.

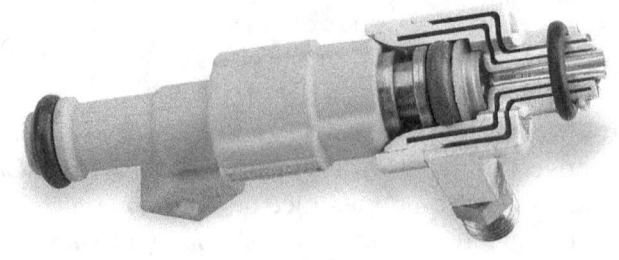

HOW TO INSTALL AND TUNE NITROUS OXIDE SYSTEMS

EFI, WET AND DRY

Project: Nitrous Express 2010 Camaro SS Single-Stage Plate Installation

The Zeta II Global rear-wheel-drive-platform 2010 Chevrolet Camaro SS runs pretty well, but with its heavy curb weight (3,800 pounds) the new Gen-V leaves many Camaro enthusiasts wanting more power. Increased performance and quick acceleration is easy to get thanks to the folks at Nitrous Express, Inc. The following steps outline the installation of the Nitrous Express LS3/LS9 2010 Camaro V Single-Stage Plate System (PN 20931-XX). Nitrous Express has combined performance, quality, and ease of installation with this Fly By Wire Stage 1 Plate kit featuring NS-patented Spray Bar-less Technology.

The NX 2010 Camaro system includes a pre-terminated wiring harness that makes installation quick and visually appealing, a 10-pound aluminum bottle, a pair of stainless-steel bottle brackets, an NX Auto Learn electronic throttle-position sensor (the TPS switch allows the nitrous to be activated at WOT), a pair of Lightning Series Stage-1 solenoids, 15-foot-long braided stainless-steel N_2O line, a direct-plug-in 3/8-10-mm Billet Fuel Rail Adaptor to simplify installation (no need to cut any factory fuel lines), one of Nitrous Express' patented stainless-steel throttle-body plates, and an assortment of nitrous jets ranging from 35 to 150 hp (there is also an optional 200-hp jet). There is also an accessory and hardware kit, which includes an arming switch, nuts, bolts, 5/8-inch fittings, and a four-color installation manual. An NX Gen-V Camaro V-8 kit retails for about $880 through participating Nitrous Express retailers.

Shown here is the Nitrous Express Energy Drink 2010 Camaro SS being prepared for the SEMA Show where the Camaro was used as the centerpiece for Nitrous Express' corporate presentation. However, this car is by no means a trailer queen. Independent dyno tests using the NX 100-hp N_2O jet produced an increase of 105 hp and 130 ft-lbs of torque over stock. The following kit installation was performed by NX National Sales Manager Mike Abney, and photographed by NX Marketing Director Randall Mathis.

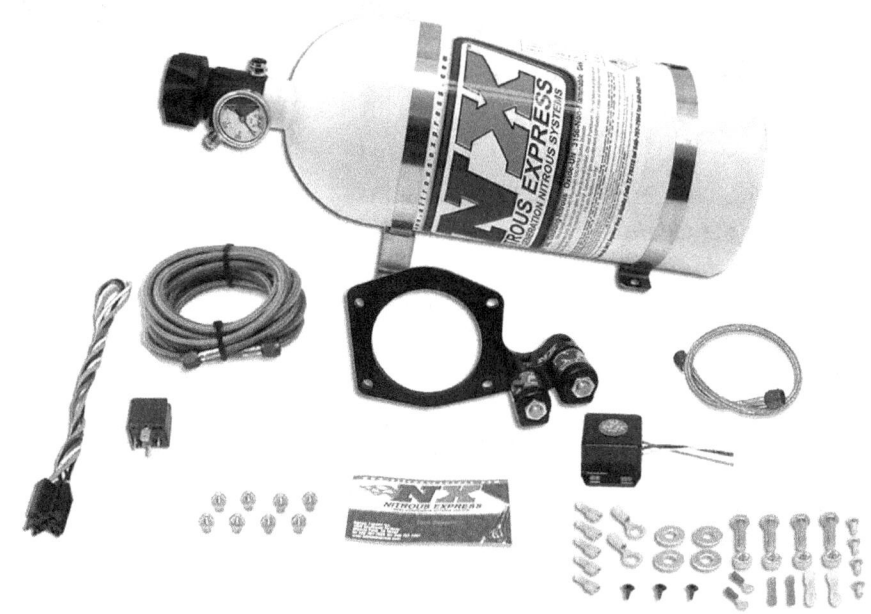

This is the Nitrous Express, Inc., 35- to 150-hp 2010–2011 Camaro Single-Stage Fly By Wire Stage 1 EFI system. The NX Camaro V-8 system includes a cutting-edge nitrous plate with integrated N_2O and fuel solenoids for maximum performance and a quick-and-easy installation.

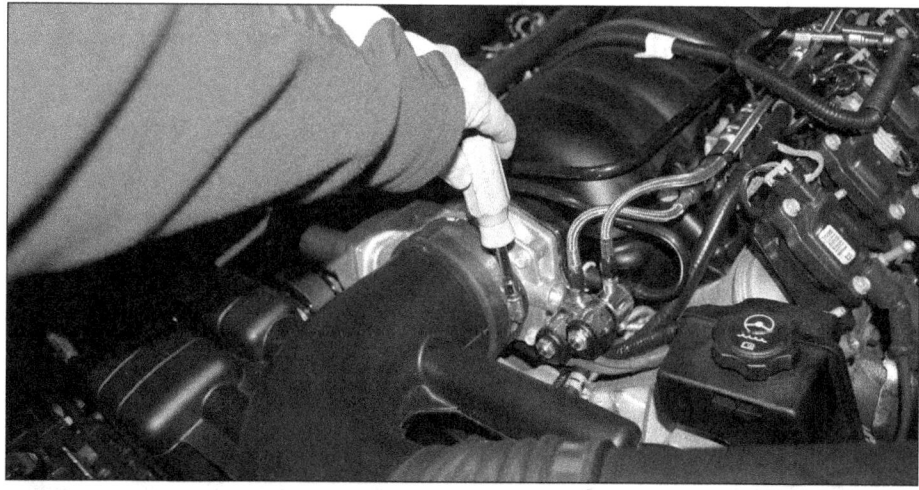

1 *Remove the engine cover, disconnect the battery, and remove the oil filler cap. Then remove the factory air intake tube from the throttle body using a common screw driver.*

HOW TO INSTALL AND TUNE NITROUS OXIDE SYSTEMS

CHAPTER 9

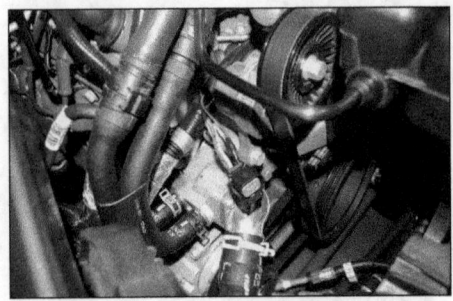
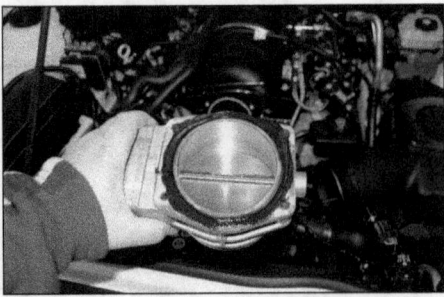
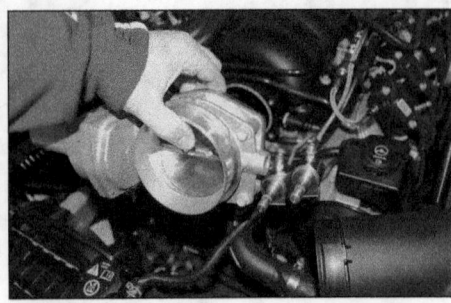

2 Unplug the electrical harness from the throttle body and remove the four 10-mm factory bolts that attach the throttle body to the upper air plenum.

3 Apply a thin bead of silicone to the throttle body mounting flange.

4 Install the NX Throttle Body Plate and dual solenoids between the LS3 throttle body and intake. Then re-install the four 10-mm factory bolts.

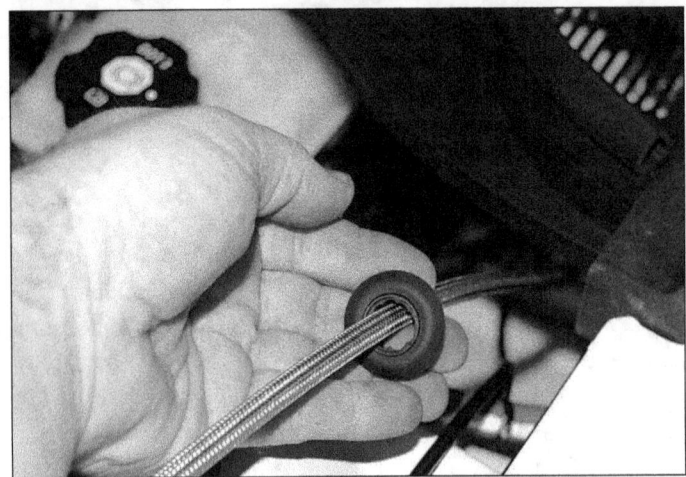
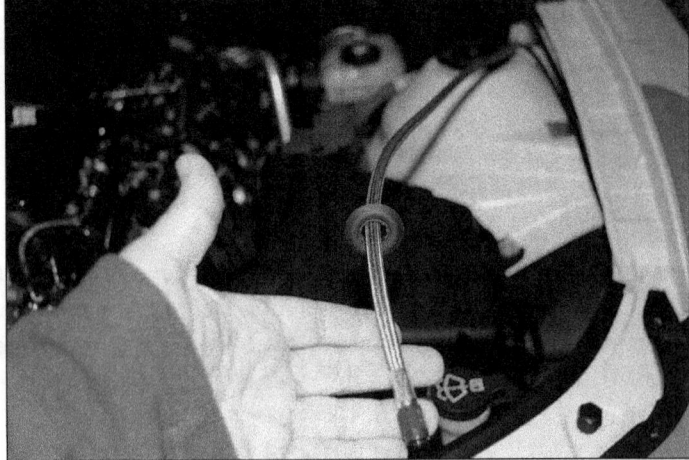

5 After the 15-foot-long braided stainless-steel nitrous supply line is run the length of the vehicle, locate the un-used rubber grommet on the driver's side of the firewall (above and to the right of the hood release cable). When the grommet is removed, enlarge the hole to 3/8 inch to accept the cable and the accompanying nitrous controller wires. To avoid any chafing or leakage, it is wise to tape the perimeter of the opening. Run the nitrous supply line from the nitrous solenoid along the top of the LS3 intake, through the firewall and insulation, and along the driver's-side plastic kick-panel/door-sill plate following NX instructions. Then route the line under the back seat cushion and out into the trunk area.

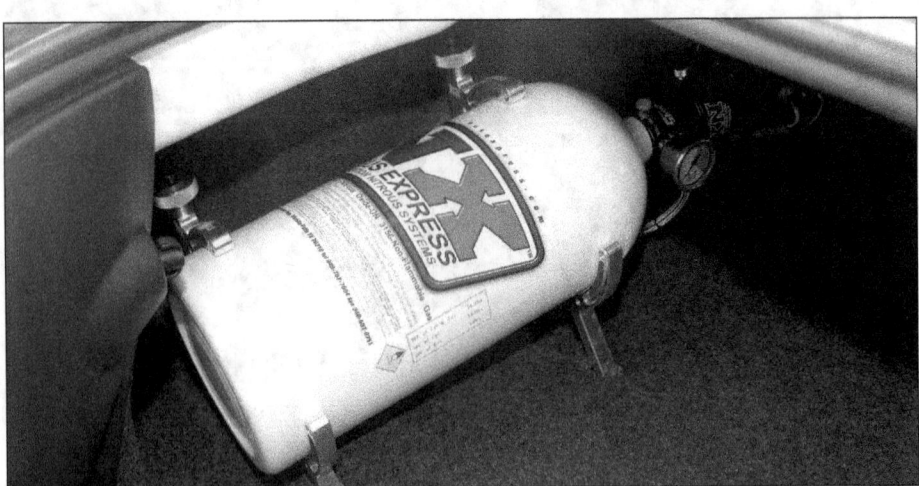

6 Bottle installation is as simple as setting up the bottle and brackets and marking the carpeting where the mounting holes are to be drilled on the driver's side of the trunk area. Drill a series of 5/16-inch holes, and then attach the bottle brackets using the supplied 5/16-inch bolts. Then attach the N_2O deliver line to the bottle using a 9/16-inch wrench.

EFI, WET AND DRY

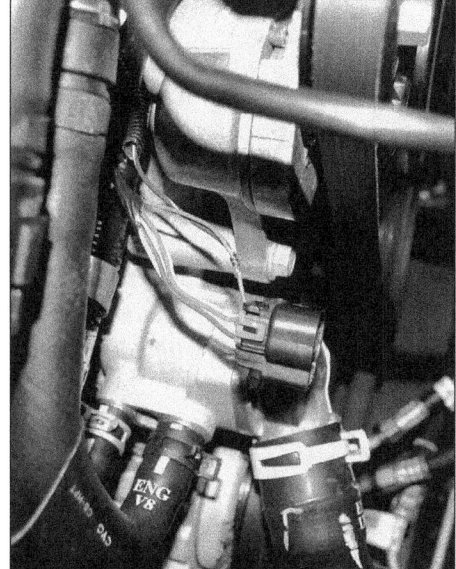

7 Now it's time to move on to the electrical hookups. Connect one ground wire from each solenoid directly to the chassis. First, run an 18-gauge wire to the purple wire on the Camaro TPS, and then route it through the previously mentioned opening made in the firewall.

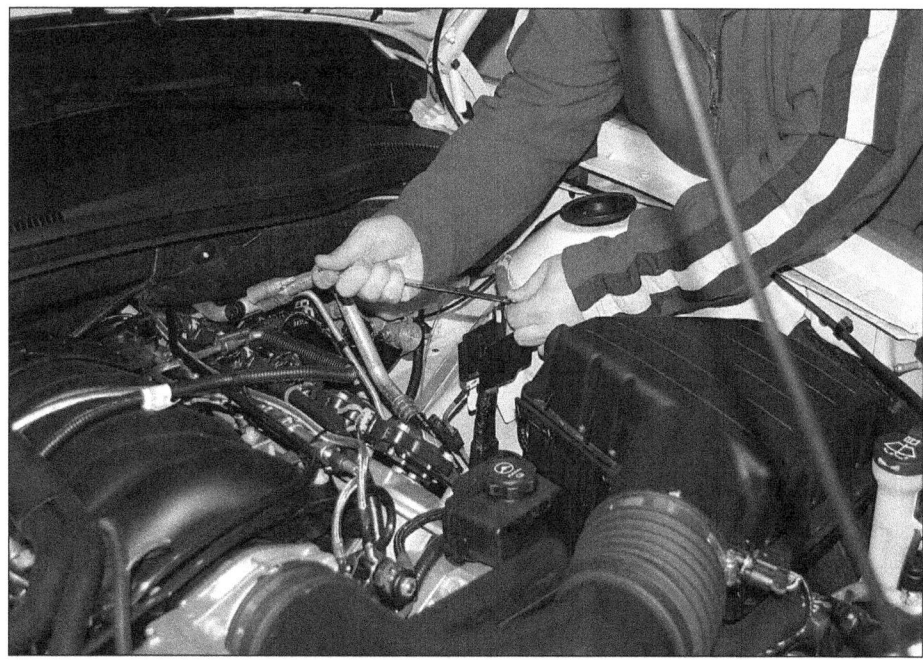

8 Wire the NX solenoid relay. Attach one ground wire from each solenoid to the green wire on the NX Relay Harness. The white wire on the NX Relay Harness goes to ground next. This can be done optionally through the Fuel Pressure Safety Switch. The black wire of the NX relay is connected to the positive battery stud on the driver's side of the engine bay, and an optional fuse link was employed.

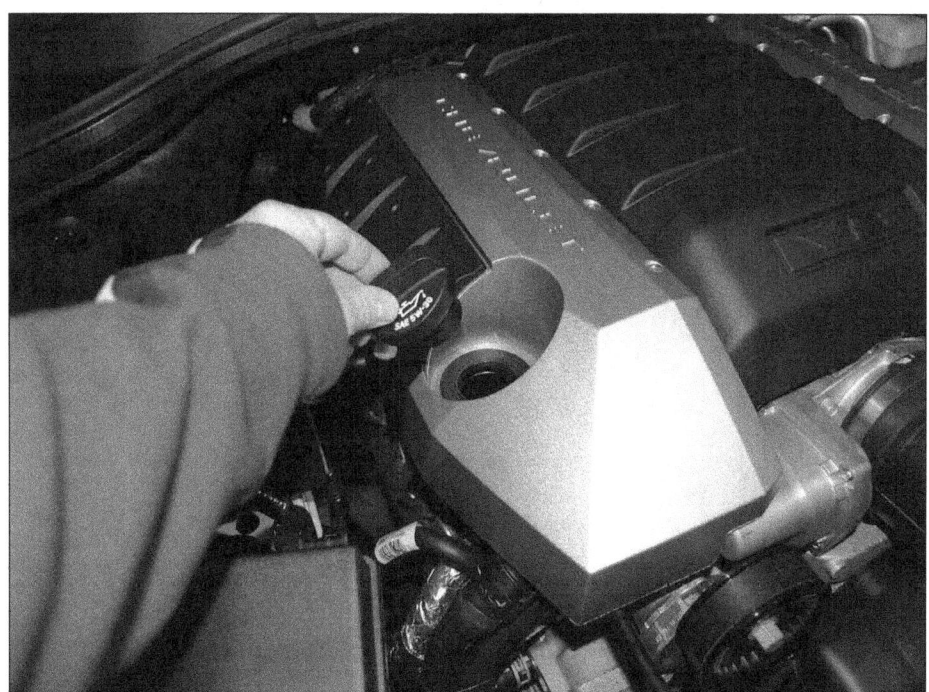

9 Next the red wire of the NX Relay Harness (the trigger wire) is run through the firewall grommet. Cover these wires with split-loom and electrical tape to achieve a clean, factory appearance. With everything done under the hood, replace the decorative LS3 plastic engine cover and oil cap.

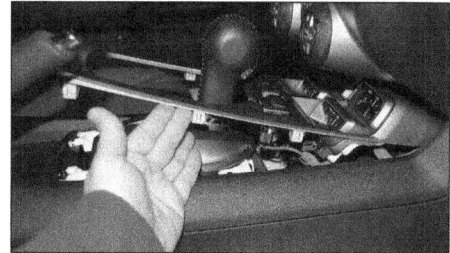

10 Moving to the interior of the car, lift the shifter trim panel to expose the factory wires leading to the electrical terminal plug for the cigarette lighter.

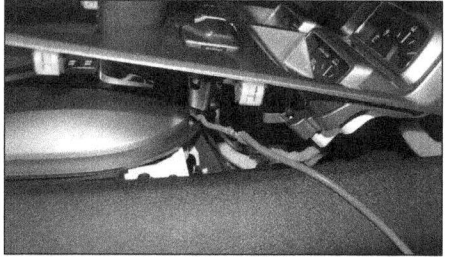

11 Splice an 18-gauge wire to the red wire leading to the cigarette lighter plug.

HOW TO INSTALL AND TUNE NITROUS OXIDE SYSTEMS

CHAPTER 9

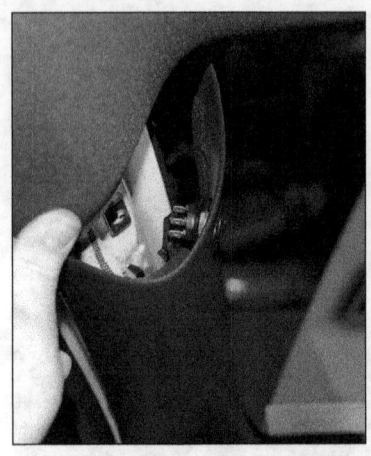
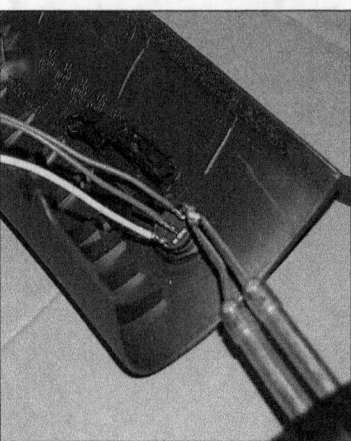

12 Route this wire behind the console and attach to the input wire of the Master Arming Switch; for this particular application our installers chose to place the actual Master Arming Switch (MAS) inside the A-pillar. The wire is run from the MAS to the red wire on the NX Throttle Position Activation Switch (TPAS). Next connect the pink wire of the NX TPAS to the red wire on the nitrous system relay and route through the firewall. Then attach the white wire on the NX TPAS to the purple wire from the TPAS. And finally, attach the black ground wire to a solid ground.

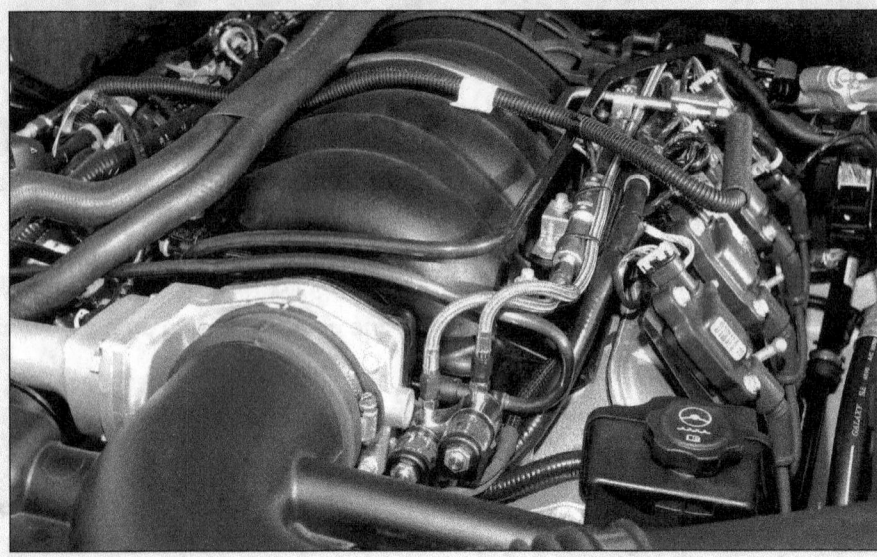

This is what the finished Nitrous Express LS3 Plate System looks like.

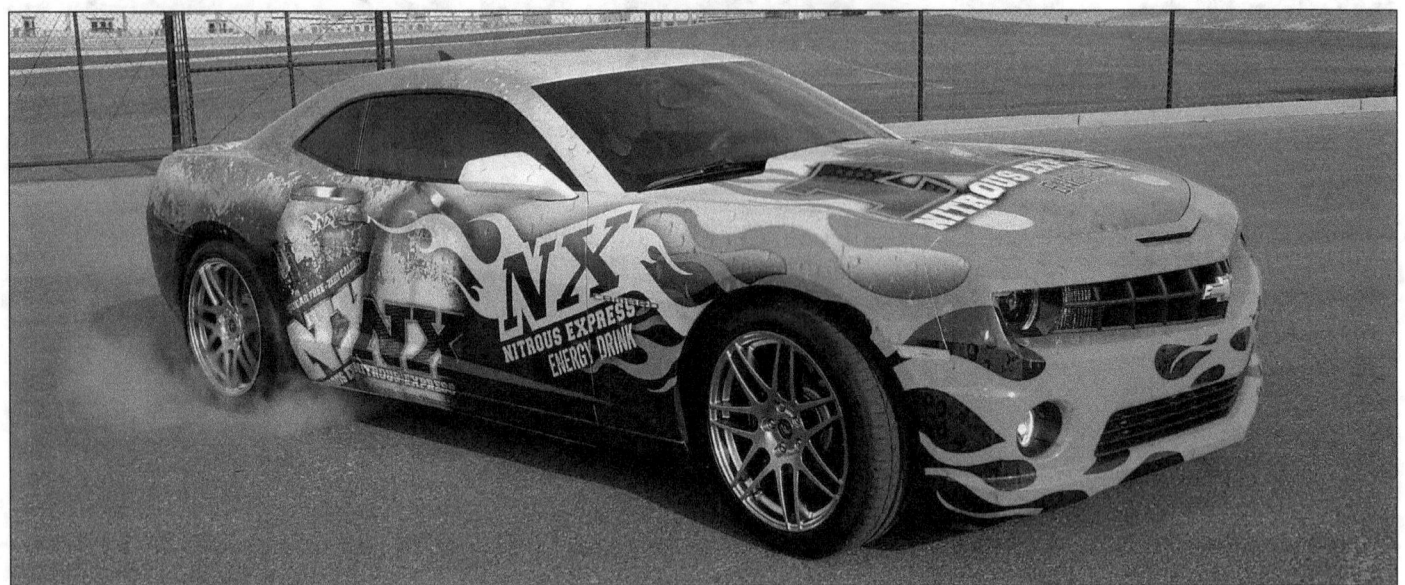

Now it's time to go out and make use of that 100+ additional horsepower!

HOW TO INSTALL AND TUNE NITROUS OXIDE SYSTEMS

Project: Bullitt Reloaded

The following is from my article that appeard in the September 2010 issue of *Mustang Enthusiast*.

When first introduced as a concept car at the 2000 Greater Los Angeles Auto Show, Ford Motor Company received such an overwhelming response from consumers that the limited-edition 2001 Bullitt Mustang specialty car was immediately rushed into production. At the time, the Bullitt was considered at the top of the Mustang food chain (SVT Mustang Cobra models excepted), with its 4.6L two-valve, twin 57-mm throttle body modular V-8 engine, which produced 265 hp (20 more than Mustang GT), and 305 ft-lbs of torque. But that was 10 years ago. Today's Mustangs easily produce that much horsepower and more. For example, the 2008 Gen-III Mustang Bullitt and 2010 Mustang GT produce 315 hp and 325 ft-lbs. The 2010 Shelby GT500 is packing 540 hp and 510 ft-lbs. Heck, even the new 2011 Mustang V-6 produces 300, and 280 ft-lbs, so the question is what can Gen-I Bullitt owners do to increase the horsepower quotient on these highly collectible Limited Edition Mustangs without spending a small fortune to modify their cars?

ZEX Nitrous Products, a division of Competition Cams, manufactures a multiple-level wet Nitrous Oxide Kit (PN 82023) for the 2001 4.6L SOHC Gen-I 2001 Bullitt Mustang that produces from 75 to 125 hp using 92-plus-octane premium fuel!

"You couldn't ask for anything more user friendly," says installed-system-owner Denny Duquette, also owner of Island Performance & Offroad. "The controller is so simplified. It's a three-wire setup and a single control box, which eliminates all the exterior mounting solenoids!"

ZEX aptly refers to this system as a plug-and-play installation. Most current nitrous systems use a throttle-actuated arming micro switch, which means you have to fabricate a mounting bracket for the switch and adjust the placement of the switch to make it work correctly. ZEX Nitrous Products' heat-resistant Nitrous Management Unit uses a 10-volt white (power) wire that you simply crimp-connect to the Throttle Position Sensor (TPS) output, which is the center terminal on the TPS input plug. In turn, the TPS voltage signal is sent to the programmable electronic switch inside the unit at a pre-determined voltage threshold. Voltage above and beyond said threshold is determined for WOT and the system activates itself. Below that threshold, it remains dormant.

Onboard features of the ZEX Nitrous Management Unit (which comes anodized in a nice purple color) include input and output nitrous and fuel line ports, along with a green light to alert the operator that the unit is functioning properly. Space is at a premium in the Gen-I Bullitt engine compartment, so installation of this unit is left to the owner's discretion. In this particular application, Island Performance & Offroad technician Shawn Voge fabricated a stepped mounting plate, which was secured to the upper lip on the passenger side of the radiator bulkhead.

According to the manufacturers, the ZEX/Bullitt N_2O system's injector nozzle is the most advanced nozzle design in today's N_2O industry. Primary features include easy-to-change metering jets, which allow for rapid fire changes in horsepower settings. The fuel transfer tube enriches the fuel mixture and injects it directly into the outer edge of the nitrous plume. This atomized, high-speed nitrous gas shears the fuel away from the tube, reportedly atomizing it to a much finer degree than competing nozzle designs. This ensures perfect distribution from cylinder to cylinder at higher horsepower settings.

The fuel transfer tube design also allows for a self-adjusting characteristic. A vacuum is created as the nitrous gas is sprayed across the tube opening. As the nitrous bottle pressure goes up, so does the gas speed and vacuum level. This increased vacuum pulls more fuel from the nozzle and ensures that the tune-up does not go into a lean stage.

As far as nitrous bottle placement goes, the passenger side of the trunk is ideal for three reasons. One, the bottle is in line with the remainder of the system because the business end of the SOHC 4.6L's fuel rail is located on the passenger side of the engine. Two, the trunk area of the Bullitt (and all SN95 Mustangs) feature a number of factory holes plugged by rubber grommets, so no drilling for the nitrous feed line is required. All you have to do is locate the hole that suits you the best, drill out the center of the rubber plug, and then run your line. Three, the 2001 Mustang Bullitt features a pair of 1x1-inch hollow rectangular subframe connectors and the passenger-side subframe connector is ideally suited for safely running the nitrous line the entire length of the car.

CHAPTER 9

Wiring the system is also easy. The red (hot) wire can be wired up to the fuse panel using a fuse tap run off the hot side of the fuse terminal. This is considerably safer than tapping into an actual wire; you're getting direct power while not drawing power off the fuse itself because the ZEX nitrous system is self-fused.

As previously mentioned, run the white wire from the nitrous management unit to the center output-voltage lead from the TPS. After those two connections are completed, you need to install the arming switch somewhere inside the interior. For this application, installer Voge located the switch to the left side of the cigarette lighter on the plastic shifter-boot cover. The black (ground) wire, in this particular case, was terminated at the radiator bulkhead.

The ZEX PN 82217 Nitrous Oxide Injection System for the Ford 4.6L SOHC costs around $660 through participating retailers. How well did this ZEX-equipped 2001 Mustang Bullitt perform? In drag tests conducted at sea level at Hilo Raceway Park, driver Denny Duquette recorded the following numbers.

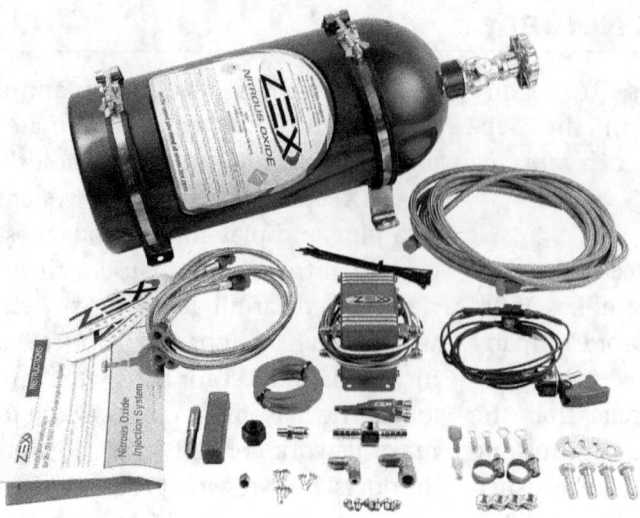

Shown is the complete ZEX Nitrous Oxide Products wet system for the 4.6L SOHC-engine, 2001 Mustang Bullitt (PN 82217). Included is the ZEX self-contained Nitrous Management Unit (NMU), a 10-pound nitrous bottle, a pair of nitrous bottle clamps, a ZEX Wet Nitrous Nozzle, a 24-inch -3 AN braided stainless-steel hose, a 16-inch -4 AN braided stainless-steel hose, and a 16-foot -4 AN braided stainless-steel nitrous delivery hose. There is also a set of .026- to .054-inch N_2O and fuel jets, the Arming Switch Harness, 10 feet of 18-gauge red wire, a switch cover, a Schrader Valve Core Tool, one fuel T-fitting, bolt packs (including bolts, nuts, washers, a tap), a 90 degree -4 AN Swivel Adaptor, ZEX stickers, and an instruction sheet, all for about $550 through participating ZEX Nitrous Oxide Products retailers.

As you can see, the ZEX 82217 Nitrous Oxide System improved this 2001 Bullitt's quarter-mile performance by approximately 1.06 seconds, with a 12.84-mph gain on the top end. Next, we wanted to see how well the Bullitt did on the dyno, so we made a quick trip to Rob Gavel's dyno facility in Hawaii and used the Dynojet Research 248 portable dyno. Based on the results, Gavel's comments included the following:

"We noticed that the ZEX N_2O system seems to be conservatively geared towards safety. When it comes to street nitrous oxide kits, that [safety] isn't necessarily a bad thing. We noticed that when the N_2O kicks in, the air/fuel ratio (AFR), goes rich, way rich; from 4,000 to 5,000 rpm it goes way off the chart—likely down in the 9.1s. The dyno AFR only reads as low as 10:1, which is extremely rich. Reading the Bullitt's 6,000-rpm redline, we were heading back toward when we would like to have been somewhere in the 11s, but by then the power band was starting to drop. It's likely the factory ECU took a bit of time to pull out the necessary fuel.

"Had we been able to control the delivery of the fuel and keep the AFRs in the mid-range 11s—an aftermarket programmer like the Diablo

2001 Bullitt Test Results

Without ZEX Nitrous Oxide

Run	60-ft Time	Elapsed Time	Terminal Speed
1	2.477 seconds	14.78 seconds	96.62 mph
2	2.323 seconds	14.51 seconds	98.33 mph
3	2.062 seconds	14.35 seconds	96.16 mph

With ZEX 100-HP Nitrous Activated

Run	60-ft Time	Elapsed Time	Terminal Speed
1	2.335 seconds	13.56 seconds	106.92 mph
2	2.071 seconds	13.55 seconds	106.08 mph
3	2.05 seconds	13.29 seconds	109.00 mph

Sport certainly would have helped—we would probably have picked up a few extra horsepower in that area. In reality, there is not really a lot of difference in peak horsepower between an engine run at 10:1 AFR versus an engine run at 12:1 AFR, and for a company producing a volatile product like a nitrous oxide kit for the street, it is much better to err and be on the safe side!"

Here are the two dyno test results:

- Without ZEX Nitrous: 216.81 hp at 5,000 rpm; 247.37 ft-lbs at 4,000 to 4,500 rpm
- With ZEX 100-hp Nitrous: 285.04 hp at 4,000 to 5,500 rpm; 353.65 ft-lbs at 3,750 to 4,000 rpm

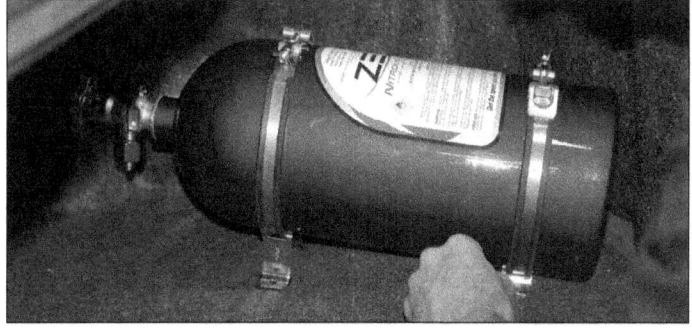

1 *In order to mount the bottle, assemble the bottle mounting clamps and place the entire assembly on the passenger side of the trunk, with both valve and bottle mounting brackets facing downward.*

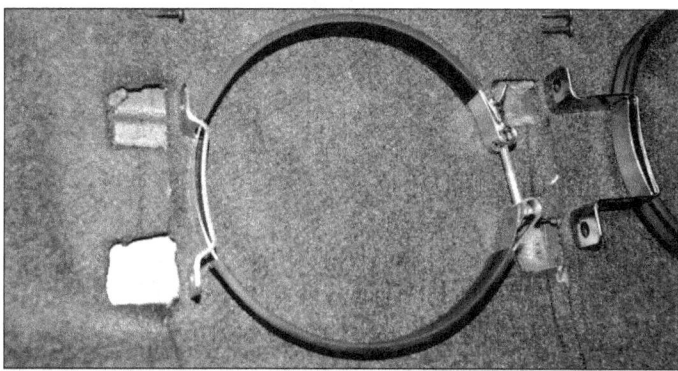

2 *After marking the location, trim away any excess padding below the carpet to avoid snagging the drill bit. Then drill a series of four holes in the floorpan where the bottle brackets are to be secured.*

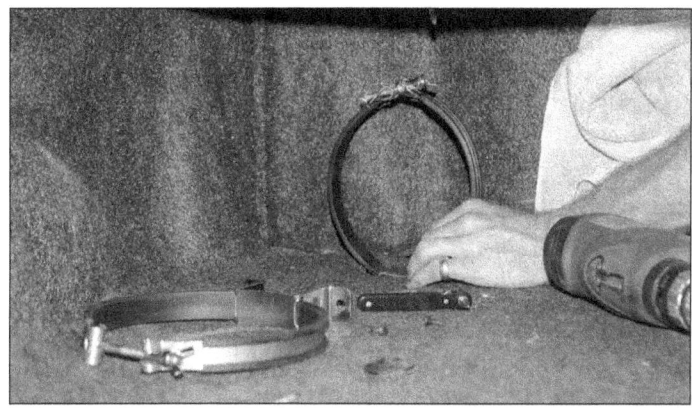

3 *Next install the bottle brackets along with the bottle using self-tapping screws.*

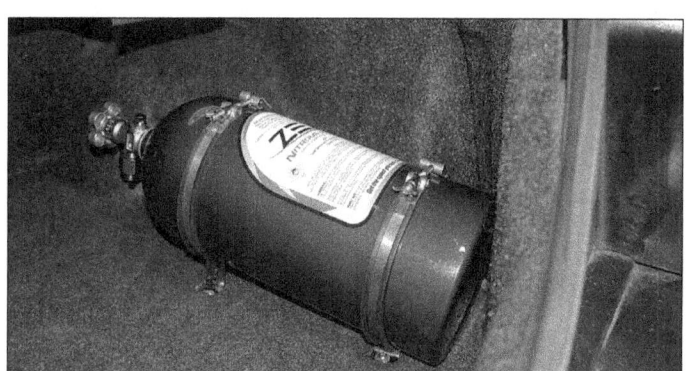

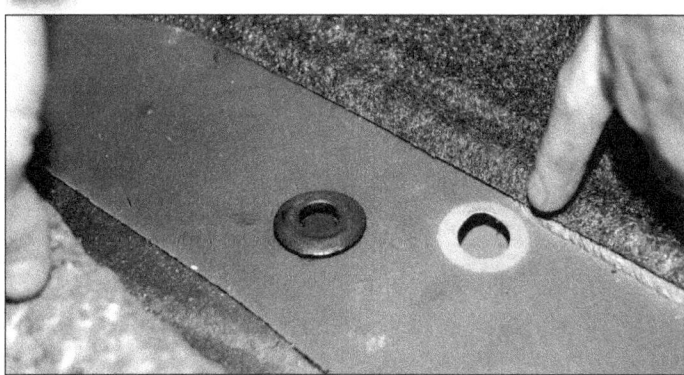

4 *All 1994–2004 SN95 Fox Mustangs feature a series of four plugged holes in the trunk pan, two per side. The plugged hole closest to the rear seatback on the passenger side is ideally suited for a nitrous delivery line.*

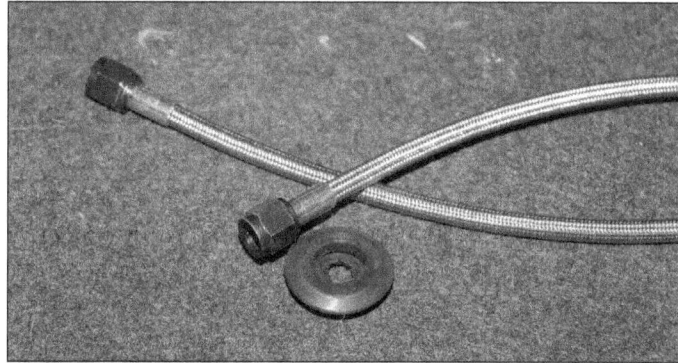

5 *All that remains is cutting out the center of the rubber floorpan grommet. Note: In order to prevent chafing the nitrous supply line, you must re-use this floorpan plug!*

CHAPTER 9

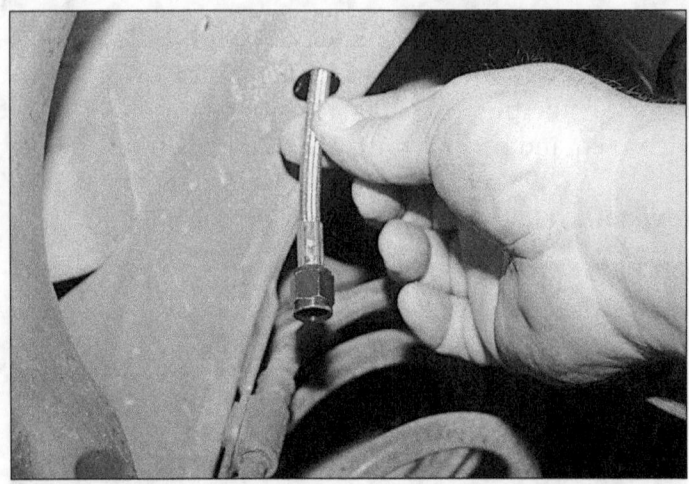

6 Run the 16-foot-long -4 AN braided-stainless nitrous line through the opening in the trunk pan.

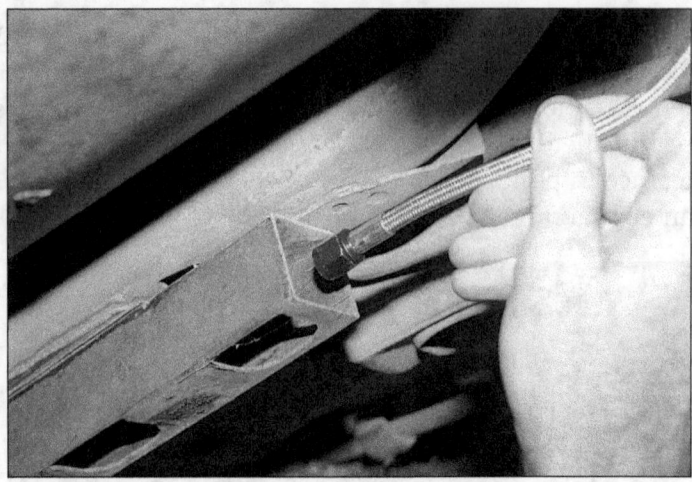

7 Route the nitrous supply line through the Bullitt's 1x1-inch hollow tube subframe connectors.

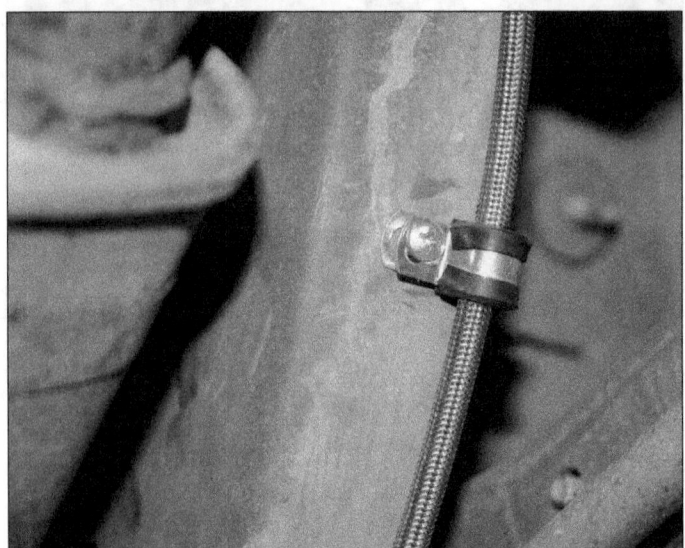

8 Secure both ends to the floorpan by rubberized crimp line connectors to keep the line from walking around.

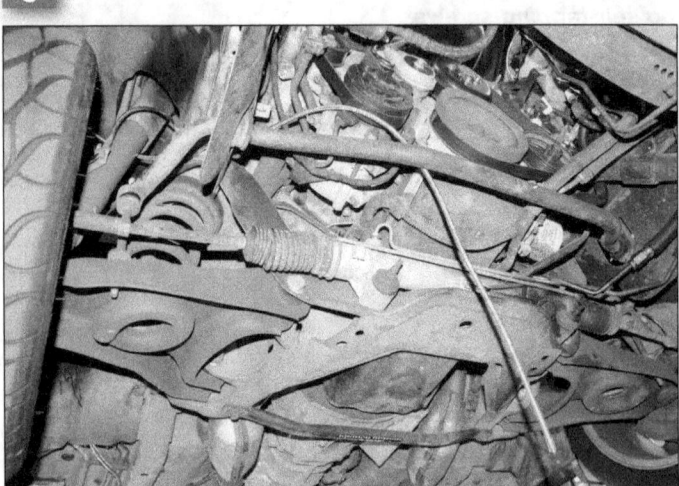

9 This is where the nitrous supply line enters the engine compartment.

HOW TO INSTALL AND TUNE NITROUS OXIDE SYSTEMS

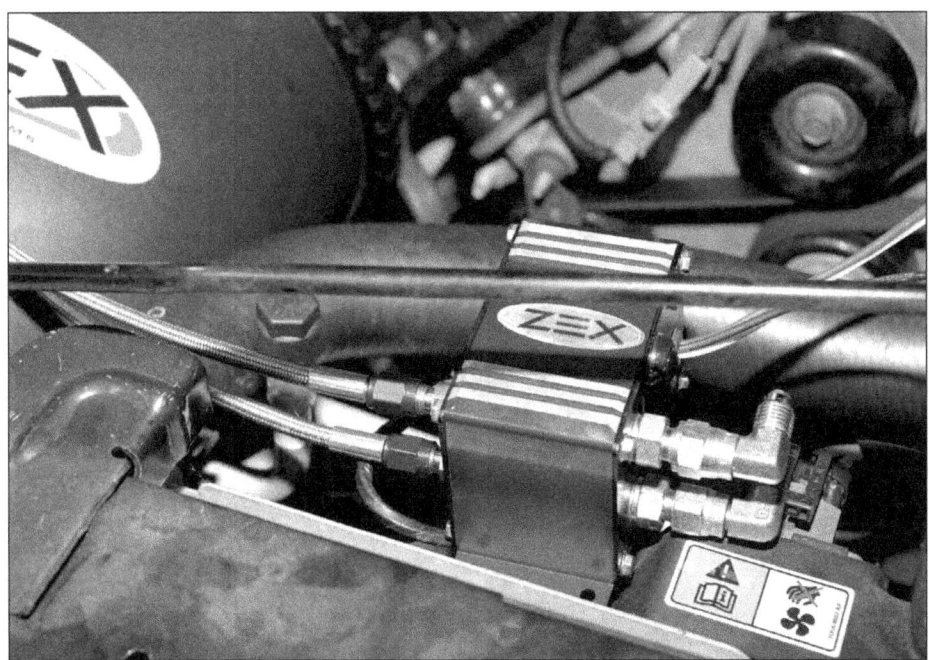

10 Trial placement of the ZEX Nitrous Management Unit comes next. For this application, it was determined that the NMU be located on the passenger side of the radiator bulkhead.

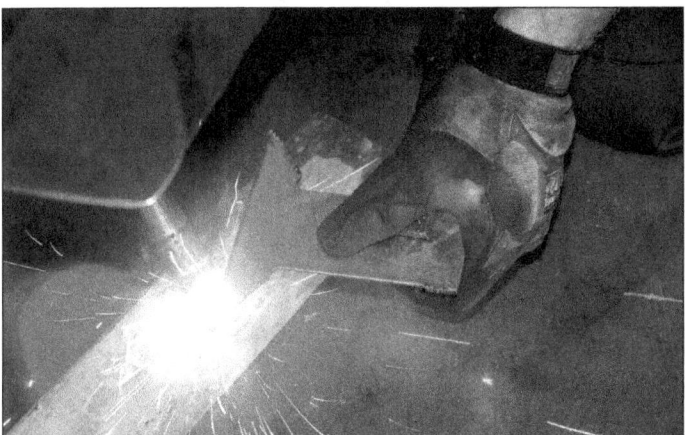
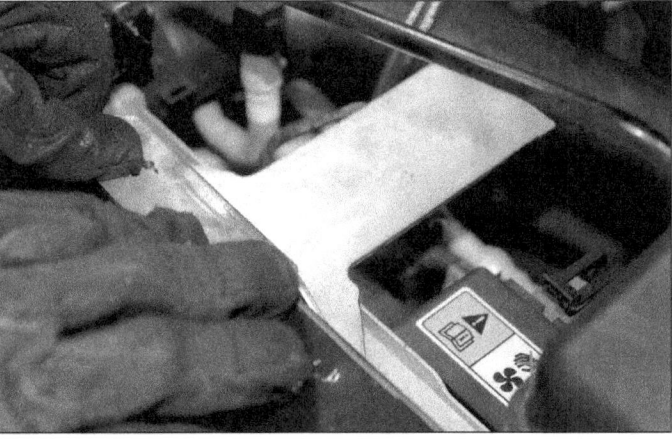

11 Fabricate a mounting bracket out of 1/8-inch steel stock, featuring a 3/4-inch stepped plate secured to the top of the radiator bulkhead, using a pair of self-tapping screws.

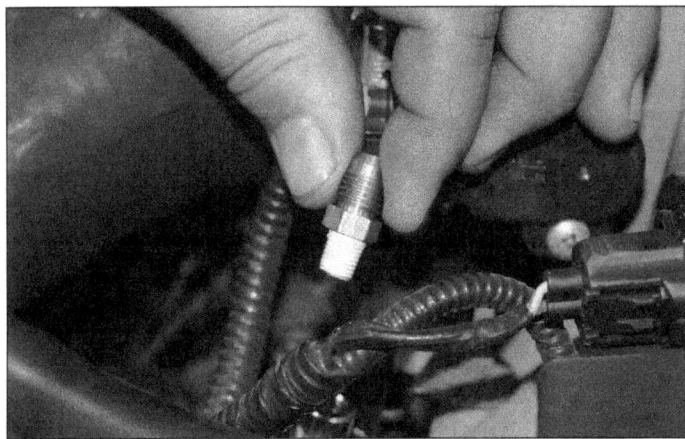
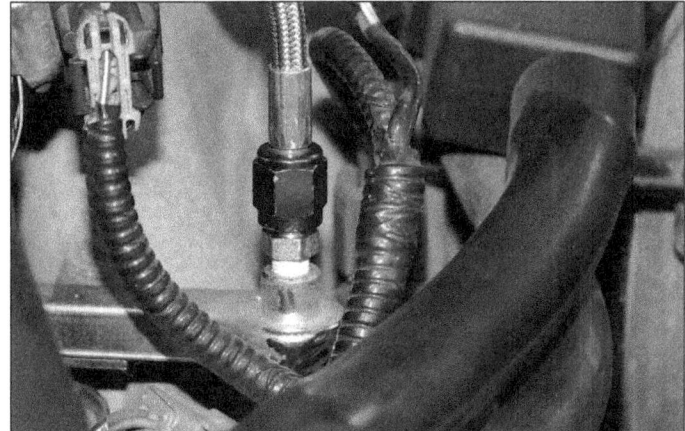

12 Install the Schrader valve onto the fuel port of the Bullitt fuel rail, then install the -3 AN braided stainless-steel fuel line. Note: Since this line is pressurized, some fuel spillage may occur.

CHAPTER 9

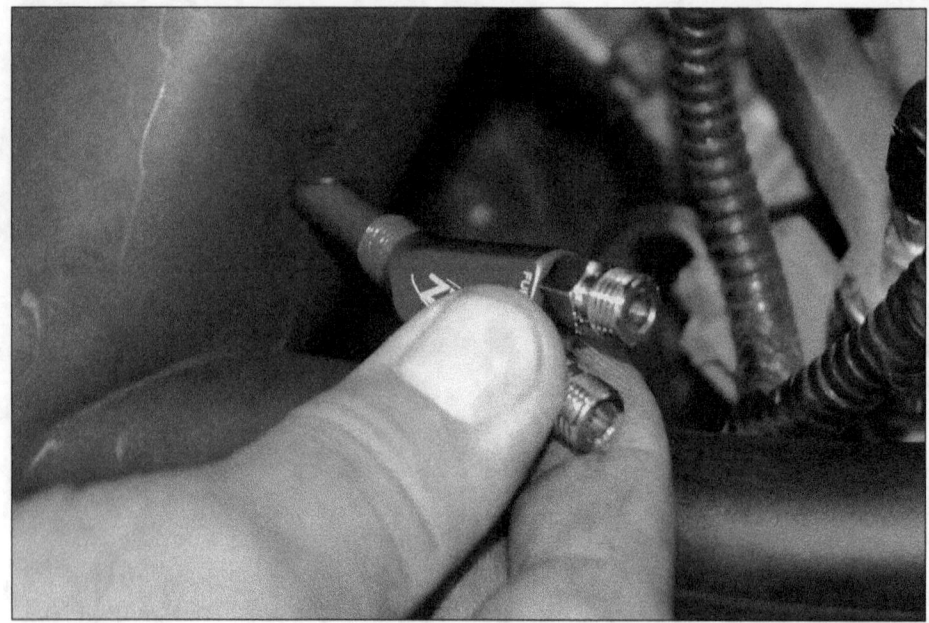

13 Place the ZEX Wet Nitrous Nozzle into the Bullitt's air intake tube. Since this is a twin-bore throttle body, you must place the nozzle far enough back in the air intake tube (approximately 2½ inches) so that the nitrous plume can spray equally into both ports and create a lean condition.

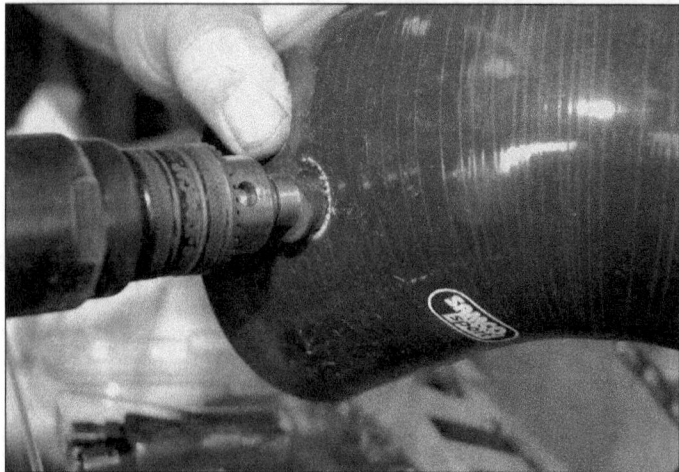
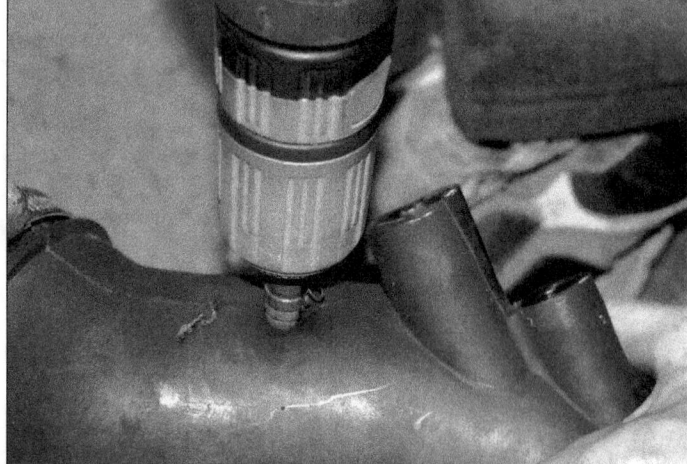

14 Use an auger bit to create an opening in the side of the 4.6L's air intake tube in order to install a threaded bung to accommodate the nitrous nozzle.

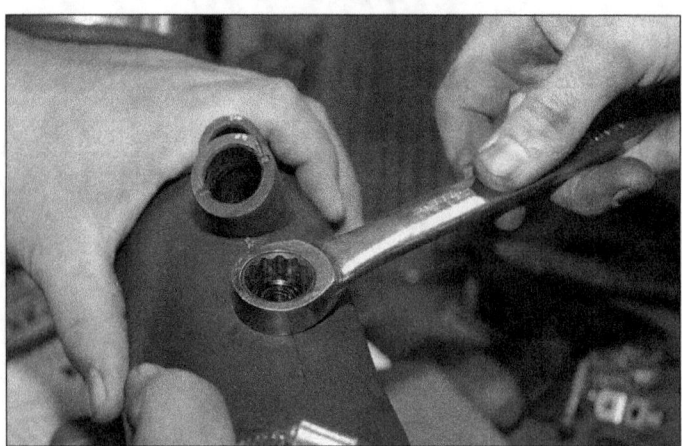
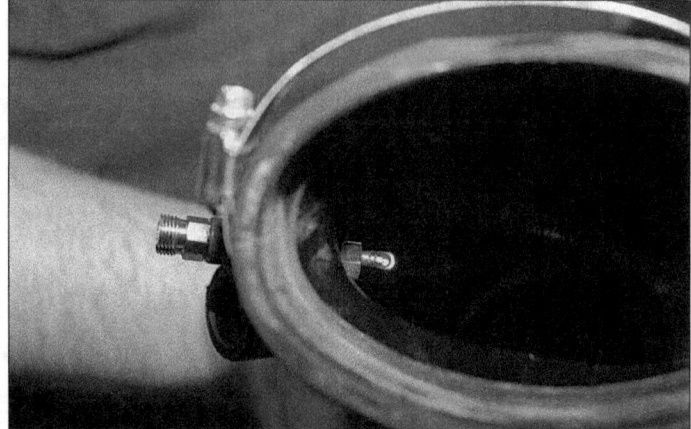

15 It's time to install the nitrous nozzle itself, all the while making sure that the sprayer is aimed directly at the Bullitt 57-mm twin-bore throttle body.

EFI, WET AND DRY

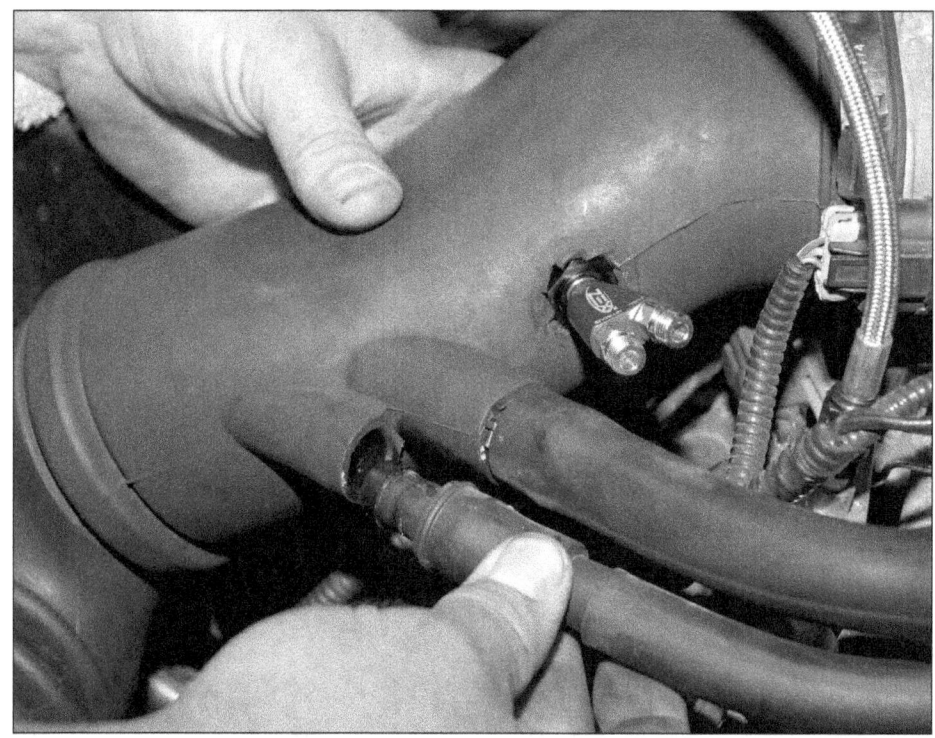

16 With wet nitrous nozzle fully installed, re-install the air intake tube onto the 4.6L SOHC Ford V-8 engine.

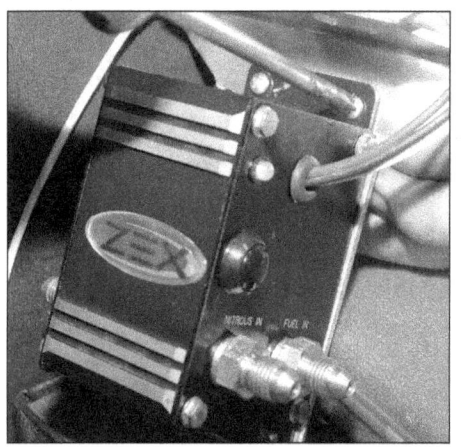
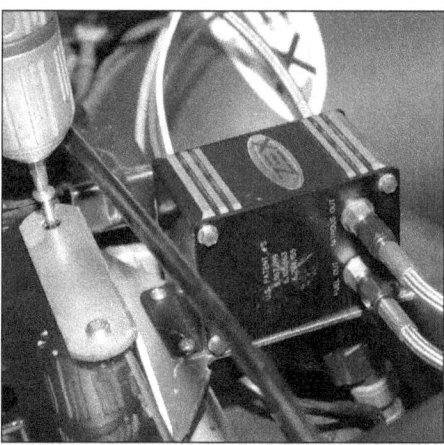

17 Secure the ZEX Nitrous Management Unit itself to the mounting bracket using a series of four self-tapping screws. Looks like a nice, clean installation.

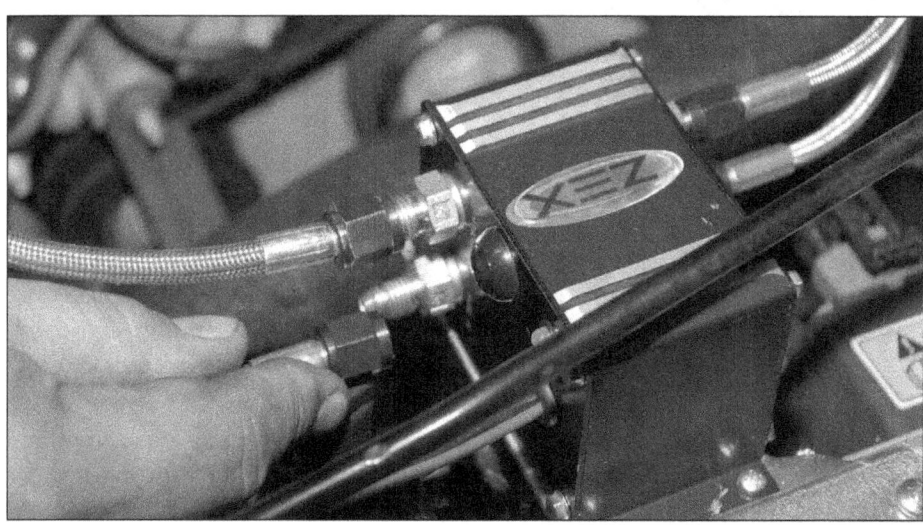

18 Attach the corresponding fuel and N_2O lines. First comes the -4 AN Nitrous In port (top line) followed by the Fuel In port (bottom line). Tighten these lines, but do not overly tighten, using a standard wrench.

CHAPTER 9

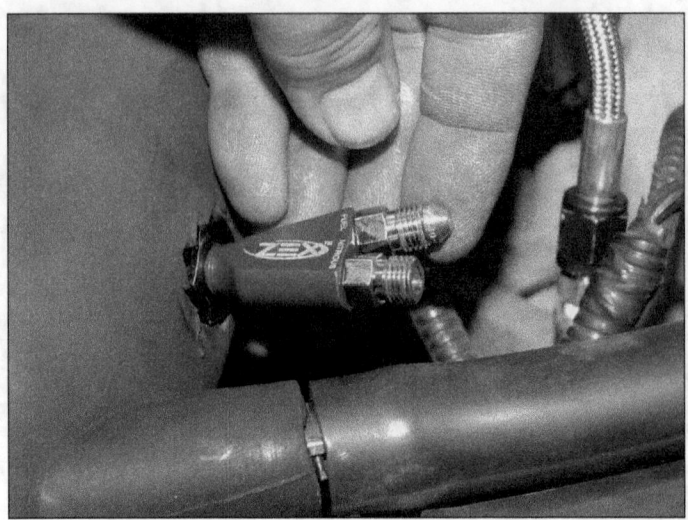
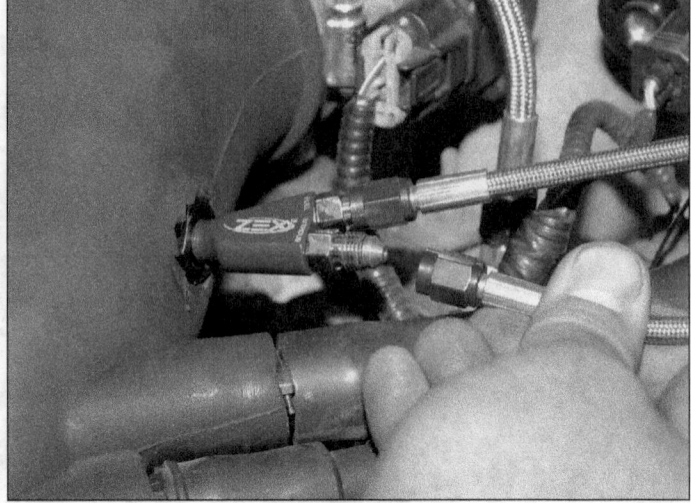

19 Install the 100-hp nitrous jets into the nozzle, followed by the Nitrous Out and Fuel Out -4 AN lines.

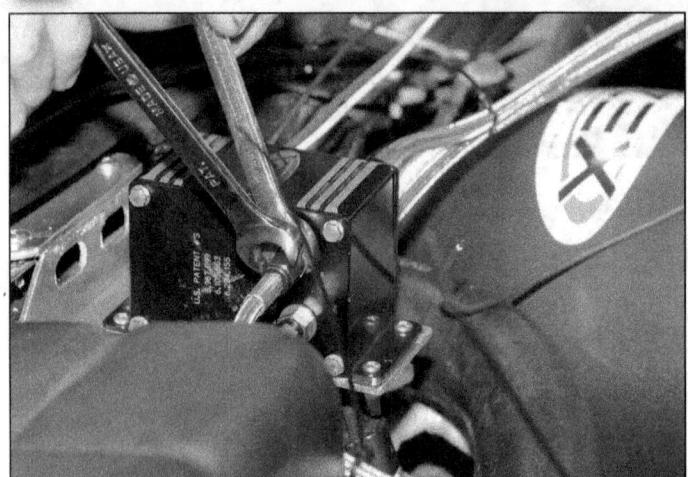
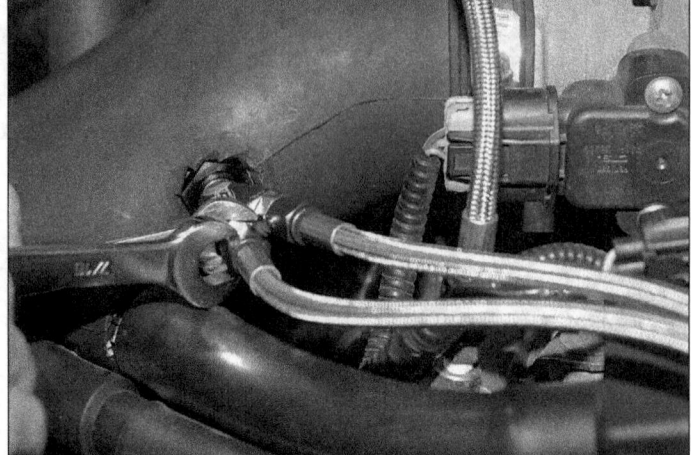

20 And finally, hook up the Nitrous Out and Fuel Out lines at the NMU. After these lines are installed, open the bottle valve and pressurize the system to check for any leaks.

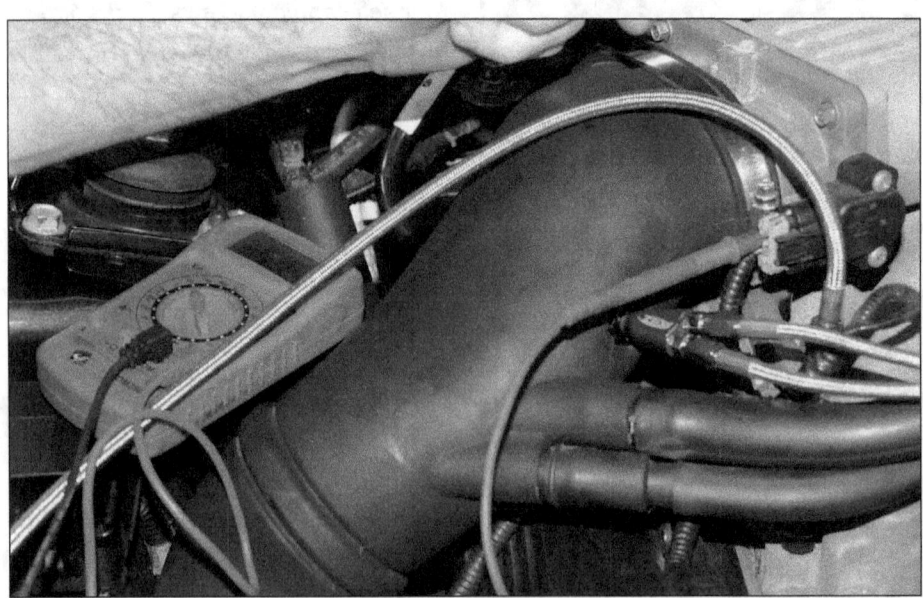

21 Perform a volt check on the TPS port. Here the installer discovered that the center electrical wire connector is the one producing the required 10 volts to operate the system at WOT. This is where the power wire will come from to activate the ZEX NMU.

EFI, WET AND DRY

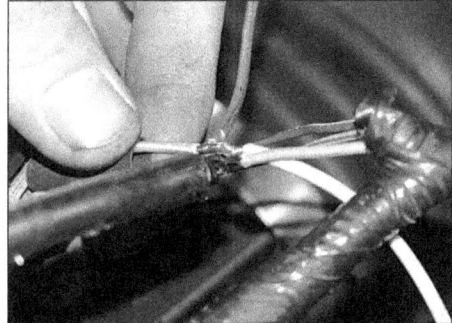

22 After locating the correct power wire on the Bullitt's TPS harness, splice the white power wire from the TPS harness to activate the XEX nitrous bottle monitoring unit. If in doubt, soldering this line is another alternative. Plug the electrical connector of the TPS back in.

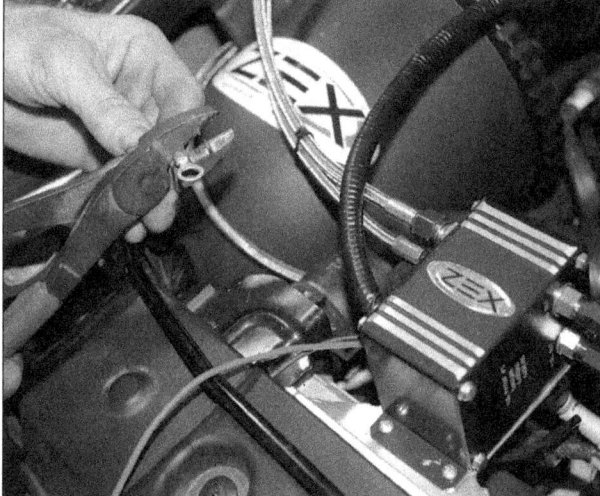

23 Next install the black ground wire onto the radiator core support, just behind the hood prop rod, using one of the supplied electrical eyelets provided in the ZEX kit.

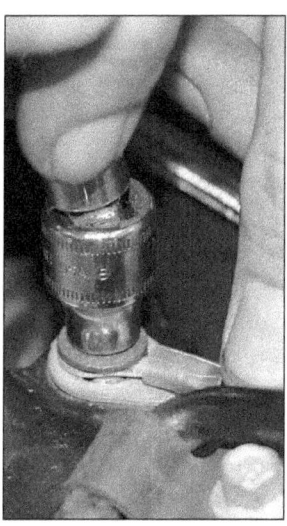

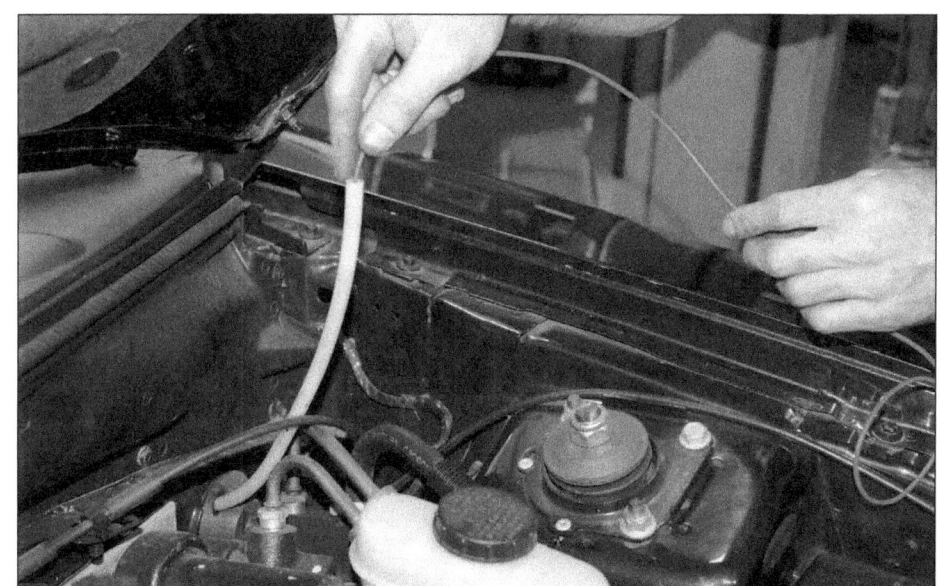

24 Locate a suitable opening in the firewall to run the Arming Switch wire using the supplied red 18-gauge wire.

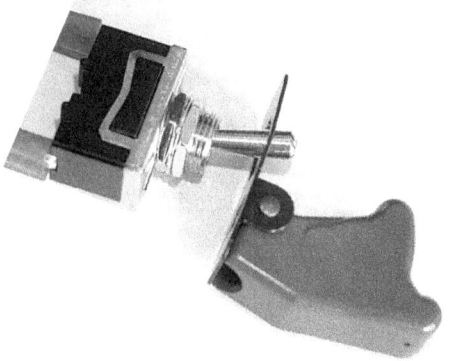

25 Part of the ZEX kit includes this Arming (toggle) Switch and spring-loaded switch cover.

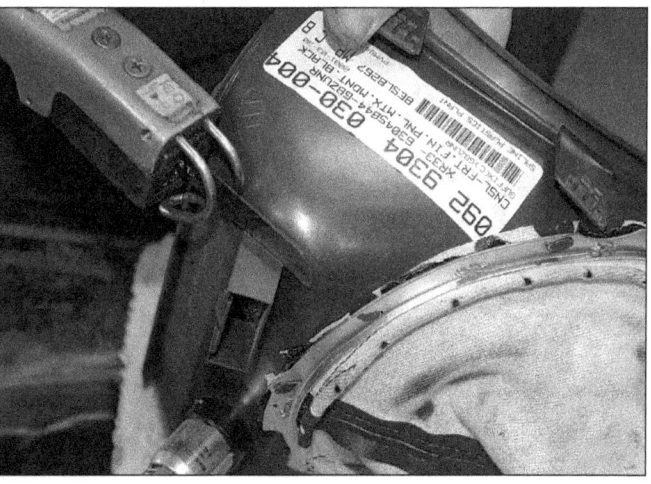

26 For this application, the plastic surround that is an integral part of the Bullitt's shifter and boot module works perfectly. All our installer has to do is trim off the plastic backing tab, center the switch, and drill the necessary hole.

HOW TO INSTALL AND TUNE NITROUS OXIDE SYSTEMS   109

CHAPTER 9

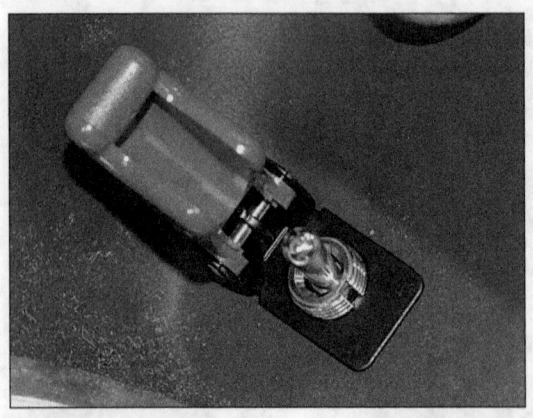

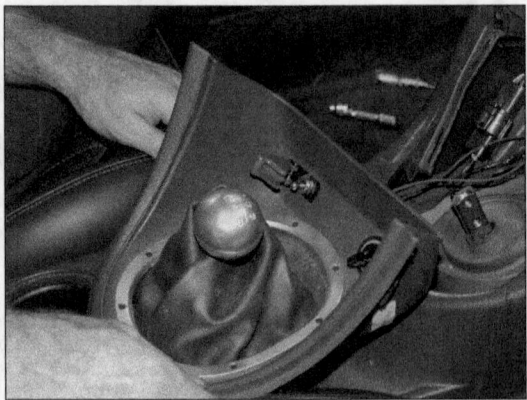

27 Looks kind of factory, doesn't it?

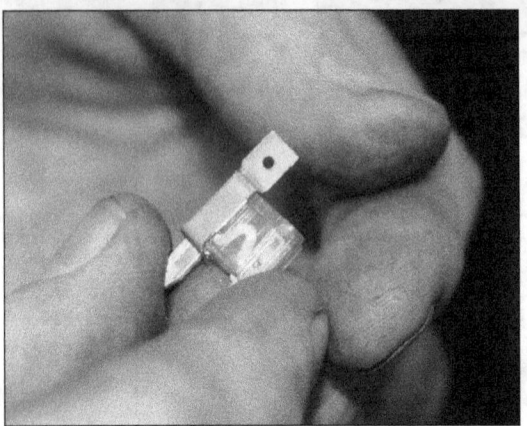

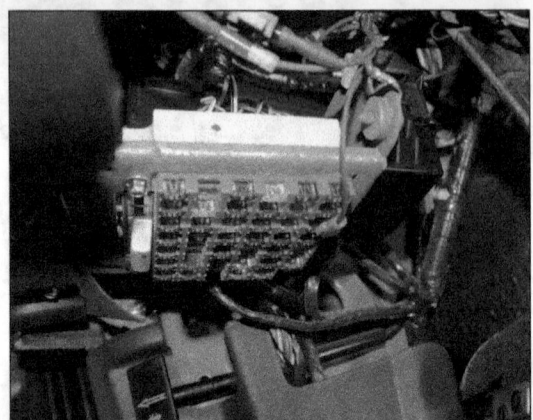

28 Energizing the system is fairly simple. The red/hot wire can be wired up to the fuse panel using a fuse link. That way, you optimize power without actually tapping into a wire, and/or drawing off the fuse itself.

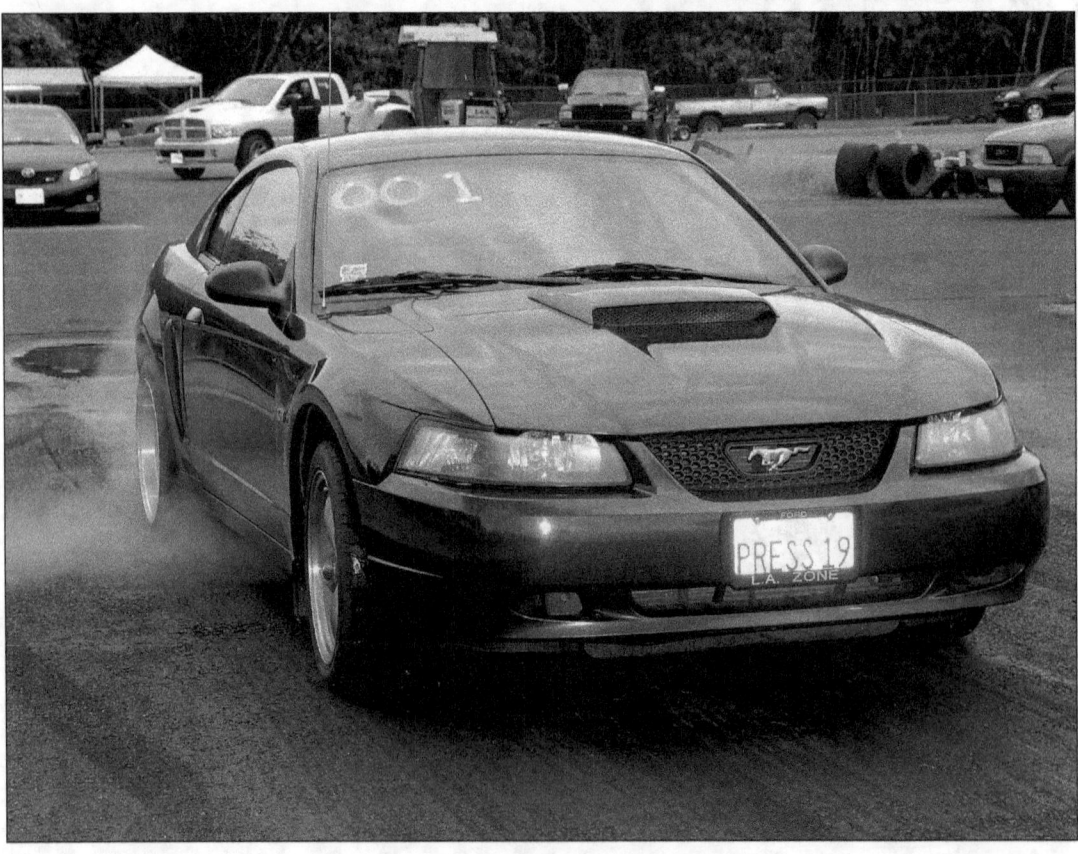

With the ZEX Wet Nitrous System energized and set to come on in second gear, the 2001 reeled off ET/MPH runs of 13.56/106.92, 13.55/106.08, and 13.29/109.00. That's a 1.16-second gain in elapsed time, and an increase of 12.84 mph on the top end!

EFI, WET AND DRY

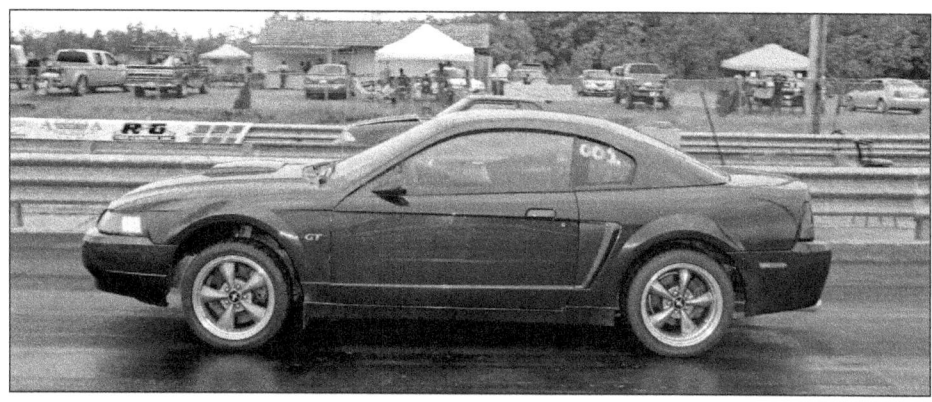

Off to the dyno shop, where Redline808.com's Rob Gavel, Jr., and C.A.R.S.S. technician Chase Augustin, recorded a best fourth-gear pull of 216.81 hp at 5,000 rpm, and 247.37 ft-lbs at 4,000 to 4,500 rpm on the engine. With the ZEX Wet Nitrous Oxides System fully activated, Bullitt number-19 produced 285.04 hp at 4,000 to 4,500 rpm and 353.65 ft-lbs of torque at 3,750 to 4,000 rpm.

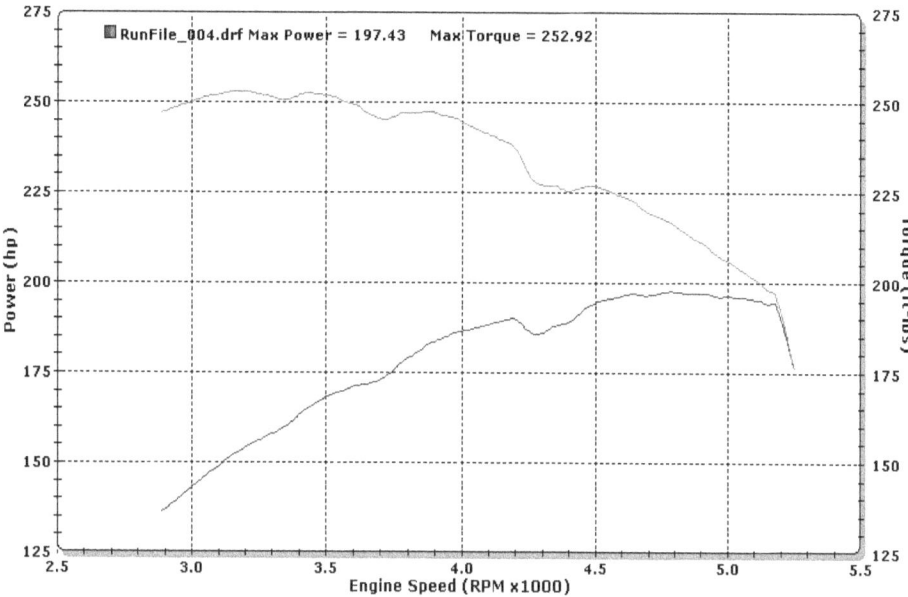

Hawaii's only portable 248 chassis dyno

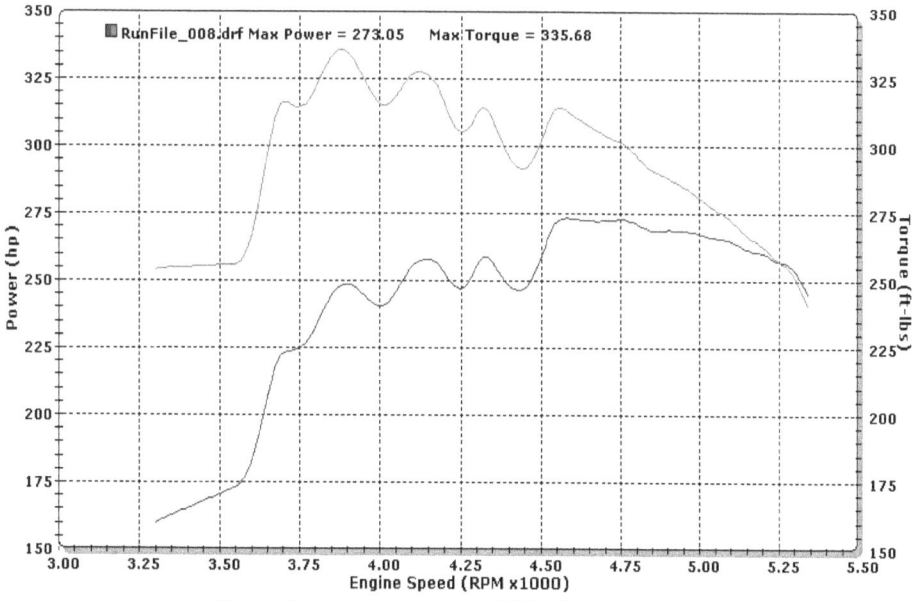

Hawaii's only portable 248 chassis dyno

HOW TO INSTALL AND TUNE NITROUS OXIDE SYSTEMS

CHAPTER 9

Project: Nitrous Express Dodge Challenger SRT8 Fly-By-Wire Stage 1 EFI Kit Installation

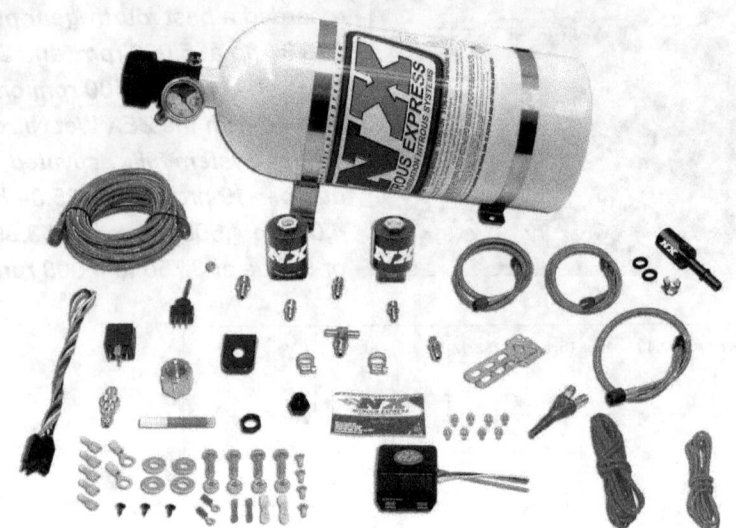

kit retails for about $450 through participating NX retailers. And how well does this kit perform? When installed on April Duquette's Hemi Orange 2008 Dodge Challenger (number 197 out of 6,200 2008s built), using a 100-jet as a baseline, dyno tests conducted at Gaspar Services using a Dynojet dyno, the following numbers were recorded:

- Before Nitrous: 354 hp at 6,200 rpm; 395 ft-lbs at 4,800 rpm
- With the NX System: 434 hp at 6,200 rpm; 500 ft-lbs at 4,500 rpm

No one can deny the fact that Chrysler Corporation's Gen-III hemispherical-head small-block V-8 engine forever revolutionized the street car and light-duty truck segments of the Mopar market. This is especially true with the introduction of the 6.1L SRT8 high-performance version, available in Dodge Challenger, Dodge Charger, Chrysler 300-C, Jeep Cherokee, and special-edition SRT8 Dodge Ram trucks. But, like everything else in life, there's always room for improvement. Factory rated at 425 hp at 6,300 rpm, and 420 ft-lbs of torque at 4,800 rpm, the quickest way to reliably increase the 6.1L Dodge SRT8's horsepower rating without having to hock the farm is the addition of an N_2O kit.

Nitrous Express offers the Fly-By-Wire Stage 1 EFI N_2O kit (PN 20918-10) for SRT applications, which effectively increases the horsepower quotient up to a whopping 250!

Using Nitrous Express' exclusive smart box technology, this is truly a plug-and-play street nitrous system. This kit comes complete with a 10-pound composite nitrous bottle, NX Auto Learn Throttle Position Sensor (TPS) switch, two stainless-steel bottle brackets, a pair of NX Lightning solenoids, and 15 feet of braided stainless-steel N_2O line. The kit also has all the necessary hardware to complete the installation, including Nitrous Express' patented Shark nozzle and a selection of jets ranging from a mere 35-hp tickle to a mind-bending 250 rear-wheel horsepower. NX's SRT8 kit lists for around $750. Installation is fairly straightforward; approximately six hours are required, using common shop tools, jack stands, and/or a hydraulic lift.

NX's GENX-2 Accessory Package, which includes an automatic bottle warmer, nitrous pressure gauge, fuel safety cut-off switch, and safety blow-down tune/fitting and purge valve, is an available option. This

Next, a series of before and after runs were made at the IHRA-sanctioned Hilo Raceway Park. The only modifications made were: a cold air intake, a 3.73:1-geared 2009 Challenger limited-slip differential, 2009 Challenger axle shafts, and a pair of Nitto Drag Radials. April's Challenger (with April driving) produced the following data at sea level:

Run	60-ft Time	Elapsed Time	Terminal Speed
1: Naturally aspirated	1.9560 seconds	12.98 seconds	107.71 mph
2: Naturally aspirated	1.9660 seconds	12.93 seconds	107.90 mph
3: 100-shot	1.750 seconds	12.01 seconds	117.94 mph
4: 100-shot	1.730 seconds	11.98 seconds	118.94 mph

Next, April's Challenger was upgraded to a 150-shot jet and produced the following data:

Run 1: 11.60 seconds at 119.00 mph
Run 2: 11.51 seconds at 120.00 mph

Now follow along as the crew from Island Performance & Offroad, Inc., shows you how easy it is to install this system.

EFI, WET AND DRY

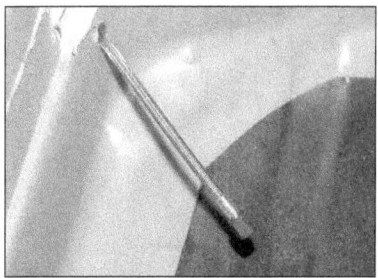

1 Nitrous bottle placement comes first. For this application, installer Denny Duquette elected to hide the nitrous bottle inside the Challenger's spare tire well, and used a 5/8-inch auger bit to open a hole large enough to accommodate the -4 AN nitrous feed line in the driver's side of the spare tire well.

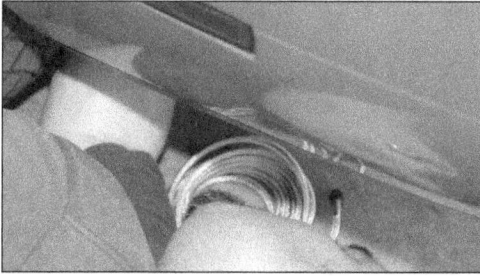

2 Run the nitrous supply line along the chassis using a series of rubber-encased crimp line connectors to secure it in place.

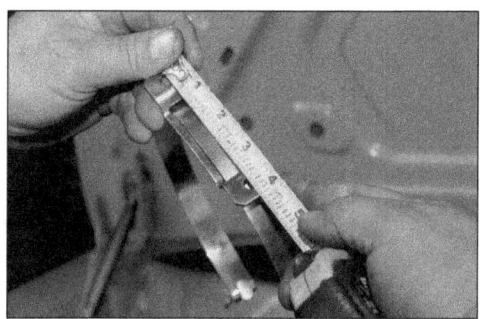

3 Measure the spread between the mounting pads (at 4 inches) on the nitrous bottle brackets.

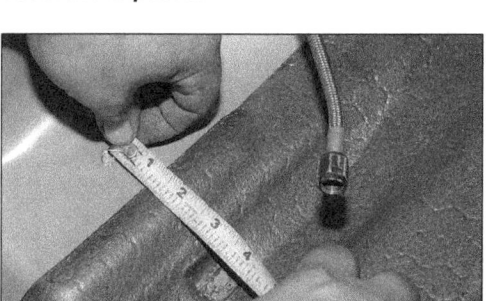

4 Transfer the measurement to the floorpan. Then drill a series of four 5/16-inch holes.

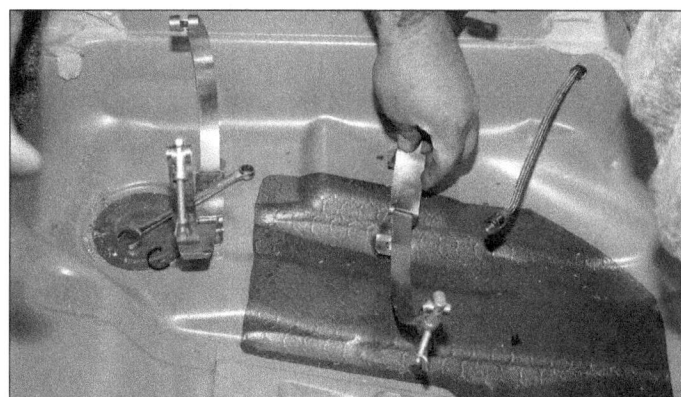

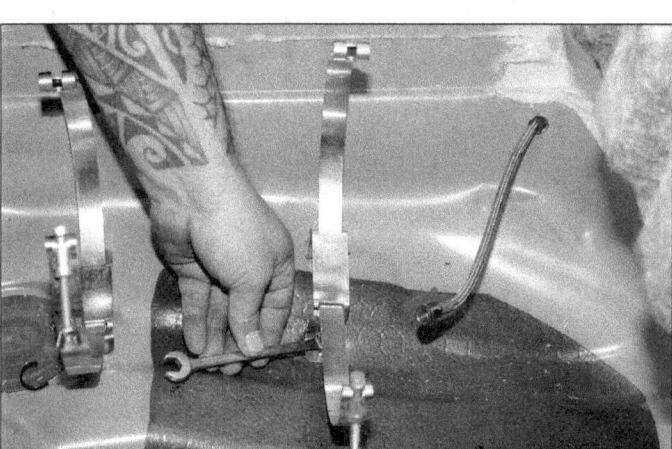

5 Install the bottle brackets using a 5/16-inch socket and driver.

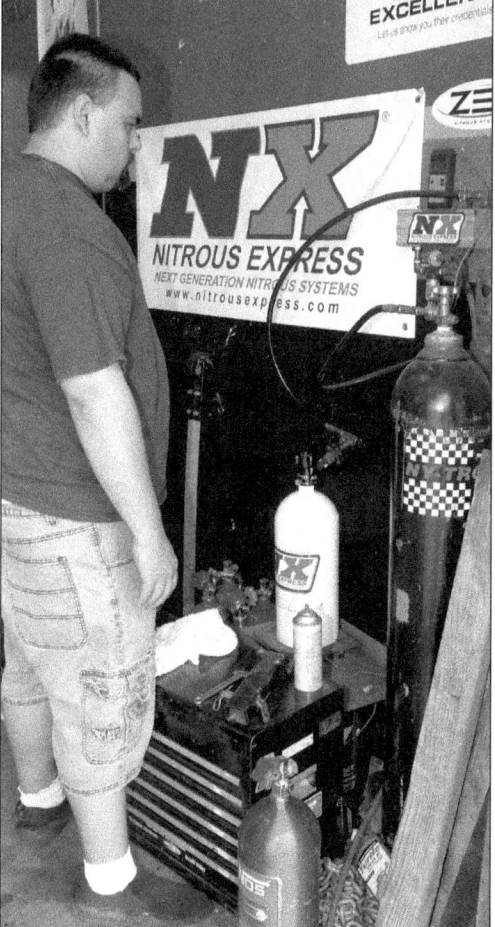

6 Prior to installing the NX 10-pound bottle, Duquette (who is an NX distributor) pumps in 10 pounds of N_2O at his nitrous filling station.

HOW TO INSTALL AND TUNE NITROUS OXIDE SYSTEMS

CHAPTER 9

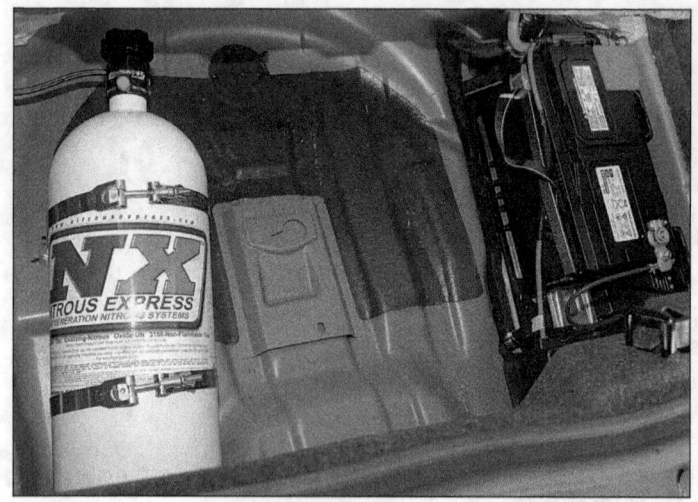

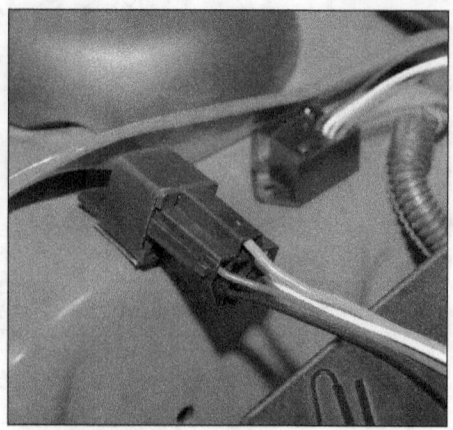

7 With bottle filled and installed with the siphon facing downward, connect the -4 AN nitrous supply line to the nozzle. Then the N_2O bottle is fully installed.

8 Install the NX Auto Learn switch and solenoid relays.

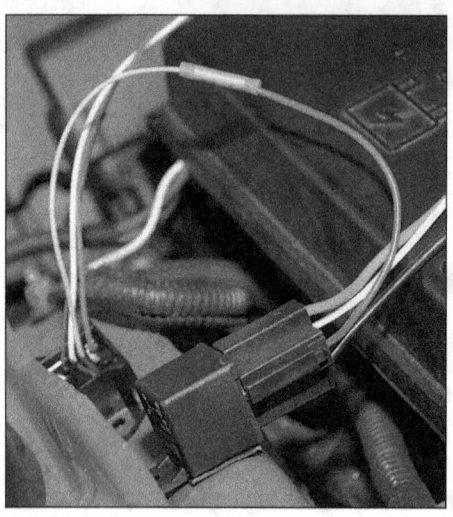

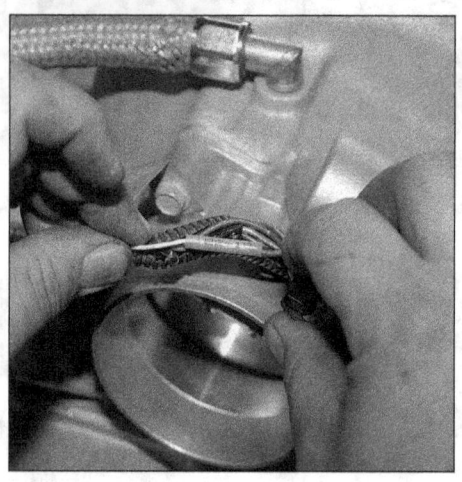

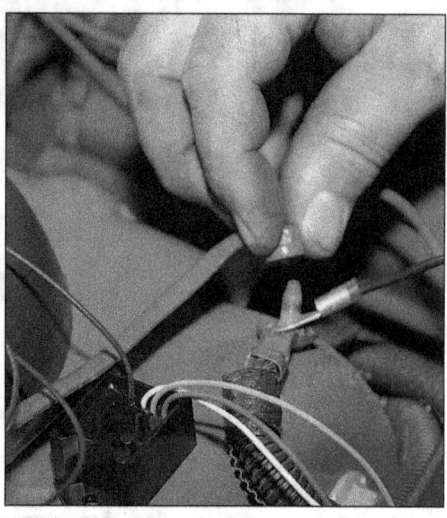

9 The red line is the positive (+) line.

10 The white line is the 5-volt throttle position sensor (TPS) lead hookup.

11 Remove the decorative plastic Hemi valve cover.

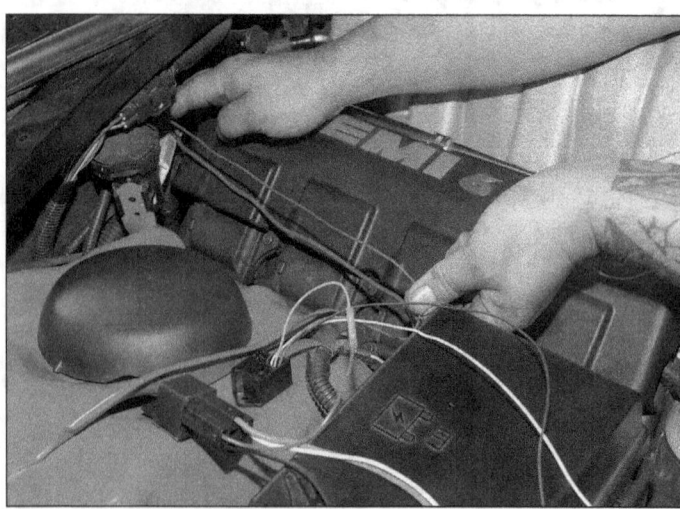

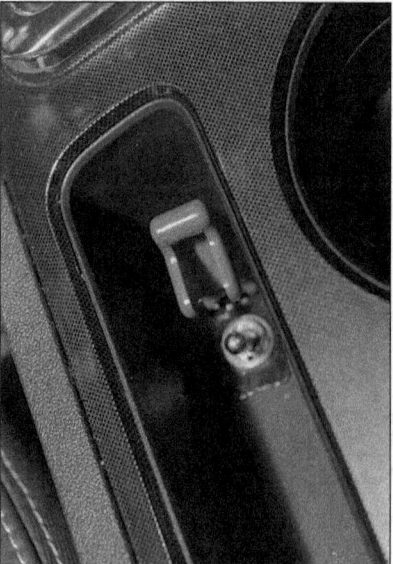

12 Hook up the black (or ground) wire.

13 The Nitrous Arming Switch has been installed inside the CD storage compartment of the Challenger's console. First, drill a 5/8-inch hole. Then mount the switch and power up using a keyed-on source at the fuse panel. Run the output wire back to the nitrous solenoids.

EFI, WET AND DRY

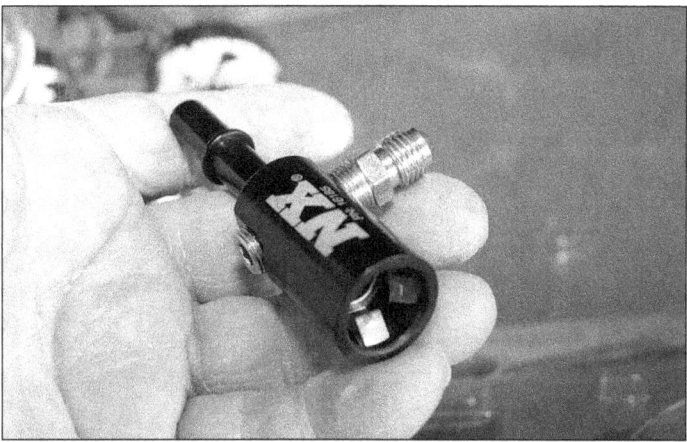

14 Disconnect the factory fuel line from the SRT8 fuel rail using a fuel line removal tool. Shown here is the NX 3/8-inch Fuel Line Adaptor, which was used to tap into the Challenger's passenger-side fuel rail.

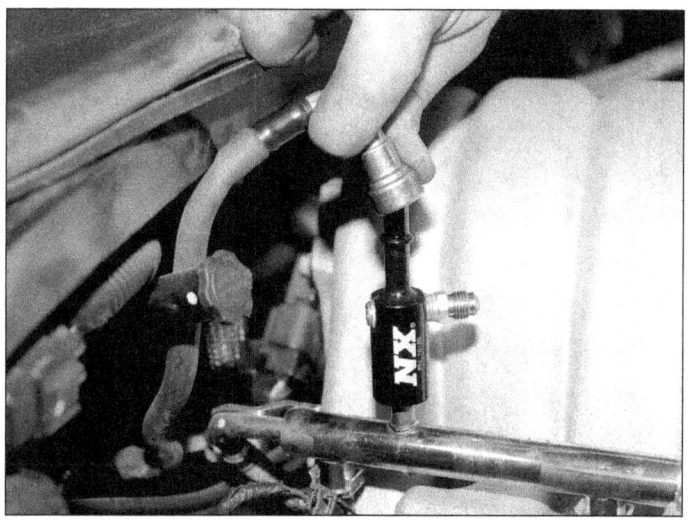

15 Attach the factory fuel line connector to the NX Fuel Line Adaptor.

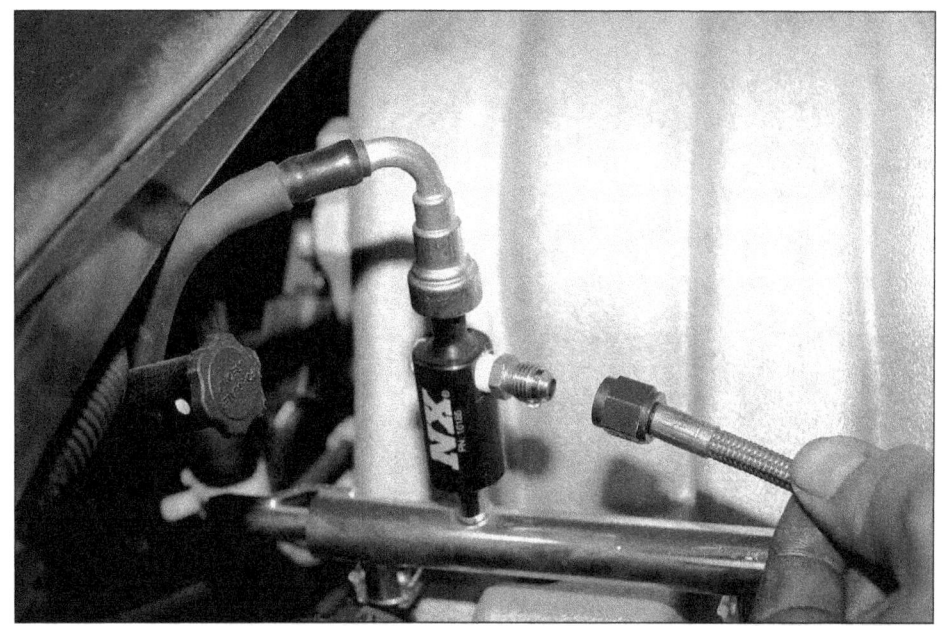

16 Attach the NX Fuel Out -4 AN fuel line to the NX Fuel Line Adaptor.

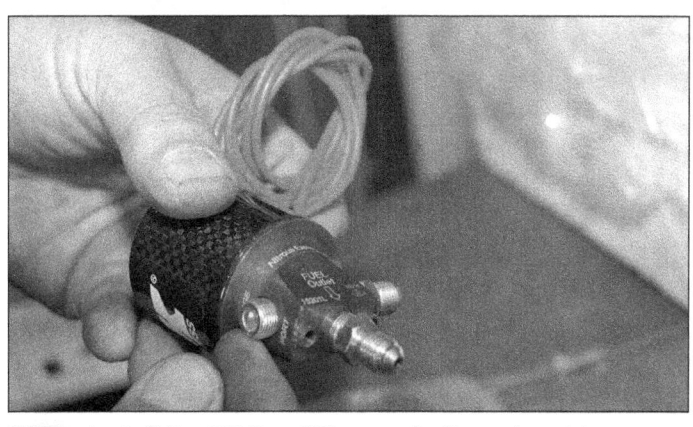

17 Install the NX line fittings onto the solenoids.

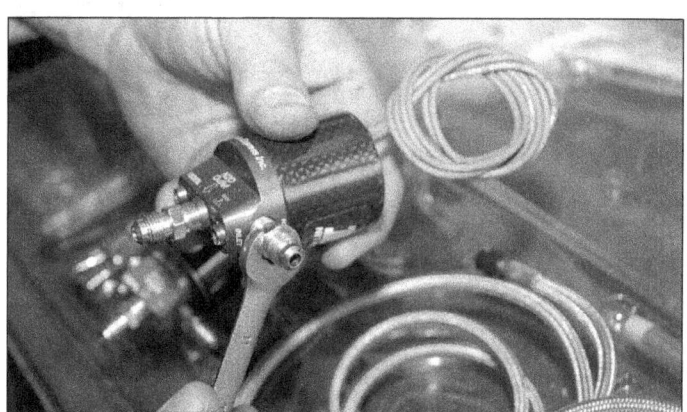

HOW TO INSTALL AND TUNE NITROUS OXIDE SYSTEMS

CHAPTER 9

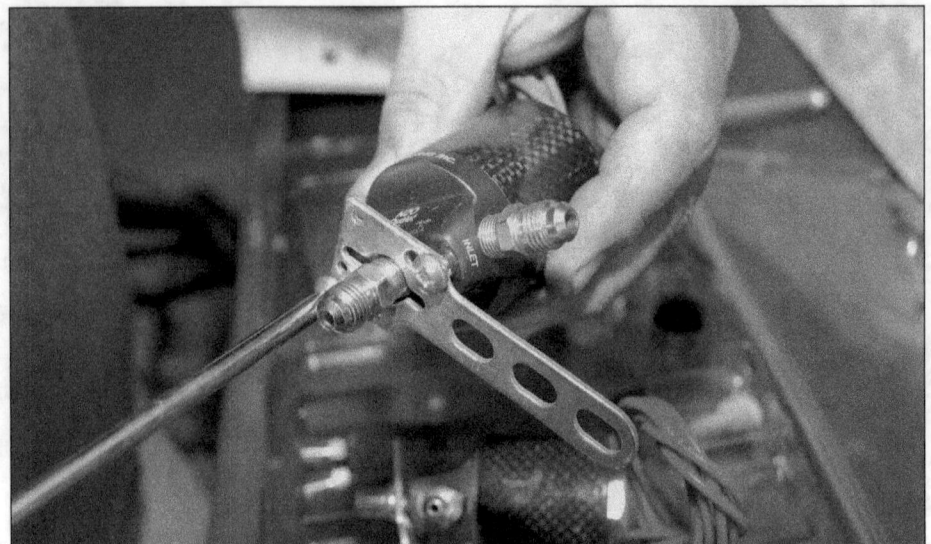

18 Install the NX solenoid mounting brackets (which can be clocked in various positions) using the supplied mounting hardware.

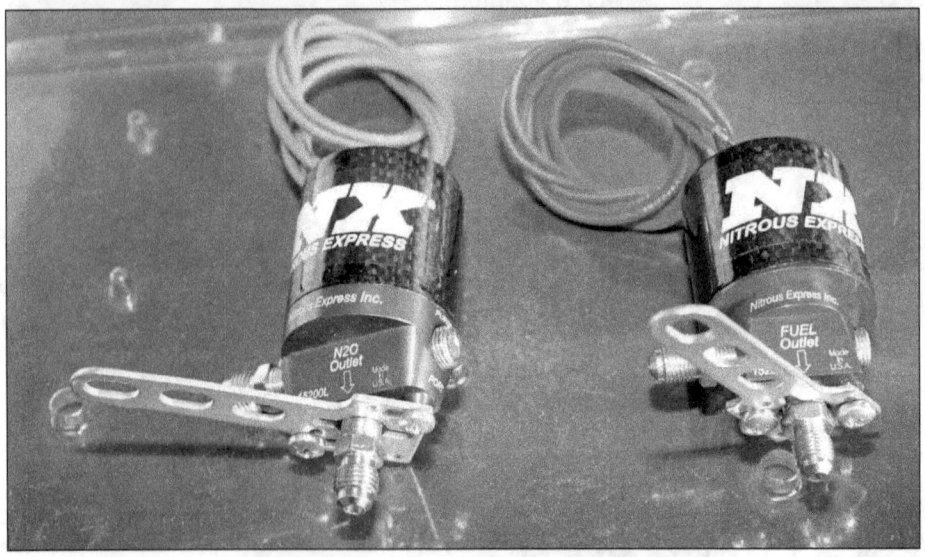

19 Here are the solenoids with mounting brackets fully attached.

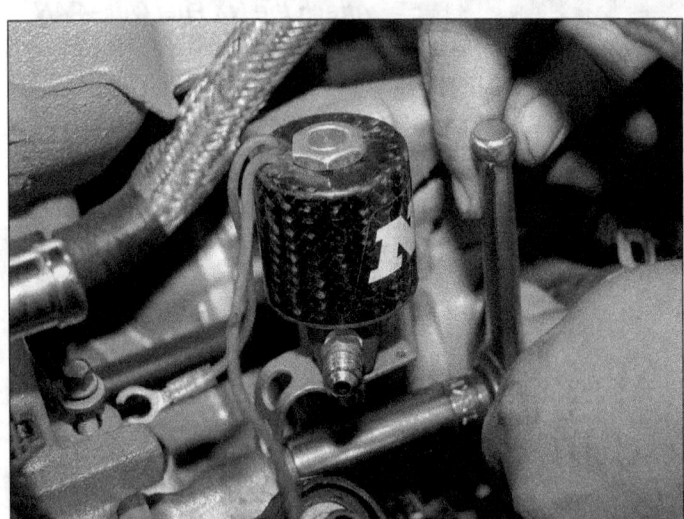
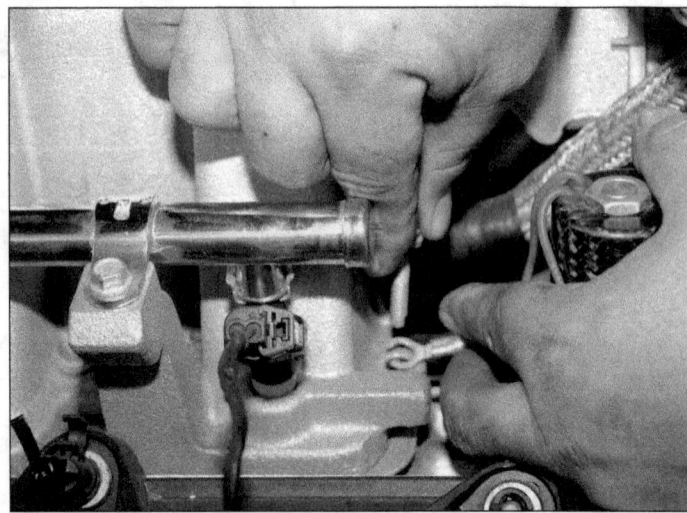

20 Installation of the fuel solenoid comes next. This unit is mounted to the driver's-side front of the SRT8 engine using a 1/4-inch bolt.

EFI, WET AND DRY

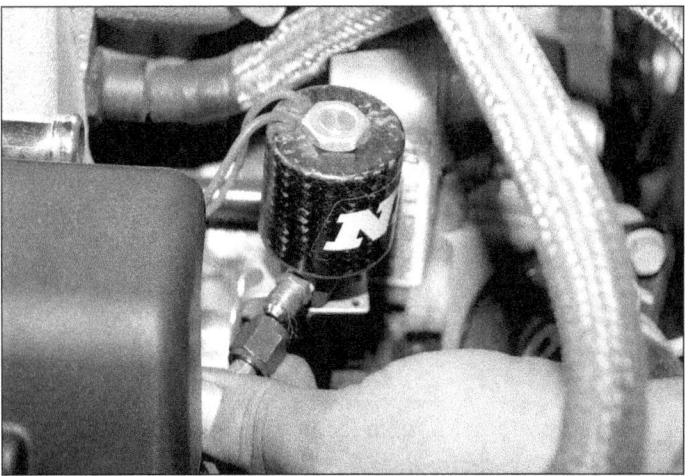

21 Attach the Fuel In -4 AN line coming from the NX Fuel Line Adaptor next.

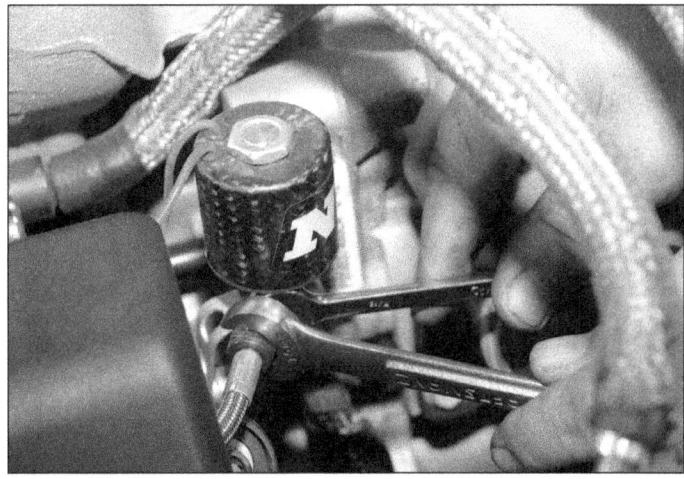

22 Use a 7/16-inch wrench to tighten the fuel line fitting.

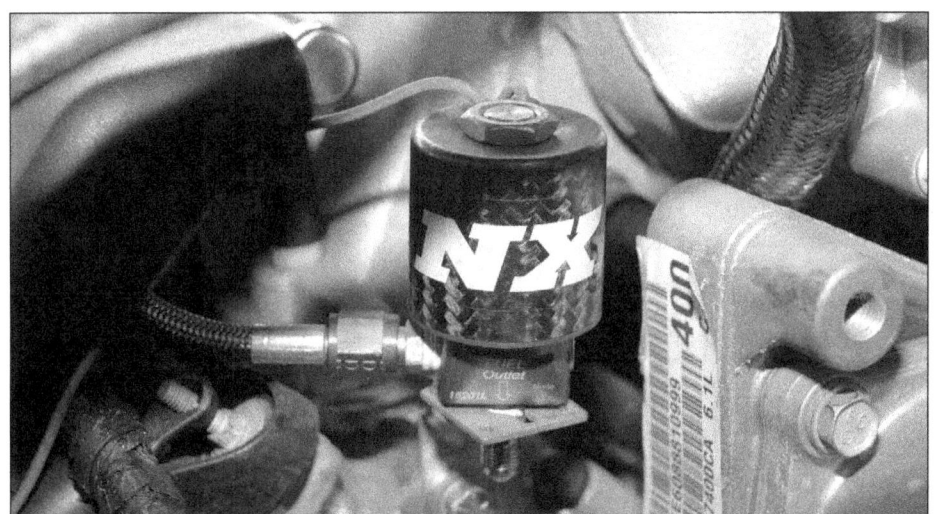

23 This is how the NX Fuel Solenoid should look once fully installed.

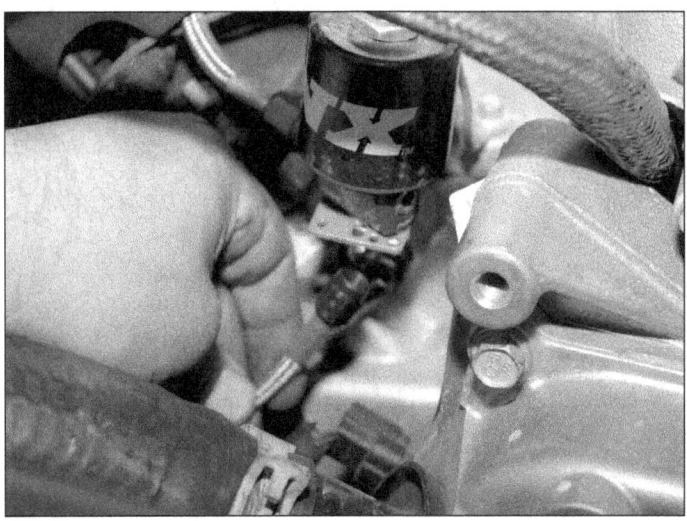

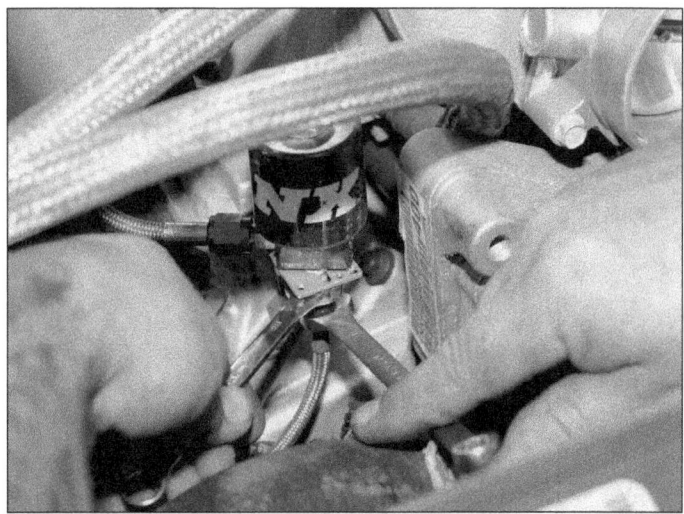

24 Hook up the -4 AN crossover line that runs from the NX Fuel Solenoid to the NX Nitrous Solenoid. This particular line is run beneath the SRT8's water filler neck at the front of the engine, and the line is tightened using a 7/16-inch wrench.

HOW TO INSTALL AND TUNE NITROUS OXIDE SYSTEMS

CHAPTER 9

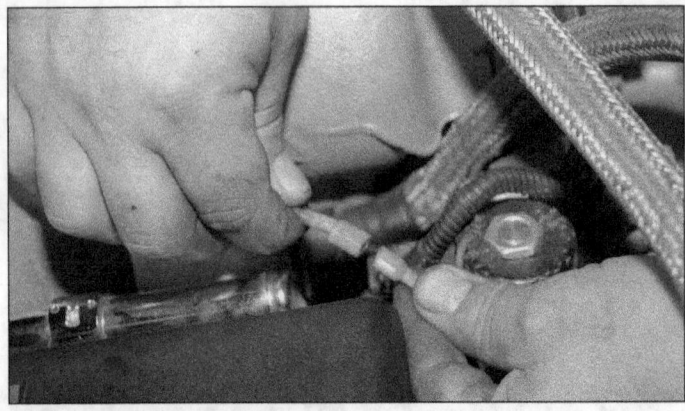

25 With the NX Nitrous Solenoid in hand, hook up the fuel and N₂O solenoid electrical wires.

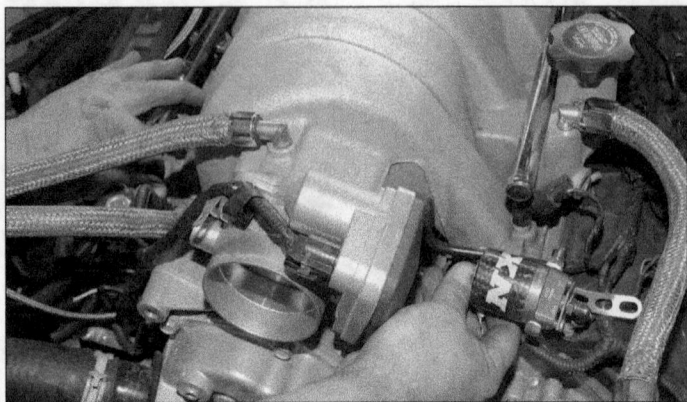

26 Search for a suitable location to mount the NX Nitrous Solenoid.

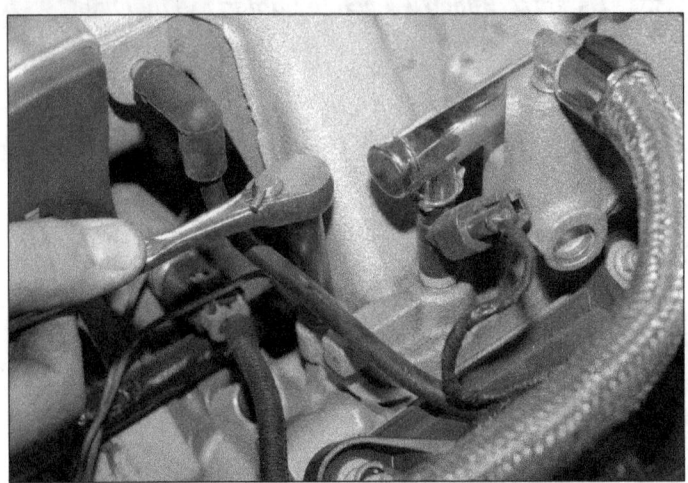

27 Locate a stud at the driver's-side front of the SRT8 intake and mount the nitrous solenoid.

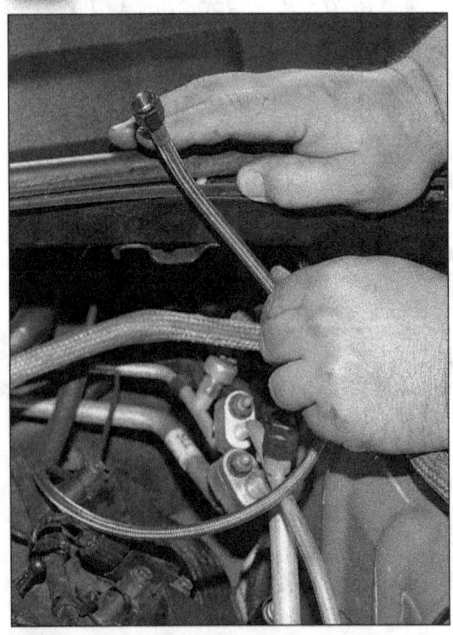

28 Hook up the -4 AN Nitrous In line to the NX solenoid.

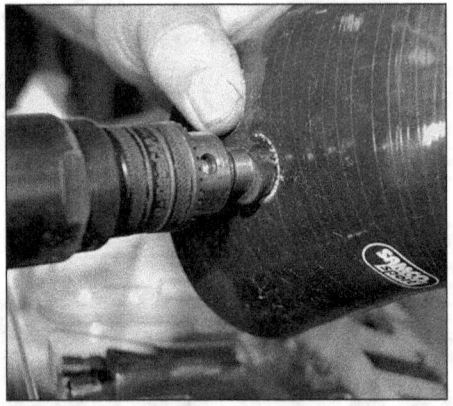

29 Installing the NX Stage 1 EFI Shark nozzle comes next. First drill a 9/16-inch hole into the SRT8 air intake tube using an auger bit to accommodate the supplied threaded nozzle-fitting adaptor. Then tighten the NX nozzle fitting adaptor using a standard 5/16-inch wrench.

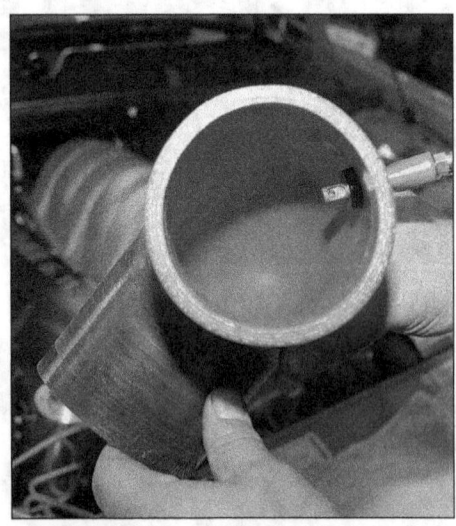

30 With the Shark nozzle fully installed, this is how it should look, keeping in mind that the sprayer must be pointed directly at the throttle body.

EFI, WET AND DRY

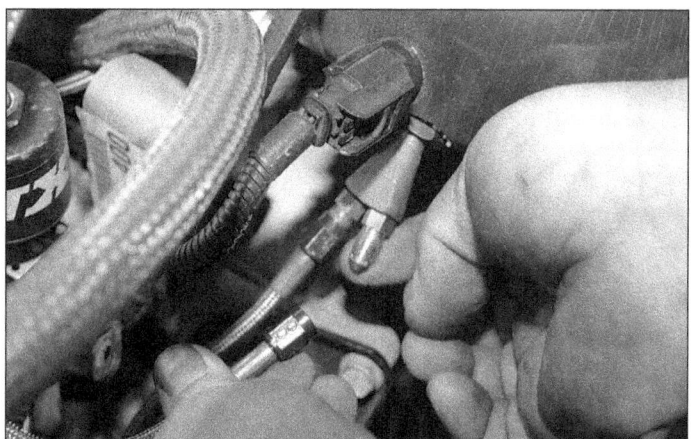
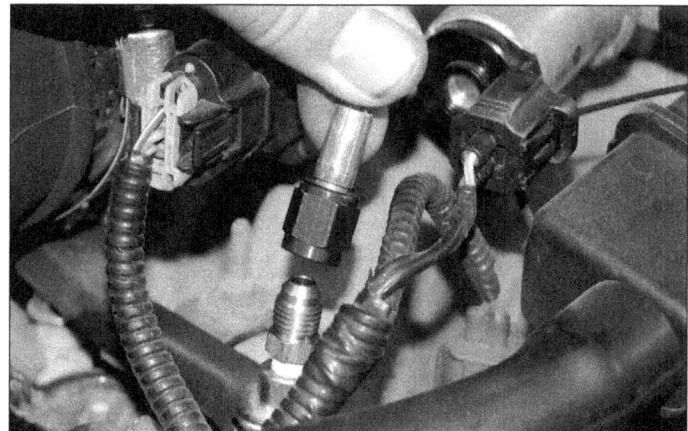

31 Hook up the Fuel In line to the nozzle. Then install the correct-size Pill (in racer's terms), or jet. In this case, Duquette used a 100-hp 6-jet, and a 7/16-inch wrench to tighten the line.

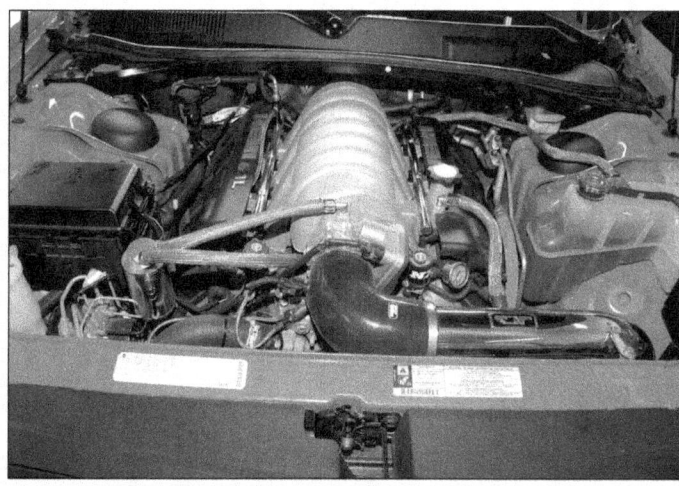

And there you have it. The complete NX SRT8 nitrous kit fully installed.

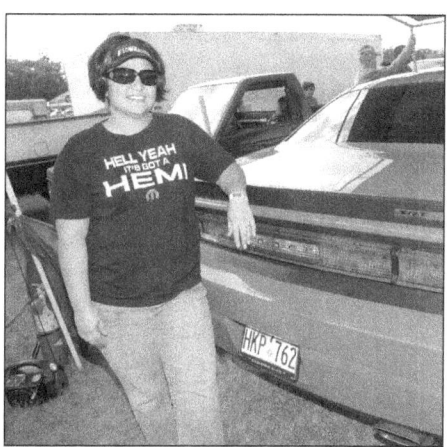

Denny Duquette's wife, April, wheels this Hemi-Orange 2009 SRT8 at the drags.

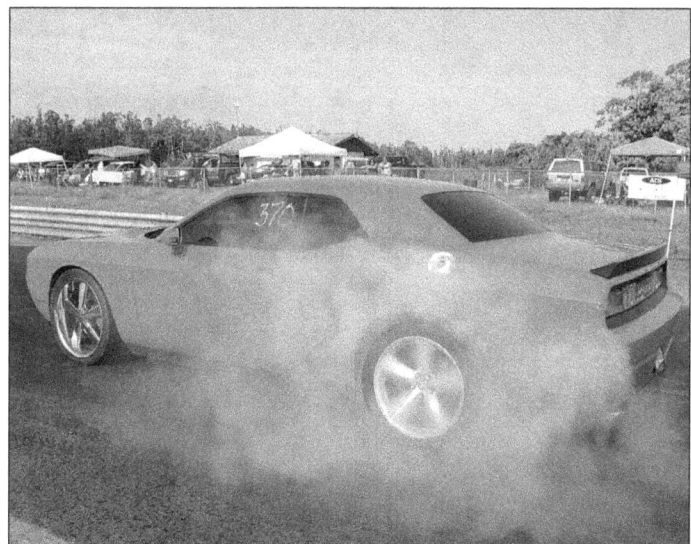

April makes a little smoke and lights up those Nitto Drag Radials.

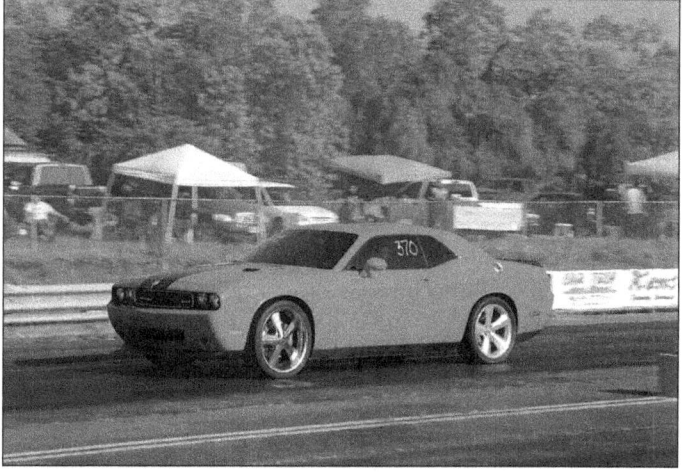

Off and running, this Challenger has run a best ET/MPH of 11.98 at 118.94 with an NX 100-Shot jet, and an 11.51 at 120.00 using the 150-Shot jet at sea level. Pretty impressive, huh?

CHAPTER 10

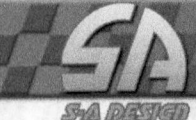

NITROUS ACCESSORIES

There are several new products and new versions of existing products that are changing the landscape of the nitrous world. These innovations might not have the many years of proven performance the typical kit parts can boast about, but in time they may become standard industry hardware.

Also, there are some goodies shown here that have been engineered for use in specific niche situations. If your project qualifies, you'll be happy to know all about these fresh new products.

At the very least, make yourself aware these parts exist. The world of nitrous is ever expanding, and the more you know about what's out there, the more effective your own system can be.

Accessory Nitrous Jetting

Most N_2O kits, carbureted or EFI, provide a limited amount of N_2O, and fuel jets, usually three to four, but you'll be happy to know that upgrade jet kits are readily available through most N_2O companies.

Aside from being turned out on a CNC machine, not all nitrous oxide jets are created equal. The proof is in the performance, and each company backs up its claims with its own test data. I wish I had the resources to conduct a nitrous jet shootout for this book; but I don't, so it's up to you to compare various products to find what works best for your application. For example:

- ZEX Nitrous Products' CNC-machined jets feature an internal taper, which minimizes turbulence and increases power. ZEX offers a Master Jet Pack containing 37 nitrous and 37 fuel jets from .125 to .014 inch.
- Nitrous Express claims that the NX accessory jets are guaranteed to be .005 inch within the specified jet size and, with its contoured inlet and multi-step outlet, outflow the competition by 35 percent.
- Nitrous Oxide Systems offers

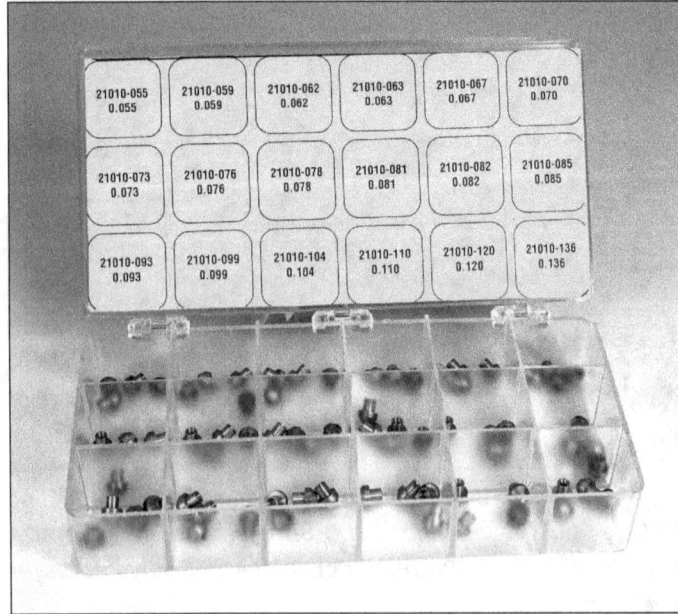

Nitrous Oxide Systems offers stainless-steel Precision SS N_2O and Fuel jets ranging from 0.014 to 0.136 inch in orifice size. NOS covers a total of 27 carbureted and EFI applications and can be purchased in 8-packs from NOS retailers.

Precision SS Flare jets, ranging from .014 to .091 inch for nitrous and from .015 to .092 inch for fuel. NOS Precision SS Funnel jets range from .051 to .093 inch for nitrous and .052 to .094 inch for fuel. These jets are touted to be accurately sized, and feature an internal taper that minimizes turbulence and increases flow and power. They can be purchased in what NOS calls Jet 8-Packs.

- Nitrous Supply's jets are available in both stainless steel and brass in both Flare and Funnel configurations in most popular sizes.

Advance-Design Nitrous Plates

Edelbrock offers the Victor Jr. nitrous plate for higher-horsepower applications. Both Wilson Manifolds & Nitrous Pro-Flow and Nitrous Supply market a Criss-Cross plate, while NX offers a Hot Plate application. Nitrous Express markets the Phase Three billet-aluminum plate. These plates can all be found on upscale 200- to 400-hp and 200- to 500-plus-hp single-stage and dual-stage 4V and 2x4V N_2O kits, or can be purchased separately for use as part of a custom-tuned system.

All the aforementioned plate designs are reported to inject more liquid N_2O into the intake with a more evenly spread pattern, while providing balanced distribution of fuel and N_2O across the intake plenum. However, most of these plates are currently being used on two- and three-stage N_2O applications. But I predict you will see some of these plates, albeit in slightly tuned-down versions, making their way into the entry-level N_2O-kit segment (with

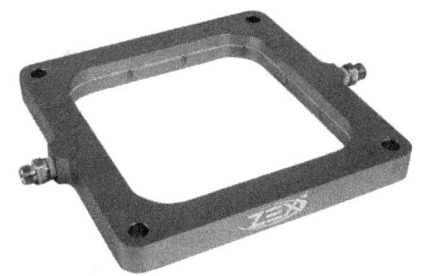

The big talk these days is ZEX Nitrous Products spray bar-less Perimeter Plate design, which creates a low pressure point in the air intake plenum for increased airflow, and provides even distribution of nitrous and gasoline for maximum power. These plates are available in square-flange (PN 82043, and Dominator-flange applications (PN 82072).

ZEX's Perimeter Plate already being an example). These assorted and sundry plates increase the overall efficiency of these systems, and competing nitrous manufacturers are determined to maintain their market share in the ever-evolving, consumer-conscious N_2O kit industry.

Super Solenoid

Nitrous Supply has recently introduced its Hi Flow N_2O solenoid, called the Slayer, for high-yield nitrous situations. Founder Mike Thermos told me: "One of the problems most racers run into when they're trying to achieve maximum flow out of a typical nitrous solenoid is that you have such a pressure differential on the topside of the plunger versus the bottom side, your electro-magnet has to really be very powerful to lift it off the seat. Of course, with some solenoids, you could increase the amperage to get them to respond quicker but it's just not safe to use that many amps on nitrous solenoids, which are currently rated at 10, 20, or 30 amps. To run that much amperage though a solenoid is just not a good policy. They get hot, the wiring gets hot, and they pull a lot of energy out of your car's electrical system. It's just not nitrous smart!"

What Mike Thermos and his technicians from Nitrous Supply have done is balance the pressure on both sides of the plunger so it doesn't have to overcome the nitrous pressure flowing in on one side from the bottle and pull through that.

"That arrangement gives us a lot of leeway," adds Thermos. "We are now able to lift the plungers up at low amperage (8 to 10 amps). Because of

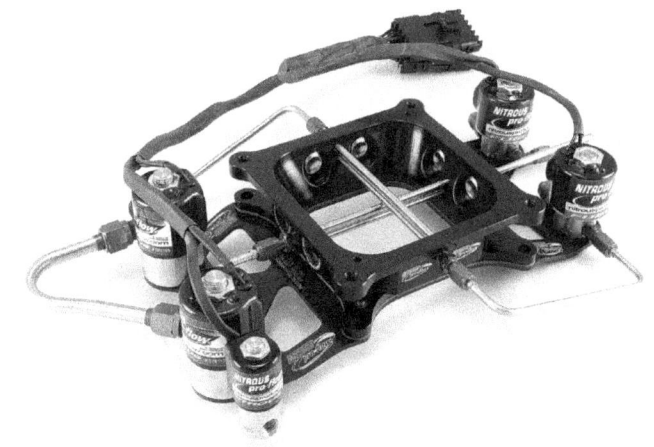

In an attempt to make more horsepower and go faster, carbureted nitrous racing has produced a number of advanced-design carburetor plates over the years. Edelbrock Nitrous has its Victor Jr. nitrous plate. Nitrous Supply has its Hot Plate, N_2O plate. NOS, TNW, and Wilson Manifolds & Nitrous Pro-Flow all offer a Criss Cross Plate (shown).

CHAPTER 10

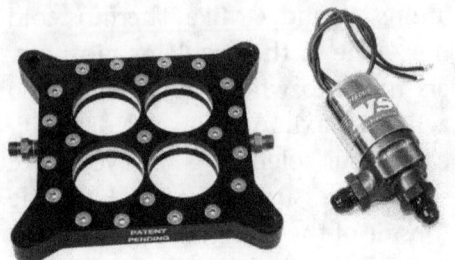

The latest power-producing plate design from Nitrous Supply is the Hot Plate, which boasts a unique stepped venturi design aided by computer designed orifices. The high pressure of the nitrous is actually used to shear the fuel, optimizing atomization of fuel and nitrous into the carburetor's air stream. This creates a halo effect that is far superior to spray-bar N_2O plates.

the balanced pressure, we can actually turn them on and off and flutter them. With the inertia of all the components in there, you can really vibrate them at a pretty high speed, and really control the flow. With a typical solenoid, without a pressure balance, you can't really get them to cycle. If you put a progressive controller on one, you'll be able to get it to go three cycles a second, which is not very good at all, and it won't have a nice flow curve to it either.

"These new solenoids can be installed on a driver, or progressive controller and you can hone them in, so to speak. A .0250-inch orifice opening is a ton of nitrous oxide volume, and with that much nitrous you certainly don't want it to come on like a light switch, you want it to come on softer, more like a rheostat."

Solenoids in a Box

ZEX Nitrous Products has a Nitrous Management Unit (NMU), available for both wet (PN 82007) and dry (PN 82008) applications. Simply put, the self-contained NMU engages and disengages the nitrous solenoids built inside its strong, heat resistant, and vibration-free aluminum housing at a pre-determined voltage threshold. Performance above and beyond that threshold is determined for WOT, and the system activates itself. For anything below that threshold, the system remains dormant.

Nitrous Express offers a similar item called the Proton Solenoid Housing, which, like the ZEX NMU, is small, lightweight, weatherproof, vibration free, impervious to heat, and works just great in tight situations. Could these products be the future of street N_2O systems?

Ignition Systems

These days, most high-intensity factory ignition systems, like Ford's EEC-IV, EDIS coil-on-plug factory ignitions, GM's distributorless Coil-Near-Plug factory setups, and Chrysler's Distributorless Coil-on-Plug ignition system, deliver more than enough voltage to light your average strip/strip N_2O system. According to MSD's Joe Pandro (Product Development/Race Teams), "When it comes to electronics, the late-model stuff is really hard to deal with. Right now, it's more important to have timing control rather than spark enhancement in terms of being able to deliver more power at the spark plug, especially with the GM products, because they use a smart coil. In other words, you can't amplify the spark because they contain a built-in driver inside of each coil. Aftermarket replacement coils become expensive because they have to have the driver built into them as well. At the present

Solenoids are as diverse as the application. For extreme high-yield situations, like big-inch carbureted gasoline and alcohol motors, Nitrous Supply's Slayer (PN 26015) operates at a safe 8 to 10 amps, yet features a quicker plunger-response time than other solenoids of its type. It boasts a .250-inch orifice, which is pretty huge when it comes to N_2O solenoids. The Slayer is currently the only solenoid of its size that can be fully modulated using a controller.

NITROUS ACCESSORIES

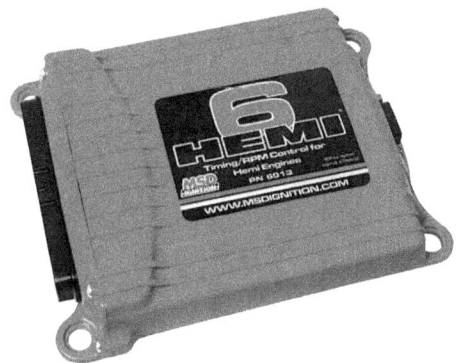

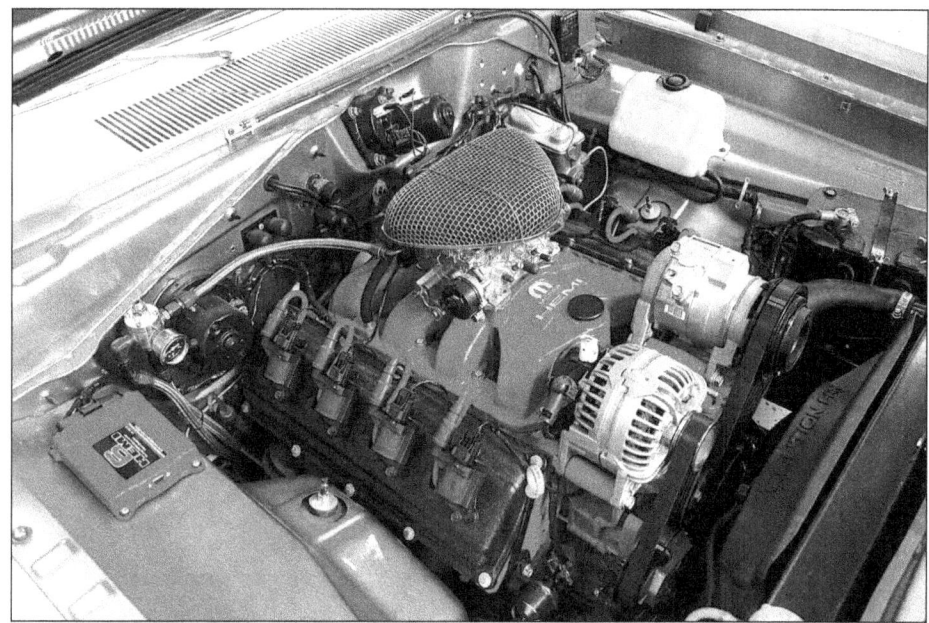

MSD's 6-Hemi Ignition Controller (PN 6013) helps control timing and keep check on detonation when used with modern computer-assisted engines like the 5.7L and 6.1L GEN-III Chrysler Hemis commonly found under the hoods of Dodge Ram trucks, Dodge Charger, Dodge Challenger SRT8, and Chrysler 300 SRT8 cars. Shown is one of MSD's 6-Hemi controllers installed inside a nitrous-equipped early Mopar, upgraded using one of Mopar Performance Part's 393-ci Gen-III Hemi crate engines.

time, there's not a whole lot to be gained there.

"Now, when it comes to the Hemis and the Fords, the only way to boost up the Ford is to add two amplifier boxes using a plug-in harness that we make. Basically, you're bolting on eight MSD boxes, so it becomes real expensive—like $600—as opposed to the cost of, let's say, a 150-hp nitrous kit.

"When it comes to the older-style stuff, like the Fords, Chevrolets, and Chryslers across the board, an MSD 6AL with a Blaster coil, which works with any distributor, is perfect. With street nitrous kits, I recommend the PN8987 Starter Step Retard Control, which is a little box that directly fits in the palm of your hand and has the ability to retard the ignition from 1 to 15 degrees. It's got a sensor wire that hooks up directly to the nitrous solenoid, so when the solenoid is activated, it pulls the timing back based on what you set the knob at. With a typical single-stage street nitrous kit, 15 degrees should be more than adequate. Once again, this box works with any type of distributor, whether it's equipped with points, is a factory electronic setup (EEC-IV or HEI), or an aftermarket setup like our MSD Pro Billet unit!"

Ignition Control Boxes and Controllers

Joe Pandro of MSD says, "MSD has control modules for the new Chryslers, such as, 6-Hemi Ignition Controller [PN 6013], the MOD-6 Ignition Controller for the Fords [PN 6011], the 24-tooth GMs 6LS [PN 6010], and 6LS2 58-tooth Ignition Controller [PN 6012], which helps you control timing, and avoid denotation. MSD's 6-Hemi Ignition Controller [PN 6013] helps control timing and detonation with modern computer-assisted, nitrous-oxide-equipped engines like the 5.7L and 6.1L Gen-III Chrysler Hemis commonly found in Charger, Challenger, and RAM trucks."

Owners of Ford modular motors can also enjoy the technological benefits of MSD technology. The company's Mod-6 Ignition Controller (PN 6011) is perfect for 4.6L two-, three-, and four-valve modular motors on nitrous or that have been transplanted into street rods.

MSD's 24-tooth Controller for the 6LS and 58-tooth 6LS2 Ignition Timing Controller helps control timing and avoid detonation with N_2O-assisted LS-Series GM engines.

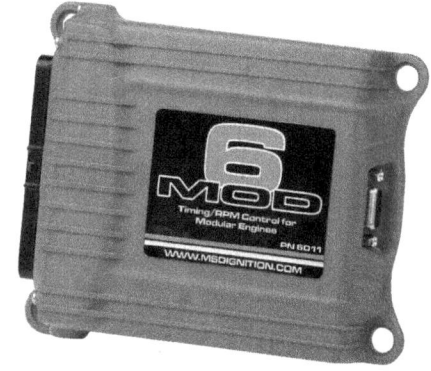

Ford modular motor owners can also enjoy the benefits of MSD technology. The Mod-6 Ignition Controller (PN 6011) is perfect for 4.6L 2V and 3V modular motors. This unit controls the flow of nitrous, features a timing retard, and controls detonation.

CHAPTER 10

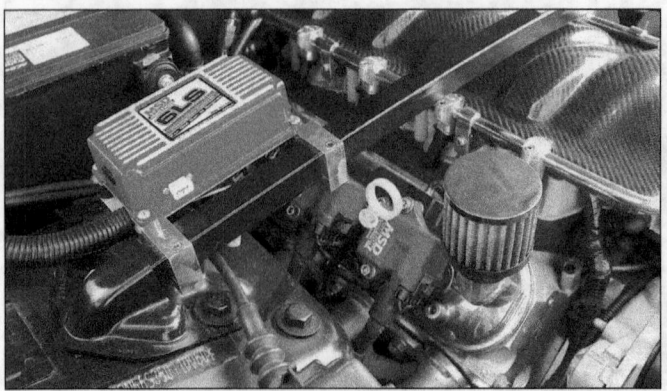

MSD's 24-tooth Timing Controller for the 6LS and 58-tooth Timing Controller for the 6LS2 (PN 6012) control nitrous delivery, retard timing, and control detonation on GMs LS1-LS7 engines. These controllers should also interface with GM's LM-Series truck engines. However, check with the manufacturer for other applications.

Nitrous Controllers

The powerful and compact Edelbrock Progressive Nitrous Controller (PN 71900) operates on the pulse-width principle and regulates the amount of N_2O being delivered over a specified period of time by the nitrous and fuel solenoids. Its easy-to-read LCD digital display and touch-switch programming, adjustable from 0 to 9.999 seconds, is about as user friendly as they come. With this unit, you have the ability to select the nitrous parameters in order to optimize traction, control the chassis, and safely ramp up the nitrous system.

From simple to serious, Nitrous Supply offers two products. The Digi-Set (PN 25835) allows you the option of activating your N_2O system's second or third stage as well as electronically time hits in increments from 1/10 second to 1 minute 45 seconds. The Progressive Controller With Brains (PN 25834) allows two separate timer programs, for changing track conditions, which can be selected via a simple dashboard switch. Six programmable

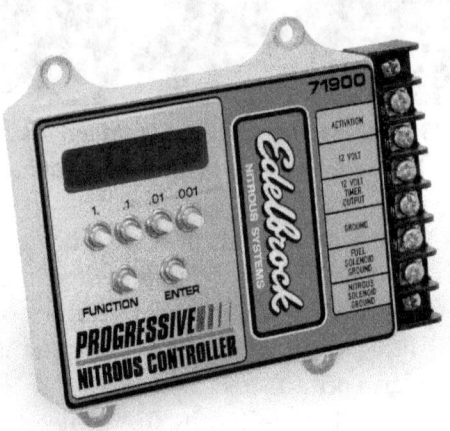

This is the Edelbrock PN 71900 Progressive Nitrous Controller. It utilizes pulse width modulation to regulate the amount of nitrous (and fuel) being delivered over a specified period of time. This way, the "hit" can be adjusted down and brought in gradually so the tires don't break loose. It also makes for less stress on the engine's internal components when the nitrous is introduced in this fashion.

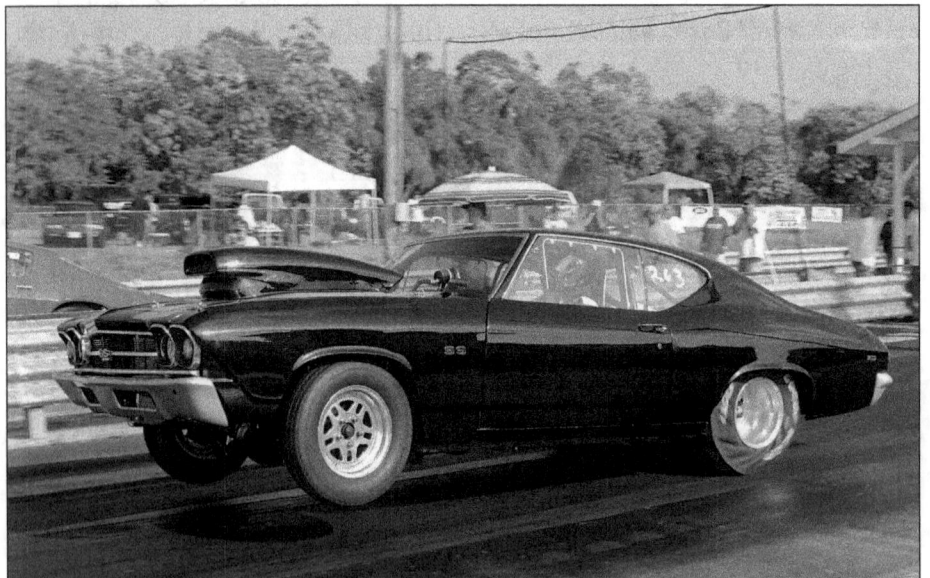

Matt Briley's Chevelle bracket car features a 502-ci big-block topped with a ZEX 150-shot single-stage system and Edelbrock Nitrous Progressive Controller (PN 71900). It leaves the line on a 75-hp shot and then turns up the wick an additional 75 hp at about 400 feet out. "The transition is so smooth you hardly feel it," says Briley. Matt's Chevelle has run an ET/MPH best of 9.70/141.00.

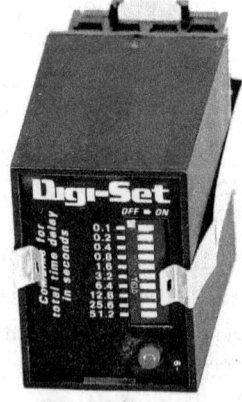

Feeling a little intimidated by all this sophisticated electronic hardware? The NS Digi Set is nitrous control simplified. The built-in time relay gives you the option of activating second or third stages as well as setting response time in 1/10-second increments to as much as 1 minute 45 seconds.

124   HOW TO INSTALL AND TUNE NITROUS OXIDE SYSTEMS

NITROUS ACCESSORIES

outputs can actuate solenoids, lock-up convertors, clutches, ignitions, turbocharger waste gates, etc.

Nitrous Oxide Systems also offers a number of N_2O timers. Right at the top of the list is NOS Programmable Progressive Nitrous Controller (PN 15834NOS). It can be programmed to control the amount of nitrous flow from 0 to 100 percent and to ramp up from first hit to full flow, delivering predetermined percentages of N_2O in a variety of seconds and enabling you to fine tune the power curve to suit track conditions. This box can also activate a retard box or second stage of nitrous.

NOS's Mini Two-Stage Progressive Nitrous Controller (PN 15974NOS) is touted to be two controllers in one case, each with its own throttle position activation switch and progressive ramps. The on/off RPM control eliminates the need for a separate window switch. The ramp time, delay time, and nitrous percentages are programmable from 0 to 9.9 seconds and the start percentage is programmable from 0 to 99 percent. A pair of programmable output features allows you to control timing retard or other devices, all done through a hand-held programmer.

Nitrous Oxide Systems' Time Based Progressive Nitrous Control System (PN 15835BNOS) starts the flow at any level you set from 0 to 100 percent, and gradually brings in the full N_2O over a period of time. This system is adjustable from 0 to 10 seconds, which allows you to start with a small shot of N_2O (say, 25 to 30 percent) to minimize wheelspin and then transition to full power when the car is successfully hooked up. One-half-second ET gains are accessible. This system features easy-to-read adjustment knobs that lock into the settings. NOS also offers the Digi-Set (PN 15838) and Time Delay Switch (PN 15838NOS).

Nitrous Express offers a series of four controllers including the Pro Traction Control Module (PN SPEED00030), the Maximizer 3 (PN 15958), Boost Reference Progressive Controller (PN NXD5000), and Octane Series Progressive Controller (PN 15835).

Pro Traction Control Module allows very aggressive nitrous setups, such as multi-stage N_2O setups, without fear of wheel-spin and tire-shake. This unit is completely adjustable and features a ramp out adjustment to correspond with the chassis, and a nitrous ramp-up feature to take full advantage of prevailing track conditions.

The Maximizer 3 features hand-held convenience, complete with a remote micro-solenoid at 40 amps per driver. Actual amp capacity is expandable by adding extra drivers. It also features integrated TPS and RPM window functions, working with the rise and fall of TPS voltage. The TPS trigger point can be set between 25 and 99 percent. A power-ramping control sets the start of nitrous flow at 0 to 1 percent, the TPS idle-voltage meter sets the idle voltage, and the TPR sets the WOT voltage. There is also an RPM Multiplier, which sets the number of cylinders, and a 12-volt Reams-Brake input that holds the N_2O during staging.

NX touts this unit as the original Boost Reference Progressive Controller, with boost-referenced or time-based power ramping, variable multi-port ramping, Ian internal window switch, built-in TPS activation, 85-psi MAP Sensor, and dual-stage capability.

The time- or RPM-based NX Octane Series Progressive Controller features an RPM window switch, WOT Detection (when used with a factory TPS or WOT switch), and supports fly-by-wire TPS rising or falling. It features five-point variable progressive ramping (time- or RPM-based), a rich/lean cutoff when used with a wideband receiver, digital/analog air/fuel inputs, bottle heater controller, first-gear lockout or delay feature, eight different viewing screens, programmable Power Up and ARM screen, multiple pressure choices, and pressure displays labeled Boost, Nitrous, Oil, or Fuel.

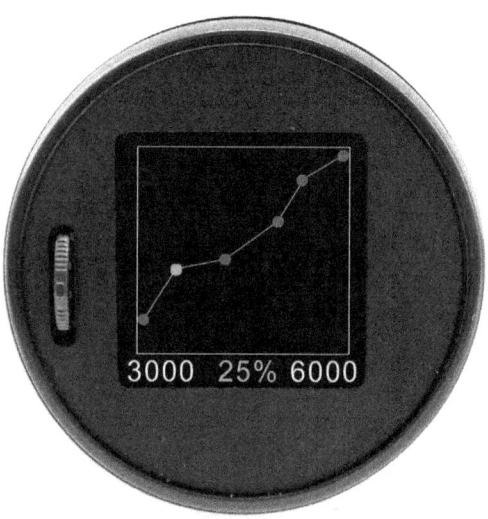

The dash-mounted NX Octane Series Progressive Controller (PN 15535) can be either time or RPM based. It features multiple wideband capabilities and rich/lean cutoff readouts when used with the wideband feature. It also features air/fuel inputs and either digital or analog display. There is also a pressure display feature for boost, nitrous, oil, and fuel. This unit can also activate bottle heater control, has five-point programmable ramping, and WOT detection when used with factory TPS or WOT switch. This is quite a toy!

CHAPTER 10

Spark Plugs

Until the introduction of nitrous oxide for the street, the average hot rodder could slap in a hotter spark plug and go for it. Gearhead mentality prevailed. It was definitely old school compared to computer-controlled, high-tech engines. With the extreme cylinder-head temperatures created with the introduction of N_2O, it certainly doesn't hurt to drop the heat range a couple points. With today's high-energy ignition systems (which actually do most of the hard work) it simply makes good sense. A colder-range spark plug safely fires in N_2O's oxygen-enriched atmosphere, while controlling detonation without creating a glow-plug effect or self-destructing entirely.

For example, a stock 215- to 225-hp, 8.5:1-compression 5.0L Mustang pushrod V-8 usually requires an Autolite 25 spark plug. But a set of Autolite 23s, which are two ranges colder, still make plenty of safe detonation-free horsepower in nitrous situations. Or, take a stock 10.7:1-compression, 376-ci, 422-hp 2010 Camaro LS-3 engine with AC Delco 41-110 plugs. Once equipped with a 35- to 150-hp shot of nitrous oxide, try switching to an NGK F13 platinum plug, which is two points colder and superior in heat transfer and conductivity. Overall, it's a much better plug.

Then too, a set of NGK A13s more than adequately fire a 6.1L, 425-hp Gen-III SRT8 small-block Hemi. But with a 100-shot of nitrous installed, a two-ranges-colder NGK TR6 platinum spark plug seems to make better sense.

By now, you're starting to get the picture—more is not always better. But there is no substitution for quality and that is why you're seeing platinum and iridium composition spark plugs (from NGK and Denso, for example) being used more frequently in high-performance applications. But what about purpose-built N_2O spark plugs? ZEX Nitrous Products' Power Tune Ignitor Core Spark Plugs are new to the market. Not platinum or iridium, which seem to have become the standard with today's computer-controlled high-tech engines, ZEX's Igniter Core uses copper surrounded by a durable nickel shell, to conduct electricity and heat five times better than platinum and almost three times better than iridium. The result is an increase in horsepower-producing spark energy and greater detonation resistance than platinum or iridium can deliver.

Another groundbreaking development is Clean Fire Technology. It uses the spark from three additional ground straps to super-clean the center electrode. This burns off excess carbon and ensures you get maximum power and superior resistance to fouling.

ZEX has developed two different types of Ignitor Core spark plugs with optimized heat ranges for your specific modifications and power levels. For engines with bolt-on performance parts and computer

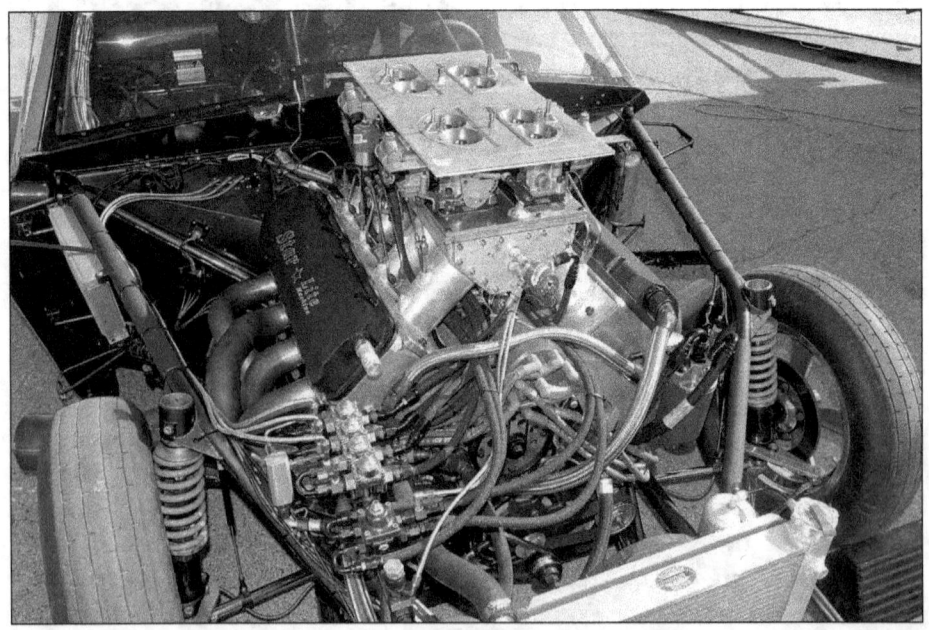

One of the most commonly used controllers by Pro Racers like Ray Vettel to time his four-stage, DART Industries/Starlight Motorsports 780-ci, 4x2 split Holley induction system Top Sportsman Plymouth Barracuda is FAST state-of-the-art XF2 controller. Vettel's 'Cuda has run a best of 6.22 seconds at 230.00 mph, using only three out of four possible stages.

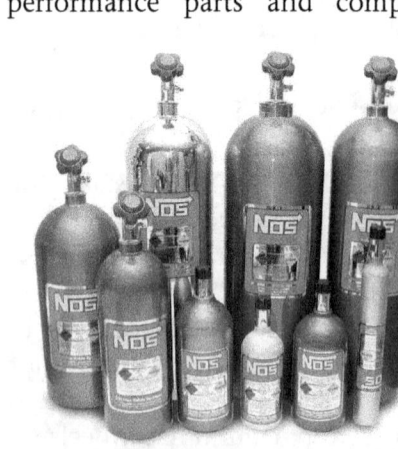

Today's N_2O bottles come in many sizes to suit myriad applications. (Photo Courtesy Nitrous Oxide Systems, Inc.)

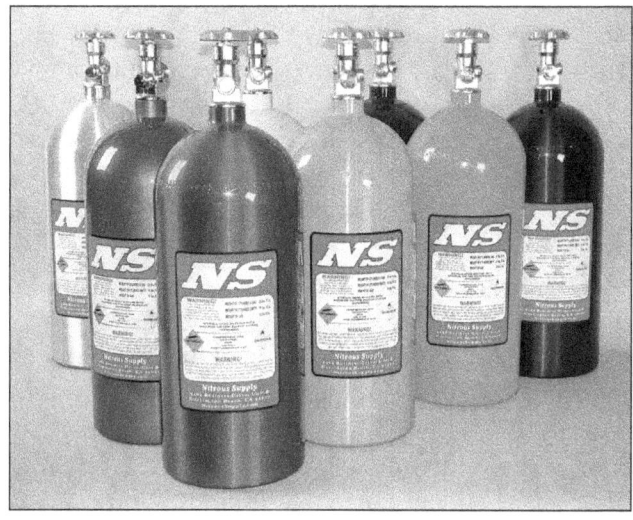

Designer N_2O bottles? Color is no longer used just to distinguish a certain manufacturer's product. Thanks to the folks at Nitrous Supply, it's possible to order these vessels in practically any color and size you want, plus polished aluminum.

tuning, up to 400 hp, the Power Tune spark plug is the right choice. In racing applications where nitrous use, supercharging, and/or turbocharging all come into play, the Power Racer spark plugs maximize performance in engines up to 700 hp. ZEX Ignitor Core plugs are available in a total of 95 applications for import and domestic vehicles, including seven Chevrolet, eight Ford, and three Pontiac part numbers.

Nitrous Oxide Bottles and Tanks

In today's nitrous marketplace bottle sizes now range from 5 ounces to 20 pounds. Colors originally distinguished one N_2O manufacturer's bottle from another. For example, Nitrous Oxide Systems' traditional blue may have once been its trademark, but now you can also get polished-aluminum versions.

Edelbrock's nitrous program offers bottles in either silver or polished aluminum. Wilson Manifolds & Nitrous Pro-Flow bottles are available in basic black, as are those used by the Nitrous Outlet, and NANO (nitrogen-assisted nitrous oxide) Systems, while Nitrous Express bottles are available in basic white. ZEX prefers to store N_2O in either a polished or candy-purple-colored bottle. But Mike Thermos' Nitrous Supply really takes the cake. At the customer's request, NS powdercoats the spun-aluminum bottles in candy-red, candy-blue, black, yellow, orange, purple, or lime green.

Forget pretty—you just want to go fast, right? Saving weight is one way of doing it, and with that thought in mind, the composite N_2O tank was invented.

The composite tank, originally manufactured for Nitrous Oxide Systems by Luxfer Manufacturing Company, was primarily designed to save weight. According to N_2O guru Wady Hammam, the composite bottle was originally field-tested by professional fire fighters who needed to be effective and move quickly!

Construction-wise, the carbon-fiber or composite nitrous tank starts out as a 1/8-inch aluminum shell, wrapped in five or six layers of carbon-fiber material. A composite nitrous bottle holds 2½ pounds more N_2O than a 10-pound aluminum N_2O bottle because of its internal construction and round bottom; and it weighs 5 pounds less. The 12.50-pound composite N_2O bottle carries certification number DOT-SP10915-2216, and is sold by Nitrous Oxide Systems, Nitrous Supply, Nitrous Express, and other top-name nitrous manufacturers.

Note: Due to DOT, federal, and state shipping regulations, N_2O bottles are shipped empty.

Bottle Valves and Openers

The standard-issue N_2O bottle valve has been taken for granted for years as being sort of a glorified throwback to the oxygen/acetylene/nitrogen bottle days. In truth, Nitrous Oxide Systems' Hi-Flow Valve

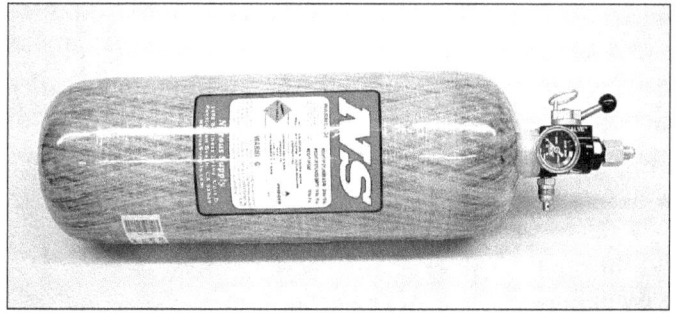

Undoubtedly the largest breakthrough in N_2O bottle technology was the invention of the carbon-fiber-wrap composite bottle, which was a joint project between Luxfer Manufacturing Company and Nitrous Oxide Systems, Inc. These bottles feature a 1/8-inch-thick inner shell and 5 or 6 layers of carbon-fiber outer material. Weight is 5 pounds less than a conventional 10-pound nitrous bottle when empty. Bottle capacity is 12.50 pounds. This Nitrous Supply bottle is certified by the DOT, and is assigned DOT- SP10915-2216.

CHAPTER 10

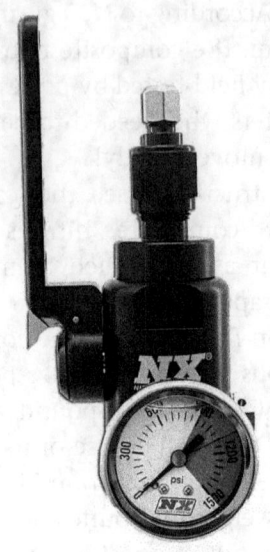

Nitrous Express Direct Flow 500 bottle valve (PN 11500) with On/Off handle is a high-flow nitrous valve featuring a .500-inch orifice, locking safety feature, and direct flow-straight flow-through design. This valve also comes with a .625-inch stainless-steel siphon tube and -8 AN hardware. NX claims this valve can handle up to 2,000 hp!

(PN 16140NOS, with built-in siphon tube) standardized the nitrous oxide bottle valve industry when it was approved by the Compressed Gas Association (CGA). Features include:

- Easy-to-turn hand wheel or knob.
- Blow-off vent/safety-disc feature designed to protect the customer from overfilling the bottle, keeping in mind that N₂O may cause severe burns on contact with the skin, at -127 degrees F, and breathing in the substance may cause respiratory damage. Extreme caution is necessary when handling a bottle around the valve area; a safety disc on the valve may release excess nitrous pressure at any time.

- The Hi-Flow Valve uses a large non-restrictive orifice that eliminates pressure drop, freezing (both of which cause surging), and a drop in horsepower. The valve was designed for serious competitors—the orifice is claimed to flow 249 percent more than the standard N₂O bottle valve. This high-flow valve is available in either 10-pound (PN 16139NOS) or 15-pound (PN 16139-15NOS) applications. The features include:
  - twin gauge ports for attaching a nitrous pressure gauge and other performance accessories
  - exclusive NOS safety venting system with -8 AN fittings for a professional in-car blow-down tube
  - standard 660 automotive connection—a must have for any serious professional

For Street

The NX Lightning 45 Bottle Valve lays claim to being the highest-flowing bottle valve on the market, and is flow-matched to complement the particular size of NX Lightning Solenoid being used. This valve also features two parts: one for a pressure gauge and one for an accessory port. Applications range from a 16-ounce motorcycle bottle valve (PN 11010) all the way up to 15-pound bottles (PN 11150). Somewhere at the top of that list is NX's most popular valve application, the 10-pound Lightning 45 valve (PN 11100).

For Pro Racers

The NX DF5 (Direct Flow 500) bottle valve with on/off handle (PN 11500) is a high-flow nitrous valve with locking safety featuring a 1/2-inch orifice, and direct-flow/ straight-flow-through design, which can handle as many as 2,000 applications. Furnished with a .625-inch stainless-steel siphon tube, -8 AN hardware, supply line, fittings, and a liquid-filled N₂O pressure gauge, this valve has to be the pro pick!

Other valve offerings are: Nitrous Supply's basic NS Powerstar CCG brass bottle valve in 5- to 20-pound-bottle applications (PN 26138), and the 250- to 560-hp NX High Flow 660 CGA Racestar bottle valve, which comes in 5- to 20-pound-bottle applications (PN 26139). NS also markets an inline high-flow/high-pressure valve (PN 26148).

Nitrous Supply's new NS Power-valve features a flow-through .500-inch orifice and a hand-activated lever that you turn to full-on or full-off position. There is a spring-loaded safety pin, a 5/8-inch stainless-steel siphon tube, two 1/8-inch gauge ports along with a racer-safety blow-off valve, and a large -8 AN outlet with supplied -6 AN adaptor. When used with one of NS's 12.9-pound carbon-fiber bottles, this combination delivers more performance than competing brands.

In a world of convenience, remote bottle openers seem to be all the rage these days. NS markets its remote bottle opener (PN 26058), which allows you the option to open and close your system with the flick of a switch from the driver's compartment.

Remote Bottle Control

Nitrous Oxide Systems' remote bottle controls are the perfect solution for when you either forget to open your bottle or forget to close it! A simple flick of the switch is all you need. This unit operates on 12 volts and fits 5-pound-and-larger nitrous bottles. The NOS Remote Bottle Control also comes with its own wiring and easy-to-follow instructions under PN 16139NOS (10 pounds) and PN 16139-15NOS (15 pounds).

Alternately, Nitrous Express' version of an automatic bottle opener is the remote bottle-valve opener in kit form (PN 11107).

ZEX also markets a remote bottle-valve opener (PN 82009), which allows you to activate the N_2O system from the driver's seat with the switch. ZEX's bottle opener kit comes with its own purple-anodized billet-aluminum housing, trouble-free modular motor (which lasts for years), wiring harness, and arming switch. It's the complete package.

NOS Pinch Valve Kit

According to the technicians at Nitrous Oxide Systems, there are a number of advantages to controlling the richness and leanness of N_2O and fuel mixture under acceleration. NOS has developed the electronically activated Pinch Valve (PN 14168NOS for the remote bottle opener; PN 16058NOS for solenoid-style remote bottle openers), which works via a simple switch. The pinch valve also facilitates exotic racing fuel use (like nitromethane and alcohol), which can be trickled into the system. A battery pack, single-action push button, solenoid, electrical wiring, and instructions are included in the kit.

Blow-Down Tube

The purpose of a safety blow-down tube is to release excessive nitrous pressure in the event that the bottle becomes overfilled or overheated. These are required by NHRA, IHRA, and independent racetracks across the country. ZEX Nitrous Products' Safety Blow-Down kits feature both externally and internally threaded safety ports that attach to the actual bottle itself. Then a blow-down tube is run from the nitrous bottle storage compartment to an outside venting area. Components can be purchased separately or in kit form (PN 82099).

Edelbrock markets its Nitrous Blow-Down Tube Kit (PN 72960), along with a Racer Safety Blow-Off Adaptor (PN 72961), which replaces the standard safety valve to allow using a hard-line blow-down tube.

Note: Many bottle warmer kits, such as Nitrous Express' GEN-X Accessory Pack and GENX2 Accessory Pack, come with a blow-down tube.

Lines–Nitrous Oxide and Fuel

For the high-pressure-rated, aircraft-quality delivery lines or hoses used in most street/strip N_2O kits, the industry standard is the Teflon-encased, braided stainless-steel -4 AN male anodized compression fitting. These lines usually measure approximately 12 to 14 feet long and use the color blue to denote N_2O.

Braided stainless-steel hoses run the gamut from -8 AN all the way up to -16 AN, with the latter being strictly custom, as in IHRA/NHRA Pro Mod, Top Sportsman, Pro 5.0, and World's Fastest Street Car Shoot-out entries.

For both nitrous and fuel delivery lines going directly to the carburetor, the color of the accompanying fitting usually denotes the application. For example, the nitrous line is blue, while the fuel line fitting is red. Because line placement varies from application to application, these lines come straight and usually measure 8 to 10 inches long.

Here's a tip: Use an old coat hanger to rough in these lines first to save a lot of headaches, and then use a tubing bender to complete the job.

Also note that N_2O hard lines measure 1/8 to 3/16 inch in diameter. N_2O kit manufacturers as well as specialty houses like Aeroquip Earl's Performance Plumbing, Russell Performance, and DMP Fasteners & Race Supplies all offer both the aforemen-

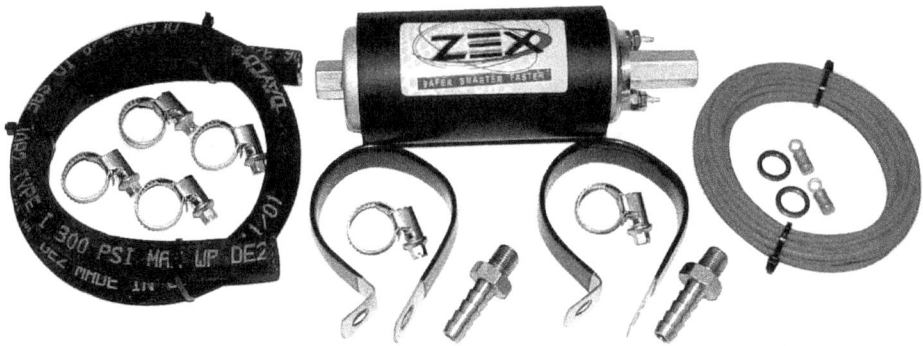

The ZEX Nitrous Products Booster Fuel Pump Kit (PN 82020), for return-line-only fuel systems, can boost your fuel capacity up to 650 hp even on a high-pressure turbocharged engine, supercharged engine, or N_2O setup. This pump is installed inline, and comes complete with all the wiring and mounting hardware.

tioned sizes of braided stainless-steel soft lines and stainless-steel hard lines.

Fuel Pumps and Systems

In high-pressure applications like EFI, two pumps may be run in series when trying to increase the flow rate just enough to handle the demands of high-performance upgrades like nitrous or an aftermarket supercharger or turbocharger. But the second (or supplementary) pump isn't usually equal to the total of the flow rates of both pumps. In most cases it is less, but just enough to handle the increase in fuel delivery. Your basic street/strip N_2O kit generally requires 4- to 10-psi extra capacity. However, note that high-volume electric or electronic aftermarket fuel pumps do not pull as well as they push, so the fewer restrictions you have before the pump, the more efficiently the system performs. Here are two examples:

- ZEX Nitrous Products Booster Fuel Pump Kit (PN 82020) can boost your fuel capacity up to 650 hp—even on a higher-pressure N_2O setup, a supercharged engine, or a turbocharged engine. This pump is also installed inline, and comes complete with all wiring and mounting hardware. Note: This product is intended for return-line fuel systems only, such as EFI.
- Electronically fuel-injected cars can also use a so-called in-tank pump, which piggybacks off the existing OE electronic high-volume electronic in-tank fuel pump.

Purge Systems

It's a necessity for serious racers, and provides a show for the fans. It's called purging the system. Nitrous oxide vapors can accumulate at the solenoids, causing a delay in response when you first activate the system. By purging the vapor, you relieve the system of trapped air or gaseous N_2O and fill the lines with pure liquid N_2O instead. The result is a system that responds quickly when activated.

But why do you see a single plume of nitrous vapor on some cars and two on others? Usually it depends on the size of the system and the setup. Inverted windshield wiper sprayers are commonly used by stock bodied racers, while others prefer to fabricate their lines. The result is still the same; the driver can actually see the system being purged.

Purge kits are available through companies like Mike Thermos' Nitrous Supply for both sport compact and V-8 engine applications (PNs 26030 and 26032, respectively).

Edelbrock offers both sport compact and V-8 purge-valve kits (PN 72176 with a -4 AN fitting and PN 72178 with a -6 AN fitting). ZEX Nitrous Products manufactures four purge kits in a total of three sizes and three LED colors.

Nitrous Oxide Systems' Ntimidator purge kit (PN 16033NOS) only features solenoids, nitrous and electrical line, and an activation button. There is also an optional LED Purge Kit (PN 16033NOS) that features a selection of white, green, red, blue, or yellow LED lights, which signal the driver when the system is being purged. You can also hook up these LEDs to signal on and off, preferably using red and green LEDs.

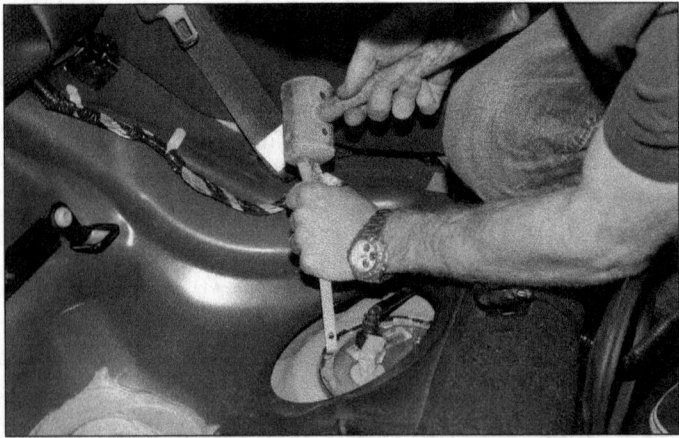 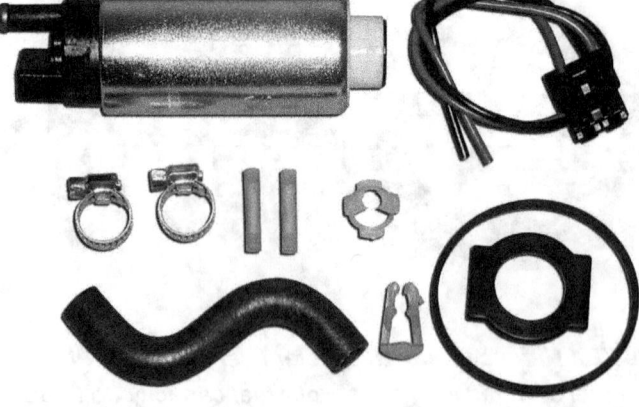

Fuel-injected cars also make use of an auxiliary in-tank pump, which piggybacks off the existing OE in-tank electronic high-volume fuel pump, like this Vortech Engineering LLC/Paxton Automotive Products (PN 8F001) unit being installed inside the tank of a 4.6L 2001 Mustang GT.

High-Flow Sprayer Nozzles

There are a staggering number of nitrous oxide sprayer nozzles to choose from. Most N₂O nozzles come standard with either 1/16- or 1/8-inch NPT screw-in threads and are made of brass, aluminum, or stainless steel. Of course, the business end of a nozzle is the tip, or orifice. These also come in different shapes and sizes, with annular, soft plume, or high flow being the most common.

When you need to determine the flow rating, or the exact amount of horsepower each design delivers, it's imperative to discuss your particular requirements with a supply company's technical representative prior to buying a set. Though they are also sellers, reps have a wealth of knowledge and experience with each design or application.

Nitrous Oxide Systems

NOS manufactures both the brass and black-anodized Fogger and Fogger 2 nozzles (PNs 13700NOS and 13700BNOS, respectively). The patented Fogger nozzle revolutionized nitrous and fuel dispersal technology in the early 1980s. But as engines got bigger and N₂O systems became more and more sophisticated, the Fogger 2 design made its debut. Fogger 2 provides more fuel and superior nitrous atomization. Note that there is also an alcohol version of both the Fogger and the Fogger 2.

The NOS Fogger stainless steel Annular Discharge nozzle (PN 13700RNOS) is touted as being the most effective annular-design racing nozzle in the world. According to NOS, the secret lies in the specially engineered annular orifices that mix N₂O and fuel in a radial pattern outside the nozzle tip. This is claimed to provide superior atomization of supplemental fuel as well as more even fuel distribution within the nitrous flow. Note that an annular-discharge nozzle shoots straight and is not a direct replacement for Fogger and Fogger 2 nozzles. The annular-discharge system requires tighter clearances (30 degrees as opposed to 90 degrees for Fogger nozzles) but is not entirely dependent on runner design. These are serious nitrous nozzles for serious nitrous racers.

The NOS stainless-steel Soft Plume 90-degree Fogger nozzles (PN 13716NOS) are ideally suited for EFI applications and provide superior fuel dispersal and atomization, particularly in smaller-displacement engines. NOS also manufactures fan spray nozzles (PN 13500NOS, in blue-anodized aluminum) or brass (PN 13503NOS) and jet spray nozzles sized at -3 AN, with a 90-degree discharge (requires jets) under PN 13656NOS or a blank jet spray nozzle that you can tailor to your specific

Here is an example of a system in action. Not only does purging a nitrous system serve a purpose, it also puts on a show for the fans.

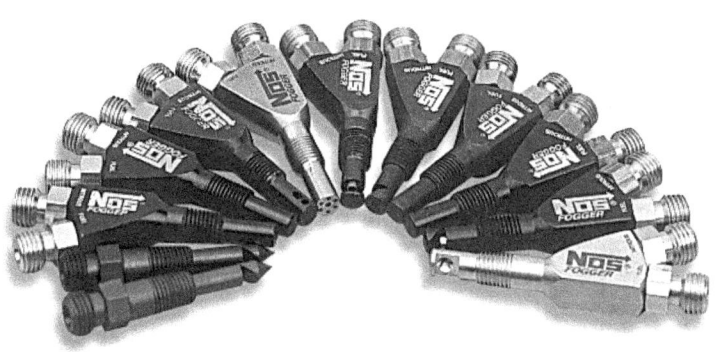

This fan photo of Nitrous Oxide Systems nozzles shows how diverse they can be. In this lineup (from left to right) the selection is led off by NOS' red and blue Fuel and N₂O annular nozzles. Next to them are Fogger, Fogger 2, and Fogger Annular Discharge Racing nozzles. And finally, NOS' selection of 90-degree Soft Plume nozzles. If you need it, they have it!

needs under PN 13600NOS. These nozzles were designed to be used independently, or in tight places where use of a fogger nozzle may prove to be impractical.

Edelbrock

Edelbrock Nitrous features four E-Series nozzles. First is the 90-degree E1 Series constructed from lightweight aluminum and anodized black. Touted for its unique fuel passage design for extremely high atomization, its 1/8-inch-NPT thread design is a direct bolt-on (PN 72560).

Second is the Billy Glidden–designed 90-degree E2 Series, which features a durable stainless-steel body with 1/16-inch-NPT threads (PN 72562).

Edelbrock's E3 Series 90-degree nozzle (PN 72563) is constructed out of titanium. Its straight-shot annular discharge design produces excellent fuel atomization, and is a direct upgrade for other brands that use a 1/16-inch-NPT thread.

And finally there's Edelbrock's

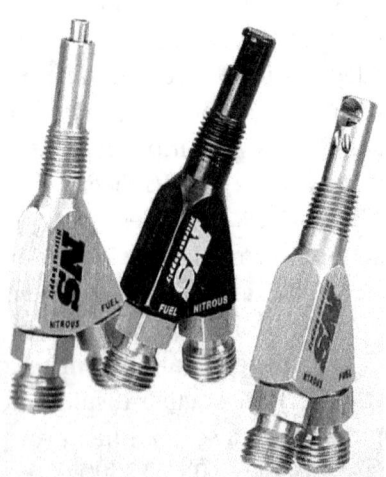

Nitrous Supply's lineup of nozzles (left to right): Fine Plume-1 (PN 23716), High Flow (PN 23700R), Fang (PN 23712), and Mutha Fogga (PN 23718), the bad boy in the NS nozzle lineup.

nitrous-nozzle-only 90-degree SS Series (PN 72556), constructed from durable stainless steel and using a 9/16-inch-NPT fitting. It's recommended for dry-system applications only.

Nitrous Express

This company markets a whole bunch of N_2O nozzles and nozzle accessory and conversion kits. Brand names include: Shark, Single-Shark, and Pro Shark nozzles, which are available in four-, six-, and eight-cylinder applications; the Piranha Nozzle (PN 70000), which is available in four- and eight-cylinder applications; the STD Standard nozzle (PN 80018), available in a number of applications; and the SSV (PN 80016), the SX2 (PN 90017), the GM NXL (PN 75001), and 1/8-NPT Dry Nozzle (no PN listed). Consult the manufacturer for specific use and applications.

Nitrous Supply

Nitrous Supply offers four different fogger-type nozzle applications. All are 1/16-inch NPT.

Leading the way is the NS Fine Plume 90-degree fogger-type nozzle (PN 23716). Versatility appears to be the key here; this nozzle is right at home with carbureted small-block and big-block engines as well as stock EFI. This unit is advertised as being un-equaled in durability and reliability.

The NS High-Flow nozzle (PN 23700R) is a straight-flow fogger nozzle design for extreme high flow of fuel and nitrous.

NS also sells the Fang (PN 23721), which is what is known as a high-intensity 90-degree fogger-type nozzle. The inner design or delivery tract is exclusive to NS, and features fuel delivery outlets on either side of the nitrous plume to ensure proper fuel atomization.

Then there's the Mutha Fogga, the only straight-shooting nozzle available that shears a full 360-degrees surrounding the fuel charge. Shearing the fuel with N_2O creates smaller droplets and ultimately creates an (advertised) fuel/nitrous fog of higher density than that of any other fogger-type design nozzle.

NS also markets three different independent nozzles, called fan nozzles, to singly deliver nitrous or fuel. These nozzles come red anodized (PN 23500), blue (PN 23502), or brass (PN 23503).

NS also sells a 1/16-inch-NPT Nozzle Tap, as well as its Nozzle Mount Kit (PN 27283), which is ideally suited for installing on EFI-type rubber air ducts or thin-wall air inlets.

Wilson Manifolds & Nitrous Pro-Flow

Wilson Manifolds & Nitrous Pro-Flow calls its line of CNC nozzles V-Force, and they are geared for all-out competition use.

ZEX Nitrous Products

The ZEX Wet Nozzle Technology program features two Power Advantage nozzles (PN 82025). The purple-anodized, CNC'd aluminum-body Power Advantage 1 features a high level of atomization, which ensures perfect fuel distribution among cylinders. This finely atomized mixture also burns more powerfully and maximizes horsepower.

ZEX Power Advantage 2 features Active Fuel Control, a revolutionary nitrous tuning and safety feature that operates on vacuum. In other words, as bottle pressure fluctuates, the speed of the nitrous discharge also fluctuates with the prevailing conditions. This causes the level of vacuum draw inside the fuel transfer tube to vary as well causing the ZEX nozzle to actually pull more or less N_2O and fuel enrichment into the engine, meaning that your tuning stays consistent and your engine never runs too lean or overly rich. ZEX also markets a Direct Port Nitrous Nozzle (PN 82155) for all-out performance applications along with a single-phase Dry Nitrous Nozzle (PN N56550) as well.

Nitrous Oxide Filling Stations

You may have seen the signs hanging in the front windows of high-performance retailers across the country, stating "Nitrous Refills Sold Here." But what is a nitrous filling station? In principle, the process is pretty much like filling a helium, oxygen, argon, or acetylene bottle, and should only be done by a professional. Here are a few words of advice about proper nitrous bottle maintainance and refilling:

- Do not puncture or incinerate an N_2O bottle.
- Do not overfill an N_2O bottle or it could explode.
- According to DOT regulations, your dealer cannot refill N_2O bottles that are out of date.

Nitrous Gauges

It's an urban myth that a nitrous oxide pressure gauge can tell you exactly how much N_2O is left in a bottle, so don't believe it! Removing the bottle and weighing it is the only effective way. Nitrous oxide performs best at optimum pressure, which should be between 950 and 1,000 psi at 92 degrees F. A nitrous gauge can tell you if the nitrous pressure needs to be increased to ensure optimum performance, keeping in mind that N_2O pressure fluctuates with atmospheric changes. If you're serious about winning races, it's a good thing to have.

Project: ZEX Bottle Pressure Gauge Installation

ZEX Nitrous Products Nitrous Pressure Gauge (PN 82005) allows precise monitoring of nitrous bottle pressure. The gauge's super-sturdy purple-anodized bottle-valve-to-nitrous-line adaptor, high-quality chrome-plated metal body with easy gauge readouts (maximum pressure, 1,500 psi), and glass lens allows for precise and vibration-free readouts. Installing one of these gauges is very easy. But because N_2O's -127 degree F temperature may cause severe burns to the skin, the following safety precautions are necessary:

- If you are installing a nitrous pressure gauge on a full bottle, be sure that the bottle valve is completely closed.
- Slowly crack the nitrous feed line to relieve it of any pressure, again being sure to keep hands, fingers, and face away from this potentially dangerous area.
- When installing the actual gauge, a single wrap of Teflon tape can be used as a seal to prevent leaks, although some N_2O manufacturers say you don't have to. Remember, if using Teflon tape, be careful not to block the flow path of the N_2O in any way.

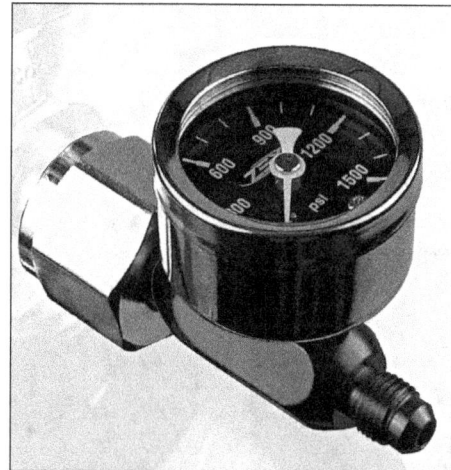

This ZEX Nitrous Pressure Gauge (PN 82005) features a purple-anodized nitrous valve-to-line adaptor and chrome-plated outer body with scratch-proof glass lens. Readouts max out at 1,500 psi. It's a real quality piece!

- After you install it, slowly open the bottle valve to slow charge the system and then check for leaks.

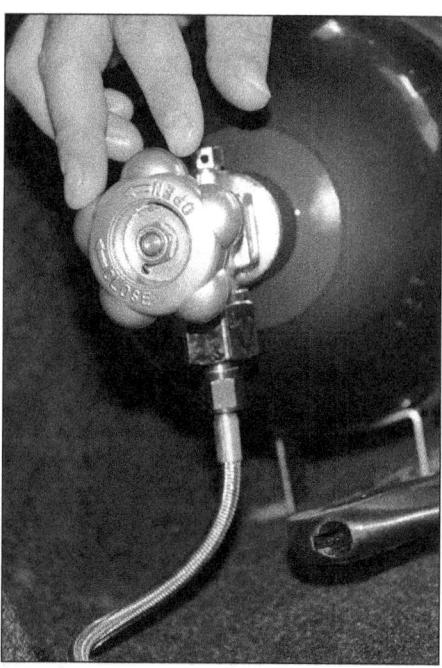

1 *ZEX bottle valve installation begins by making dead certain that the bottle valve is completely closed, to prevent a -127-degree F nitrous burn.*

CHAPTER 10

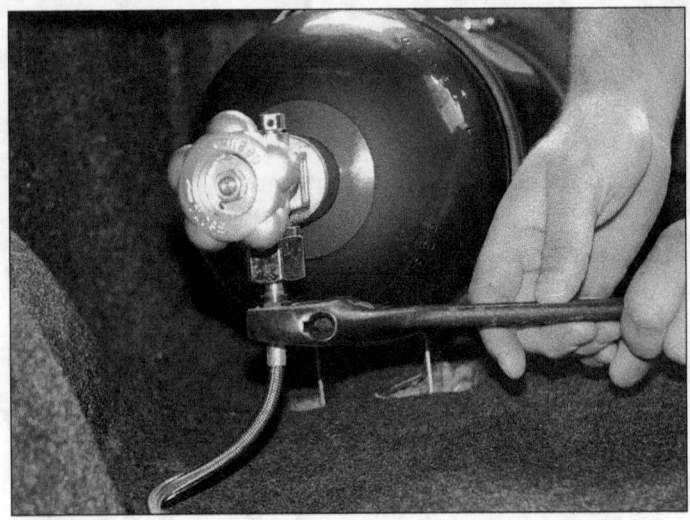

2 Slowly crack the -4 AN fitting on the nitrous line directly connected to the ZEX bottle valve/adaptor using a wrench, gradually releasing any excess pressure.

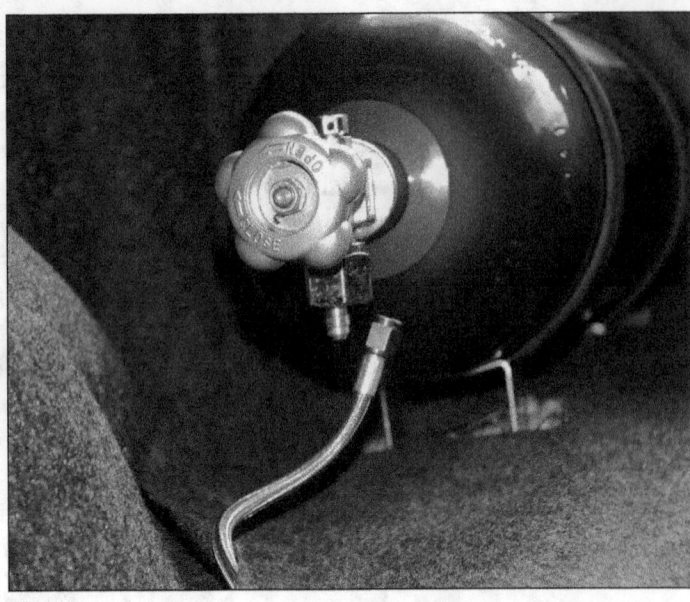

3 Here's what the disconnected nitrous delivery line looks like.

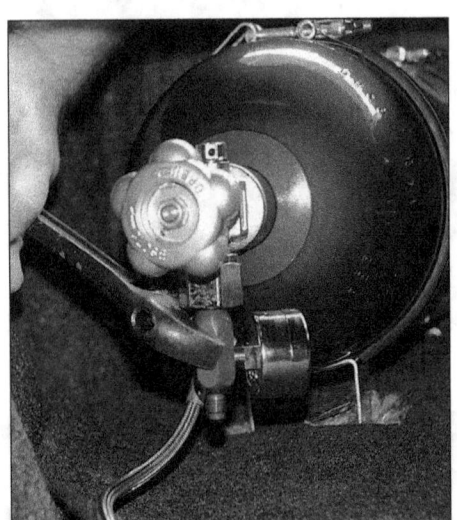

4 Wrap the nipple on the gauge adaptor with Teflon tape, install the ZEX 1,500-psi Nitrous Pressure Gauge, and carefully tighten counter-clockwise with a wrench.

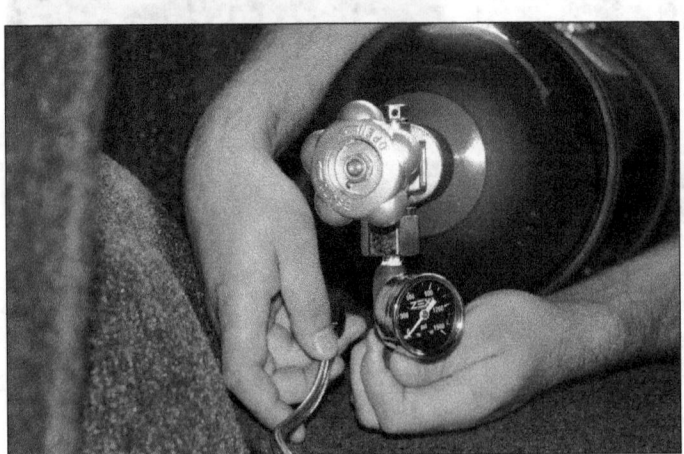

5 Now attach the N$_2$O supply line. After it's installed, energize the system and check for any leaks.

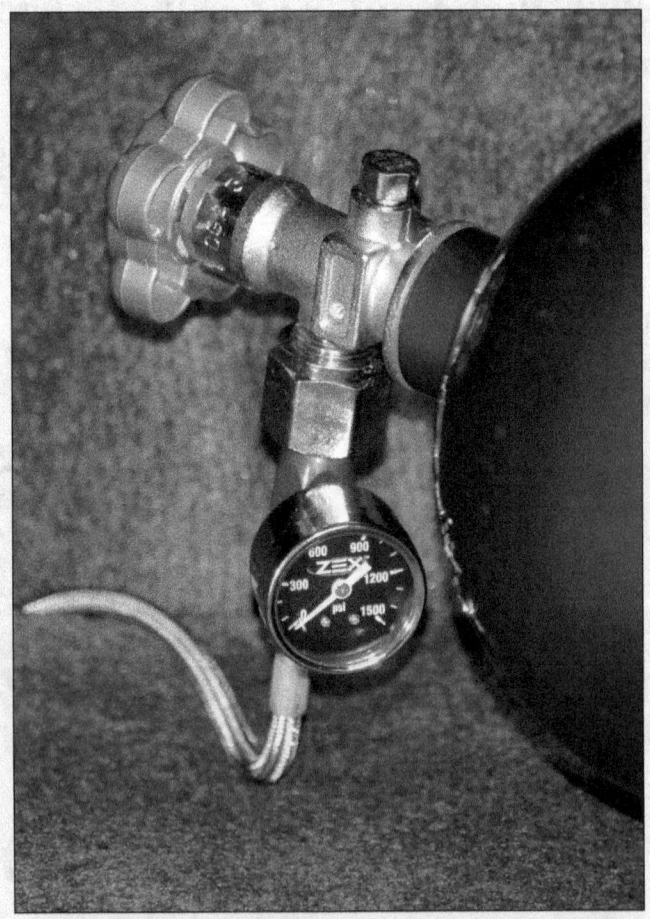

Here's ZEX's Nitrous Pressure Gauge installed, pressurized, and ready to give faithful service.

HOW TO INSTALL AND TUNE NITROUS OXIDE SYSTEMS

NITROUS ACCESSORIES

Bottle Blankets

Bottle blankets were originally intended to stabilize the temperature of N_2O because it is contained under extreme pressure (800 to 1,000-plus psi) and is extremely susceptible to atmospheric changes. This is especially true when a bottle is installed inside various late-model street cars with little or no trunk, and huge back windows. In any car, parked with closed windows, temperatures can often exceed 120-plus degrees F in some parts of the country. This is dangerously close to N_2O's flash point; so the question is, do you want to share the same space with a potential missile? I think not!

Bottle blanket design varies from a simple black-velvet cloth bag like ZEX Nitrous Products offers, which mainly protects the painted or polished surface of the N_2O bottle, to insulated and nylon-wrapped bottle bags like the ones NOS and Nitrous Express offer. Heat Shield Products, manufacturers of high-temperature thermal wrap for headers, thermal blankets, and other heat-resistant products, has just introduced its SEMA-SFI-approved high-temp wrap. It features an inner layer of fiberglass insulation to regulate inside temperatures, and a reflective aluminized fiberglass outer wrap to deflect heat. These bottle bags are claimed to reduce temperatures as much as 60 to 70 percent. Remember, safety is as safety does!

Project: Nitrous Express GENX2 Bottle Warmer Installation

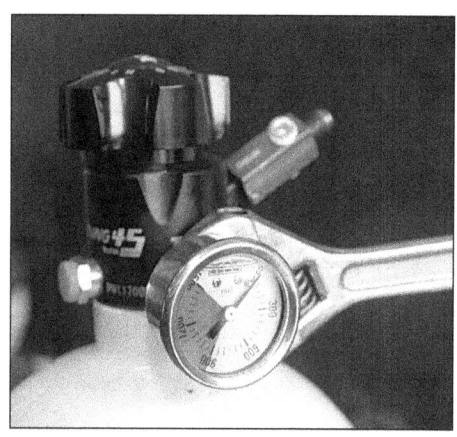

You can install an NX liquid-filled nitrous bottle pressure gauge using an adjustable wrench.

Wait a minute! Didn't I just explain about reducing the temperature of N_2O using a bottle blanket? No, this further discussion is not redundant. Bottle warmers and blankets ensure safe and insulated storage of N_2O when it is not in use. With more than 60 square inches of surface area, the Nitrous Express Bottle Heater automatically turns itself on via a pressure transducer when bottle pressure drops below 900 psi, and turns itself off at approximately 1,050 psi. This permits a warm-up time of only minutes! Again, there are some safety rules that you must follow:

- Danger! Bottle heaters are not recommended for use with carbon-fiber N_2O bottles.
- Never operate a bottle heater with the bottle valve closed. The pressure transducer cannot sense the internal bottle pressure when the valve is closed.
- The surface temperature of the NX bottle warmer can reach as high as 400 degrees F. Do not touch it while it's in operation!
- Never operate your bottle heater unless the heating element is tightened firmly against the bottle and completely flat, or else you could run the risk of burning out a heating element.
- NX also advises that (with its bottle warmer) you do not attempt to operate the heater without the heavy-duty relay properly installed per the provided wiring diagram. Failure to do so results in premature transducer failure.

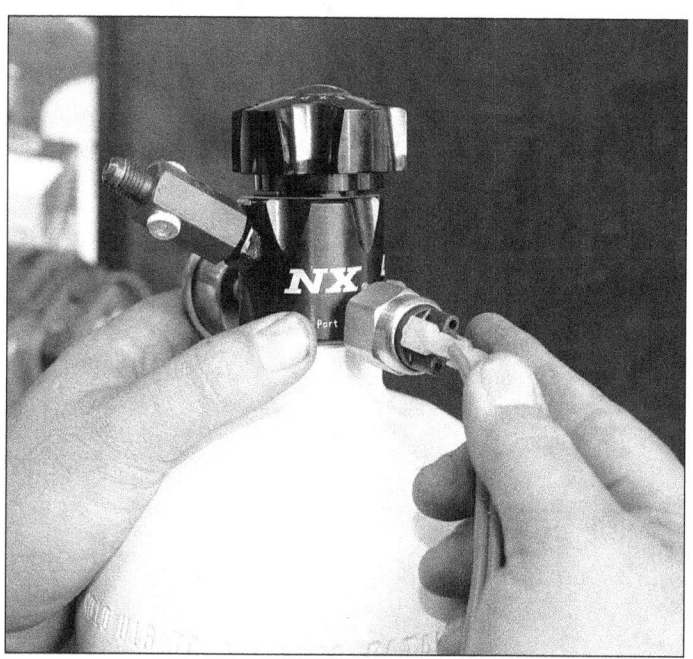

1 Install the NX Pressure Switch on the opposite side of the bottle valve.

CHAPTER 10

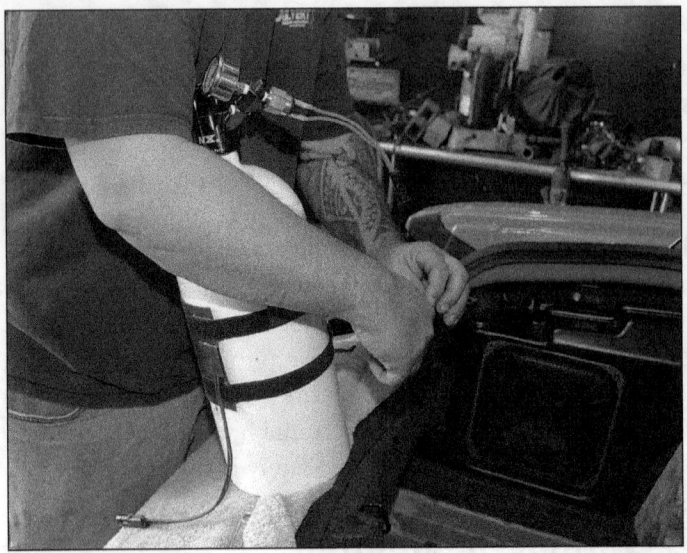

2 Wrap the NX bottle heater around the 10-pound NX aluminum N₂O bottle.

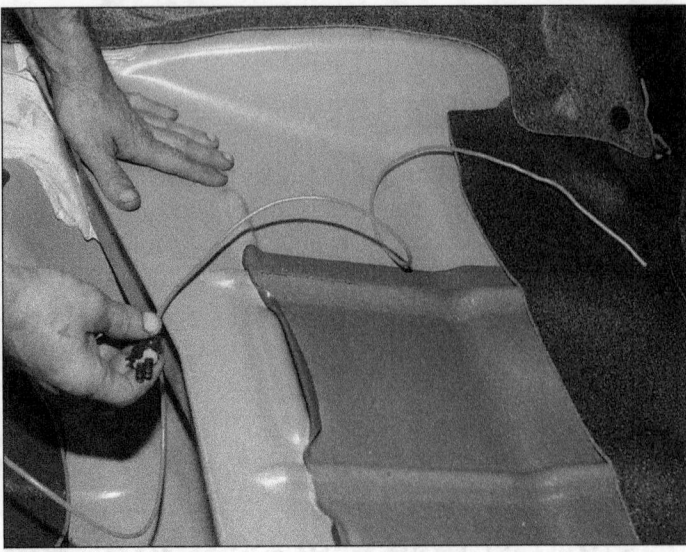

3 Run the switch relay wire through the bottom of the floorpan.

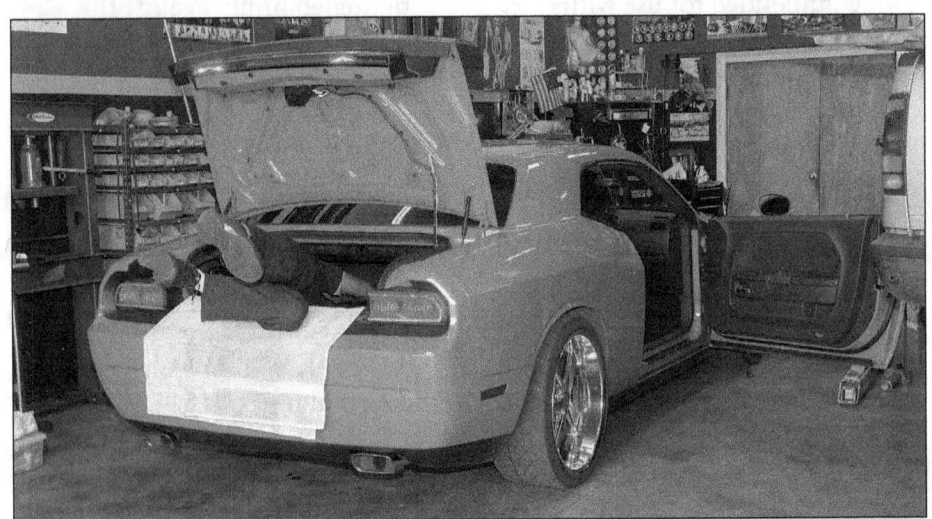

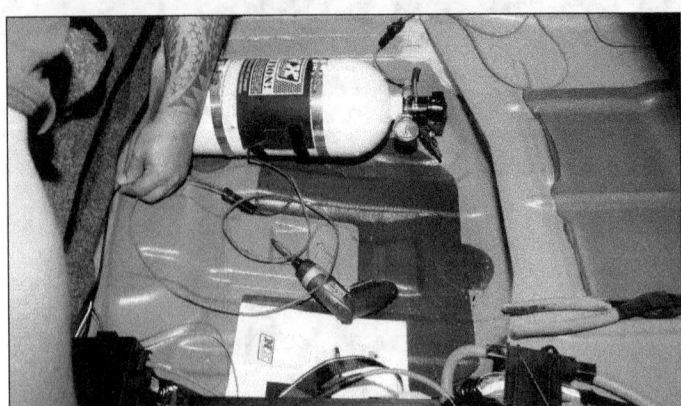

4 As you can see, this may take a little bit of crawling around inside the trunk.

5 Place the actual bottle and NX nitrous warmer inside the car with all the fittings and hookups in place. Then run the NX bottle heater power wires to the battery relay.

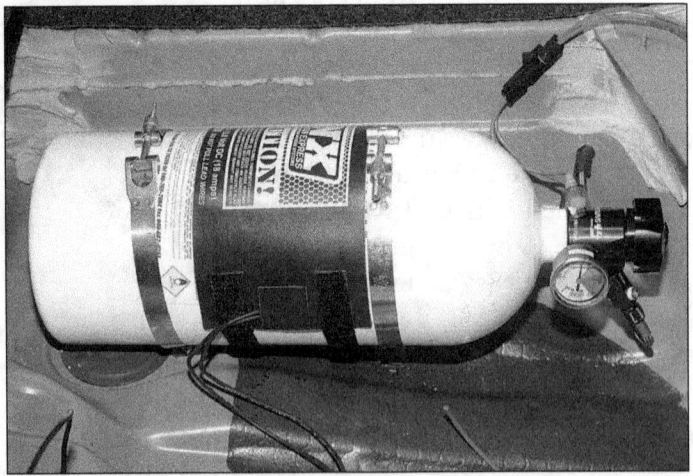

6 This is how the N₂O bottle and bottle heater should look when completely installed.

NITROUS ACCESSORIES

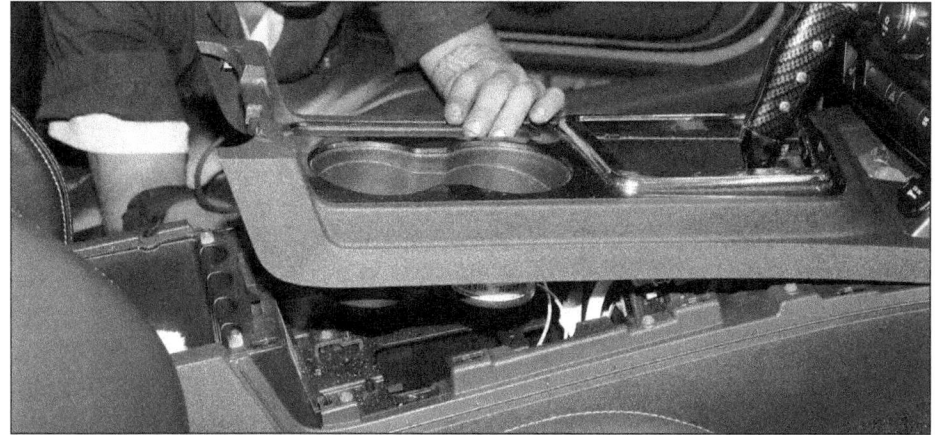

7 Locate a power wire and hook up and arm the bottle warmer heating switch. For this application, a Power Point Hot lead, normally used to charge a cell phone, was found on the Challenger console. It worked out perfectly!

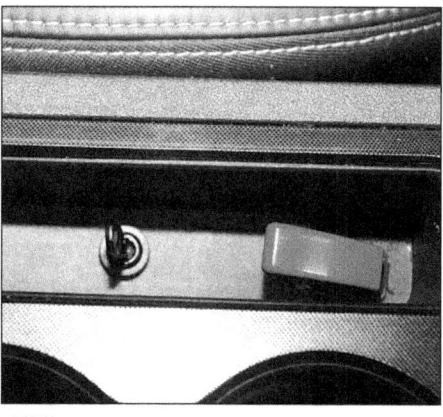

8 The NX bottle heating switch was located just 1½ inches away from the NX's 250-hp Arming Switch previously installed in this car.

Another Way of Doing It

The concept of nitrogen-assisted nitrous oxide (NANO) is a patented technology invented by Thomas E. Darnell, general manager of NANO Nitrous, LLC. High-pressure nitrogen, which is lighter than N_2O, is used to pressurize the bottle. This forces the N_2O to the bottom of the bottle, allowing a siphon to collect and disperse every bit of its contents.

Another byproduct of this action is consistent nitrous pressure and delivery for the life of the bottle in all kinds of atmospheric conditions—no more worrying about N_2O temperatures and bottle pressure. It was lab tested using an automated flow bench. A NANO Nitrogen-Assisted Nitrous Oxide system was compared to a standard, non-siphon 10-pound N_2O system and bottle heater. Results were plotted and horsepower calculated using a 5.2:1 N_2O/fuel ratio. According to the manufacturer, this data was simultaneously backed up by Dave Koehler's Nitrous Wizard software. The NANO system was reported to develop 25-percent-more average horsepower, or mass flow, than a standard N_2O system using the same jetting. Horsepower on mass flow of N_2O reflected a 180-percent increase using the NANO system. Ramp-up time versus a bottle heater was also notably significant.

Factory literature states that NANO automatically adjusts to any nitrous tune from 50 to 500 hp, and the system works perfectly with any N_2O controller. Furthermore, a NANO nitrous bottle (available in 10-, 15-, and 20-pound bottles) can be refilled at paintball stores and dive shops. The manufacturer offers four Power Solutions, ranging from 250 to 850 hp.

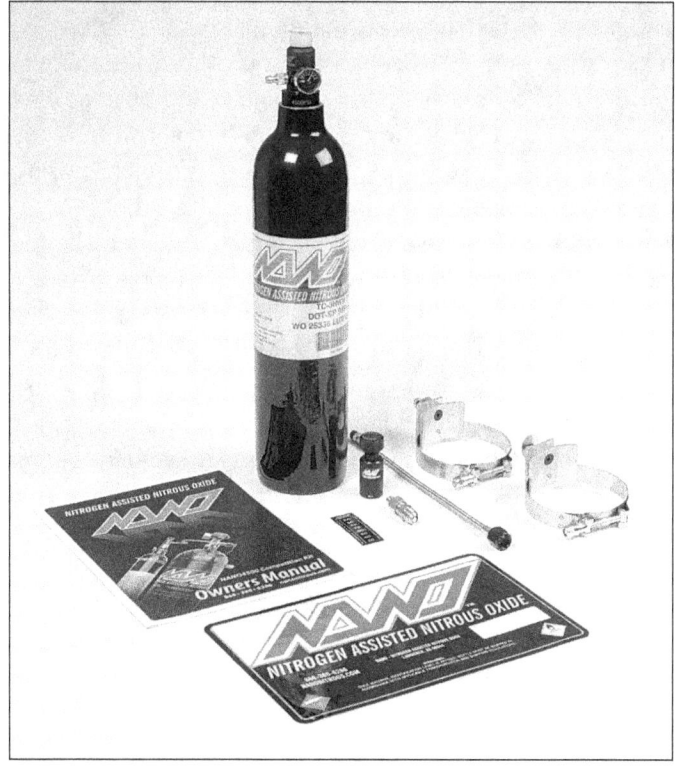

NANO's 250-hp Nitrous Oxide Universal Kit, which can be adapted to any popular aftermarket N_2O kit.

CHAPTER 10

Pelech Brothers' NMCA Nitrous Camaro

Could this be the ultimate NMCA Stage-1 street-legal nitrous car in the land? Ted Pelech of Pelech Bros. Racing holds the distinction of having been the two-time National Street Car Association (NSCA) Elapsed Time and MPH record holder for 7.62 seconds at 182 mph. This Jeff Prock–tuned 465-ci street-legal 1990 Chevrolet Camaro, with Applied Nitrous Technology's nitrous assistance, has recently posted a time slip of 7.22 seconds at 191 mph, so draw your own conclusions.

"As a kid, I guess I watched the NHRA USA Nationals on ABC's Wide World of Sports far too many times," says Pelech, an OE design engineer. "Then, I read about the 'World's Fastest Street Car Shootout' in *Hot Rod* magazine, and I instantly knew what I wanted to do! I love all things mechanical, and so does my brother Tim."

The Pelech brothers first burst on the scene by taking the win with a 1978 Chevrolet Camaro Z28 at the 1990 All Star Chevy Weekend held at Milan Dragway. Pelech's next brush with victory came exactly one year later at the Martin, Michigan, U.S. 131 Super Chevy Show, where Ted Pelech went all the way to the semi-finals in a tough 80-car field before being eliminated. These early successes planted the seed to compete in the NMCA's Heads Up Street category, and the remainder of that first decade was spent re-engineering the Pelech's beloved Z28 until he and his brother Tim had taken the car to its limits. Next, around 1995, Team Pelech ordered a new Camaro from Competition Motorsports.

"Over the years," Pelech continues, "my brother Tim and I have updated the Camaro on several occasions. Essentially this is a back-half car, which has now been converted to a nearly-full-tube-chassis car, and it was awarded the NSCA's Best Engineered Race Car award at Columbus, Ohio, in 2002."

Ted's Camaro is currently certified to compete in the NMCA, where Pelech hopes to continue his winning ways.

Out back, the 103-inch-wheelbase hot rod features a Competition Motorsports/Tim Pelech–prepared, Koni-coil-over-suspended, and Mark Williams 4.56:1-geared Ford 9-inch rear end. A set of Mark Williams Enterprises 35-spline rear axles turn a set of 16x15-inch Weld Aluma Star rear wheels wrapped with a pair of 33x10.5x16-inch Mickey Thompson slicks. Stopping is provided by a pair of Strange Engineering 11-inch-diameter carbon-fiber racing brakes. Also along for the ride are a Competition Motorsports-constructed wishbone locater, a Pelech-fabricated anti-sway bar, and Jerry Bickel–constructed titanium wheelie bars.

Up front, Ted and Tim's Camaro makes use of a Santhuff-constructed coil-over-strut front suspension featuring Jerry Bickel Race Cars (JBRC) rack-and-pinion steering, Strange Engineering 11-inch-diameter carbon-fiber front disc brakes, and a Wilwood Engineering dual master cylinder. Front wheels and tires consist of 15x3.5-inch Weld Aluma Star front wheels rolling on 28x4.5-inch Hoosiers. Also located up front in the frame rails is a plastic 2.5-gallon fuel tank.

Probably what makes this Camaro unique is the fact that Pelech's three-stage dry fuel-injection system was designed and tuned by Jeff Prock, son of pioneer Funny Car driver Tom Prock, and younger brother to Jimmy Prock. Jimmy Prock was the mechanical mastermind behind the Robert Hight–John Force Racing car that won the NHRA Full Throttle Drag Racing Series Funny Car championship. In single-stage configuration, the 465-ci version cranked out 1,500-plus hp on the Holbrook Racing Engines dyno.

"This has been three years in the making," says Ted. "We just didn't stumble into this. We worked real hard, and obviously relied on the right components to reach this point. You've got to admit that 1,500 [hp] on a single-stage is pretty amazing, and it really shows how Jeff Prock knows his product."

Internally, the Pelech's 465-ci billet-aluminum Dart block features a deck height of 9.25 inches. Inside, the cam location has been raised .600 inch and the cam tunnel has been equipped with a set of encased needle roller bearings. The lifter position has also been relocated, using Trend Performance, Inc., bronze lifter bushings to ensure correct valvetrain geometry. One of Sonny Bryant's steel-billet crankshafts (riding on a set of Speed Pro main bearings) hooks up to a set of GRP aluminum-alloy connecting rods with a set of Hell Fire-ringed, 12.5:1 compression Diamond Racing Products coated pistons pressed onto the opposite end. The cams are proprietary grinds, and all feature 1 inch of gross valve lift to work with the nitrous.

A set of CNC-ported Dart Big Chief 11-degree-valve-angle cylinder heads makes use of a set of a 2.400-inch-diameter Exceldyne titanium intake. The 1.900-inch-diameter Exceldyne exhaust valves use PAC Racing valvesprings, Competition Cams retainers, and Jesel shaft-style rocker arms riding on a Pelech-designed mounting bar. All engine fasteners are either ARP or A1 Technologies, and the valve covers are Moroso. Ignition uses an MSD belt-driven distributor, MSD HVC-II coil, MSD 8-mm ignition wires, either Autolite or NGK spark plugs, and an MSD Digital-7 individual-cylinder-control module working in conjunction with a FAST XFI Engine Management Control System.

The exhaust system on the Camaro consists of a set of Performance Welding–designed three-step stainless-steel headers. Getting all that power to the pavement is a Reactor billet-aluminum flex plate hooked up to a Hutch's Transmission Service/Dedenbear-case manual-valve-body 2-speed Power Glide. The final link in the Camaro's powertrain is an aluminum metal-matrix composite 62-inch-long drive shaft by Drive Train Specialists (DTS).

Although considered a street car, very little other than the roof, quarter panels, and rear sail panels remain of the original steel 1990 Camaro. Weight-saving components include polycarbonate windows and carbon-fiber front fenders, front and rear fascias, hood, hood scoop, doors, and rear spoiler mounted to a hand-fabricated aluminum rear deck. Charlie Vickery (of Paint by Chaz) painted the Camaro in Matador Red.

Inside, the interior also features extensive carbon fiber, including the seats, and features a Racepak LCD dash display, a Pelech-fabricated steering column, and RJS Safety Equipment. Acting crew are crew chief and tuner Jeff Prock, his brother, Tim Pelech, Todd Betts, Mike Flosky, Nick D'Agostino, and Ted's wife, Karin.

Ted had noted on his tech sheet that the team also has a bigger (468-ci) big-block. This is only speculation, but I'm sure that that's the engine that makes good use of Jeff Prock's three-stage X4 throttle body from Applied Nitrous Technology. This setup leads with nitrous only at the injector nozzle, and then introduces large doses of nitrous and fuel via the FAST XFI computer and FAST XFI fuel injectors. "This combination," in crew member "Nitrous" Nick D'Agostino's words, "should be able to produce close to 2,000 hp with all the candles lit!"

Ted Pelech purges the system on the starting line to ensure a fresh shot of nitrous is fed to the 465-ci big-block Chevy engine. The powerful 1990 Camaro routinely runs low-7-second passes at more than 180 mph in NMCA competition on relatively small, 10.5-inch-wide rear tires. The engine's peak power is approximately 1,500 horses with the single-stage nitrous system flowing at full capacity.

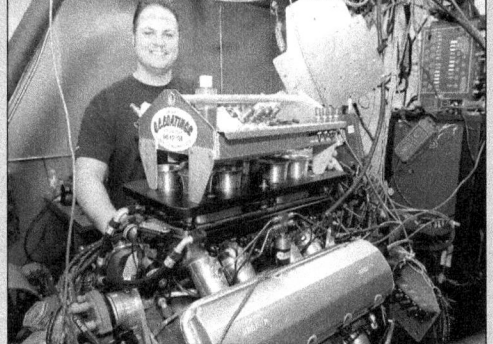

A 468-ci engine with a three-stage system is waiting in the wings with 2,000 hp on tap.

CHAPTER 11

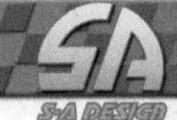

COMMONLY ASKED QUESTIONS ABOUT NITROUS OXIDE

By Mike Thermos, CEO of Nitrous Supply

Q: How does nitrous oxide work?

A: Nitrous Oxide is made up of two parts nitrogen and one part oxygen, or 36-percent volume by weight. During an engine's internal combustion process, at about 572 degrees F, N_2O breaks down and releases oxygen. It is this extra oxygen that allows more fuel to be burned, thus creating additional horsepower. Also, N_2O entering the intake manifold at -127 degrees F creates an intercooling effect that drops the inlet charge temperature by 60 to 70 degrees—every 10 degrees of decrease in inlet charge is a 1-percent horsepower gain.

Q: Is it a good idea to use an aftermarket computer chip in conjunction with nitrous oxide?

A: Only if the computer chip has been designed specifically for use with nitrous oxide. Most aftermarket chips use more aggressive timing-advance curves to create more power. This can lead to potential detonation. You may wish to check with the manufacturer of the chip before installing it. All the top aftermarket chip manufacturers make special chips for use with nitrous oxide.

Q: Is it necessary to upgrade the ignition system?

A: Most late-model ignition systems are well suited for N_2O applications. In some higher-horsepower applications, it may be advisable to look into a high-performance ignition system with retard capacity.

Q: How does nitrous oxide affect engine reliability?

A: The key to engine reliability when using N_2O is to choose the proper horsepower increase for a given application. Kits using the correct factory calibrations do not usually increase wear. Increased cylinder pressures also places more load on supporting components. If load increases exceed the load capacity of the supporting components, the result is increased wear. Nitrous oxide kits are designed for use on demand only at wide-open throttle, making N_2O extremely advantageous in that it is used only when needed, not at all times. Kits are designed for maximum power with reliability for a given application.

COMMONLY ASKED QUESTIONS ABOUT NITROUS OXIDE

Q Does nitrous oxide raise cylinder head pressures and temperatures?

A Yes, due to the ability to burn more fuel; this is exactly why N_2O makes so much power.

Q So, is it possible to bolt a nitrous induction system onto a stock engine?

A Yes! However, you should choose the correct system for the given application, such as: four-cylinder engines normally allow horsepower increases of 40 to 50 hp; on six-cylinder engines, 75 to 100 hp; on small-block V-8 engines up to 400 ci, up to 140 hp; and on big-block V-8s up to 454 ci, 125 to 200 hp. These suggested ranges provide maximum reliability from most stock displacement engines using cast pistons and a cast crankshaft with few or no engine modifications.

Q Is carburetor jetting necessary when adding nitrous oxide?

A No; nitrous systems are independent of—placed below—the carburetor and a system injects its own mixture of fuel and N_2O into the cylinders of an engine.

Q What are some of the rules for even greater horsepower gains?

A Generally, forged-aluminum pistons are a prerequisite for large horsepower increases with nitrous induction. Generally, ignition timing should be retarded by 1½ to 2½ degrees per each 50 hp gained. In many cases, a high-flow fuel pump may be necessary, along with 100-plus-octane fuel, and spark plugs that are two ranges colder than normal with gaps closed to .025 to .030 inch. Horsepower gains over 250 may require additional modifications such as a forged-steel crank, forged-steel connecting rods, a high-output fuel pump to supply additional fuel demands, and racing fuel with a high specific-gravity rating and an octane rating of 110 or more.

Q Are there any benefits to chilling a nitrous bottle?

A No! Chilling a nitrous bottle lowers bottle pressure dramatically and lowers the flow rate of the nitrous, causing a fuel-rich condition and reducing horsepower. For optimum running conditions, keep bottle pressure at approximately 900 to 950 psi. An N_2O pressure gauge allows you to monitor this. If you live in or operate an N_2O system in colder climates, it may also be a good idea to purchase a bottle heater kit. Generally, ambient temperatures of 70 to 90 degrees F allow for optimum power potential from an N_2O kit.

Q When using the same nitrous oxide kit and jetting, will the degree of performance increase in a highly modified engine when compared to a stock engine?

A Not really. In most cases the amount of increase is greater from a stock engine because it is not as efficient as the modified engine in a normal non-nitrous mode. However, since the effects of N_2O magnify the output of any engine, the total power output is much higher in the modified engine.

Q Can high-compression engines successfully utilize nitrous oxide?

A Absolutely! High-compression or low-compression ratios can work quite suitably with nitrous, provided the proper balance of N_2O/fuel enrichment is maintained. On Pro-Modified–type race motors, which often exceed a 15.0:1 compression ratio, more ignition retard and higher-octane fuel is required. Speaking with one of the technicians from the company whose kit you are purchasing is always a wise idea.

Q Is nitrous oxide flammable?

A No. Nitrous oxide by itself is non-flammable. However, the oxygen present in N_2O causes combustion of fuel to take place more rapidly.

Q Does the use of nitrous oxide produce a negative effect on a catalytic convertor?

A No. The increase in oxygen present in the exhaust may actually increase the efficiency level of a catalytic convertor. Because the continuous use of N_2O is normally limited to 10 to 20 seconds, there is usually no appreciable effect. Temperatures are usually well within acceptable standards.

Q Where is the best position to mount a nitrous oxide bottle?

A Most N_2O bottles come with siphon tubes and, in order to maintain proper nitrous pickup, it is important to mount the bottle correctly. I recommend mounting the bottle at a 15-degree angle, with the valve end higher than the bottom of the bottle. The valve end of the bottle should point to the front of the vehicle and the valve knob and label should face up.

Q What are the advantages of using nitrous compared to other performance options?

A Dollar for dollar, you can't buy more performance with less money than with nitrous. The cost of many high-performance options can put you in the poorhouse. With an N_2O system, performance and reliability can be had for a much more reasonable price while still retaining the advantages of a stock engine during normal driving. And nitrous offers tremendous gains in torque without having to rev the engine to excessive RPM. These factors help your engine last longer than any other method of boosting horsepower.

Q What is the function of the blow-off safety valve on an N_2O bottle?

A It is very important not to overfill a nitrous bottle. For example, a 10-pound-capacity bottle should not be filled with more than 10 pounds of N_2O by weight. Overfilling and/or too much heat can cause excessive bottle pressures, forcing the safety seal to blow and releasing all the contents of the bottle.

Q Can pump gas be used for street/strip nitrous oxide use?

A Yes. Use a premium-grade-type leaded or unleaded fuel of 91 octane or greater. But when using higher compression or horsepower levels, a racing fuel with an octane rating of 100 or more must be used.

Q How much improvement in performance can one expect with the introduction of nitrous oxide?

A For many applications, expect an improvement from 1 to 3 seconds in elapsed time and as much as 10 to 15 mph in the mile. Factors such as engine size, rear-end gearing, tire size, and jetting influence the final results.

Q When is the best time to use nitrous?

A Unless a controller is being used, nitrous is best suited at wide-open throttle due to the tremendous increase in torque. Traction permitting, you generally find the best results with early activation. A good rule is that N_2O can safely be applied above 2,500 rpm under full-throttle conditions.

Q What type of nitrous oxide induction system is best, a plate system or a direct-port-injection system?

A The advantages of a plate system are the ease of installation and removal, the ability to transfer easily from one vehicle to another, the ability to change jetting combinations quickly, and it usually provides all the extra horsepower you need—75 to 350 or more. In some cases, such as inline engines with long intake runners, a direct-port-type system is advisable for maximizing distribution. In applications where more than 350 hp is desired, a direct-port or fogger-type system provides the ultimate in distribution at more than 500. Direct-port systems are also desirable when the system is hidden underneath the intake manifold.

SOURCE GUIDE

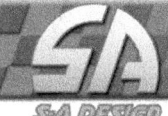

10,000 RRM Speed Equipment
42541 6th Street E.
Lancaster, CA 93535
www.1000rpm.com
(661) 942-1312

Applied Nitrous Technology
1018 Gateway Drive, Suite A
Mooresville, NC 28115
(704) 660-5060
www.appliednitroustechnology.com

ARP Fasteners, Inc.
1863 Eastman Avenue
Ventura, CA 93003
(800) 826-3045
www.arp-bolts.com

ATI Performance Products
6747 Whitestone Road
Gwynn Oak, MD 21207
(866) 379-4632
www.atiperformanceproducts.com

Braswell Carburetion
7671 N. Business Park Drive
Tucson, AZ 85743-9622
www.braswell.com
(520) 579-9177

The Carburetor Shop
1461 E. Philadelphia Street
Ontario, CA 91761
(909) 947-3575
www.customcarbs.com

C.A.R.S.S., LLC
69 Railroad Avenue, Bay A-13
Hilo, HI 96720
(808) 969-9819
www.carss808.com

Compucar Nitrous Oxide Systems
614 Atomic Road
North Augusta, SC 29841
Tech Hotline: (803) 444-9206
Order line: (800) NITROUS
www.compucarnitrous.com

Diamond Racing Products
23003 Diamond Drive
Clinton Township, MI 48035
(586) 792-6220
www.diamondracing.net

DMP Fasteners & Race Supplies
9620 Owensmouth Avenue, Unit 2
Chatsworth, CA 91311
(888) MR BOLTS
www.DMPfasteners.com

Edelbrock Corporation
2700 California Street
Torrance, CA 90503
Tech Line: (800) 416-8628
www.edelbrock.com

Ferrea Racing Components
2600 N.W. 55th Court, Suite 234
Ft. Lauderdale, FL 33309
(888) 733-2505
www.ferrea.com

Heatshield Products
27354 Valley Center Road
Valley Center, CA 92082
(800) 750-3978
www.heatshieldproducts.com

Hogan's Racing Manifolds
303 N. Russell Avenue
Santa Maria, CA 93458
(805) 928-8483
www.hogansracingmanifolds.com

Holley Performance Products, Inc.
1801 Russellville Road
P.O. Box 10360
Bowling Green, KY 42102-7360
(800) HOLLEY1
www.holley.com

Induction Solutions
16121 Flight Path Drive
Brooksville, FL 36404
(352) 593-5900
www.inductionsolutions.com

Island Performance, LLC
73-5617 Maiau Street, Suite 7 & 8
Kailua-Kona, HI 96740
(808) 331-0770
www.islandperformance.com

Jesel Valvetrain Products, Inc.
1985 Cedar Bridge Drive, Suite A
Lakewood, NJ 08701
(732) 901-6777
(732) 905-6517
www.jesel.com

SOURCE GUIDE

Lucas Oil Products, Inc.
302 N. Sheridan Street
Corona, CA 92880-2069
(800) 342-2512
www.LucasOil.com

Lunati Power, Inc.
11126 Willow Ride Drive
Olive Branch, MS 38654
(662) 892-1500
www.lunatipower.com

Meziere Enterprises, Inc.
220S. Hale Avenue
Escondido, CA 92029
(760) 746-3276
www.meziere.com

Milodon, Inc.
2250 Agate Court
Simi Valley, CA 93065
(805) 577-5950
www.milodon.com

Moroso Performance
80 Carter Drive
Guilford, CT 06437
(203) 453-6571
Tech Hotline: (203) 458-0542
www.moroso.com

MSD Ignition
1490 Henry Brennan Drive
El Paso, TX 79936
(915) 856-2472
www.msdignition.com

Nano Nitrous
811 E. 28th Street
Lawrence, KS 66046
(785) 331-2390
www.nanonitrous.com

Nightmare Motorsports
906 W. 18th Street
Nevada, IA 50201
(515) 238-1024
www.nightmare-motorsports.com

Nitrous Express, Inc.
5411 Seymour Highway
Wichita Falls, TX 76310
(940) 767-7694
www.nitrousexpress.com

Nitrous Oxide Systems
1801 Russellville Road
Bowling Green, KY 42102-7360
Tech Line: (270) 781-9741
www.nosnitrous.com

Nitrous Supply
5482 Business Drive, Unit D
Huntington Beach, CA 92649
(714) 373-1986
www.nitroussupply.com

QMP Racing Engines
9530 Owensmouth Avenue, Unit 2
Chatsworth, CA 91311
(818) 576-0816
www.qmpracing.com

Quick Fuel Technology
129 Dishman Landing
Bowling Green, KY 42101
(270) 793-0900
www.quickfueltechnology.com

Racetrans.com
10953 Tuxford Street, Unit 15
Sun Valley, CA 91352
(818) 767-3021
www.racetrans.com

Slover's Porting Service
10953 Tuxford Street, No. 14
Sun Valley, CA 91352
(818) 768-0155
www.sloversportingservice.com

Trend Performance, Inc.
23444 Schoenherr
Warren, MI 48089
(800) 326-8368
www.trendperformance.com

Vortech Engineering
1650 Pacific Avenue
Oxnard, CA 93033-9901
(805) 247-0226
www.vortechsuperchargers.com

Wilson Manifolds &
Nitrous Pro-Flow
4700 NE. 11th Avenue
Fort Lauderdale, FL 33334
(954) 771-6216
www.wilsonmanifolds.com

World Products
51 Trade Zone Court
Ronkonkoma, NY 11779
(613) 737-0467
www.theengineshop.com

ZEX Nitrous Products
3418 Democrat Road
Memphis, TN 38118
(888) 817-1008
www.zex.com

www.ingramcontent.com/pod-product-compliance
Lightning Source LLC
Chambersburg PA
CBHW051414070526
44584CB00023B/3417